Cancer Genetics for the Clinician

Cancer Genetics for the Clinician

Edited by

Gail L. Shaw

H. Lee Moffitt Cancer Center and Research Institute
at the University of South Florida College of Medicine
Tampa, Florida

Springer Science+Business Media, LLC

Library of Congress Cataloging-in-Publication Data

Cancer genetics for the clinician / edited by Gail L. Shaw.
    p.   cm.
Includes bibliographical references and index.
ISBN 978-0-306-46194-1   ISBN 978-1-4615-4699-3 (eBook)
DOI 10.1007/978-1-4615-4699-3
1. Cancer--Genetic aspects.   I. Shaw, Gail L.
[DNLM: 1. Neoplasms--genetics Congresses. 2. Genetic Counseling
Congresses. 3. Genetic Predisposition to Disease Congresses.   QZ
200 C2151517 1999]
RC268.4.C354 1999
616.99'4042--dc21
DNLM/DLC
for Library of Congress   99-37279
                                                         CIP

Proceedings of the symposium, Cancer Genetics for the Clinician, held March 6–8, 1998, in Clearwater
Beach, Florida

ISBN 978-0-306-46194-1

© 1999 Springer Science+Business Media New York
Originally published by Kluwer Academic/Plenum Publishers in 1999

10 9 8 7 6 5 4 3 2 1

A C.I.P. record for this book is available from the Library of Congress

PREFACE

The field of cancer genetics has evolved rapidly during the last five years. The ability to accurately identify patients whose cancer could be attributed to specific inherited alterations in cancer susceptibility genes has empowered physicians at a time when we are still forced to feel inadequate in being able to provide recommendations related to this specific information. While heritable cancers account for between five and ten percent of all cancer cases, these molecular alterations may give us important clues into the mechanism by which cancer occurs, not only in these predisposed individuals, but also for sporadic cases of cancer. Recognizing these clues in the mechanism of carcinogenesis is critical for being able to utilize this very valuable information.

The importance of understanding the genetics of cancer, and particularly inherited cancers, has been emphasized at every level. Patients and their families are becoming increasingly aware that it is important to identify the etiology of cancer within their family and to further elucidate the risks of family members who have not developed cancer. More and more clinicians find patients insisting on being advocates of their own health care and surveillance practices for cancer. The issue has stressed physician accountability in recognizing the importance of heritable cancers. A surgeon in Florida who operated on a woman for medullary thyroid carcinoma was successfully sued for failing to advise his patient that this could be part of an inherited cancer syndrome when the patient's daughter subsequently developed a medullary thyroid cancer. This book provides a reference for individuals who wish to increase their knowledge on heritable cancers.

Physicians are now finding it necessary to be able to provide their patients with information regarding their potential risk for cancer, which may at least in part be related to their family history. The components of a genetic cancer risk clinic, including guidelines for documenting a comprehensive family history, can be assembled in an oncological or primary care setting. There are many critical issues related to genetic counseling for individuals with inherited cancer susceptibility as well as their family members. While certified genetic counselors have been formally trained to provide this type of information, in many settings this can be successfully accomplished with nurses with specific adjunctive training. Counseling can be supplemented with cancer risk estimation using one or more models available. While the models incorporate family history to varying degrees, an important aspect of the counseling process is to put a person's risk into perspective. Follow-up data has enabled clinical recommendations for screening and cancer treatment to be developed for heritable malignancies.[1,2]

At least three founder mutations in BRCA1 and BRCA2 have been identified in the Ashkenazi Jewish population. Further study of this subset is important not only for testing purposes, but also in further defining the level of breast cancer risk associated with each mutation. Hundreds of mutations associated with hereditary breast or breast/ovarian cancer have been identified.

Testing minors for inherited cancer risk remains a controversial issue. Prior to the discovery of cancer susceptibility genes, genetic testing was primarily used in pediatric cancers where early interventions were critical. However, cancer is a disease of adulthood. Although some forms of cancer, such as familial adenomatosis polyposis and its related colon cancer do have specific guidelines and interventions that should begin early in life, hereditary breast and ovarian cancer, and hereditary non-polyposis colon cancer occur well into adulthood. Currently there is no standard preventative available and no recommendation to start any type of surveillance in childhood.

The laboratory methodology used to identify mutations in cancer susceptibility genes is important in interpreting results. It is critical for the ordering physician to understand that the current state-of-the-art of laboratory analysis is still evolving with a continuing rate of discovery of new mutations in these genes. In addition, more genes continue to be discovered, which are important in identifying highly susceptible populations. Many clinicians naively believe that these tests are as straightforward to interpret as a test for serum cholesterol. As we close the twentieth century, results of genetic testing still have many findings of uncertain significance.

Options for the person with an identified inherited cancer susceptibility are still limited. Prophylactic surgery remains an option and prophylactic mastectomy has been recently demonstrated to reduce the risk for breast cancer in women with a strong family history.[3] However, as discussed in the accompanying editorial, this is still a less desirable option. Another possible option is that of chemoprevention. While the Breast Cancer Prevention Trial demonstrated that tamoxifen reduced breast cancer incidence by 45% in a high-risk population as compared to placebo,[4] this is still not generally regarded as standard care for all high-risk women. In addition, the analysis of the effectiveness of tamoxifen versus placebo in women with a predisposing mutation is not yet available. Prophylactic oophorectomy is also an option in hereditary ovarian cancer or breast/ovarian cancer families, but does not afford 100% protection given reports of peritoneal carcinomatosis after surgery in these families.

Hereditary non-polyposis colon cancer is associated with mutations in MLH1, MSH2, PMS1, and PMS2. Founder mutations have been identified in HNPCC families also. Specific management recommendations for affected individuals have been defined.[2]

The impact of genetic testing on insurability is still an area of concern. While there has been some progress with legislation to protect patients from genetic discrimination, life and disability insurance still could be potentially adversely affected by documentation of an inherited cancer predisposition. The ethical and legal implications of genetic testing remain poorly resolved and it is extremely critical that individuals understand the current state of protection of this data before embarking on this important process.

We hope to provide the clinician with a useful reference for addressing some of their patients' questions. Physicians are increasingly called upon to address diverse issues with their patients and their family members. The ability to recognize family cancer syndromes is important for all clinicians. An understanding of how genetic counseling and testing can be important both to the patient and the family is an important step in providing patients with the information they need to be able to make informed decisions.

REFERENCES

1. Burke W, Daly M, Garber J: Recommendations for follow-up care of individuals with an inherited predisposition to cancer. II. BRCA1 and BRCA2. JAMA 277:997–1003, 1997
2. Burke W, Petersen G, Lynch P: Recommendations for follow-up care of individuals with an inherited predisposition to cancer. I. Hereditary nonpolyposis colon cancer. JAMA 277:915–919, 1997
3. Eisen A, Weber BL: Prophylactic mastectomy—the price of fear. New Engl J Med 340:137–138, 1999
4. Fisher B, Costantino JP, Wickerham DL, et al: Tamoxifen for prevention of breast cancer: report of the National Surgical Adjuvant Breast and Bowel Project P-1 Study. J Natl Cancer Inst 90:1371–1388, 1998

CONTENTS

COMPONENTS OF A GENETIC CANCER RISK CLINIC

June A. Peters,[1,2] Jennifer Graham,[3] Mona Penles Stadler,[1,4] and
Kate Sargent[5]

[1] UPMC/UPCI Magee-Women's Hospital Cancer Genetics Program
[2] University of Pittsburgh Graduate School of Public Health
  130 Desoto Street, Crabtree A300, Pittsburgh, PA 15261
[3] Arthur G. James Cancer Hospital and Research Institute
  Clinical Cancer Genetics
  300 W. 10th Ave, Columbus OH 43210-1240
[4] 300 Halket St, Room 3522, Pittsburgh PA 15213
[5] Barbara Ann Karmanos Cancer Institute
  Cancer Risk Assessment Service
  Harper Professional Building
  Suite 612, 4160 John R., Detroit, MI 48201

INTRODUCTION

Because of wide publicity, many oncologists are aware of the availability of genetic susceptibility testing to detect mutations in cancer susceptibility genes such as *BRCA1*. One might innocently assume that the genetic test is as easy to order as filling out your standard requisition form for a blood count. This is not consistent with current practices. The daunting ethical, medical, legal, social, and technological challenges must be addressed. In order for a genetic test to benefit your patients, it should best be undertaken in the context of a well-organized, comprehensive Familial Cancer Risk Counseling program. Establishing such a program is the focus of this chapter.

[1,2] 412-624-7854, fax 412-624-3020, e-mail: jpeters@helix.hgen.pitt.edu
[3] 614-293-6694, fax 614-293-2314, e-mail: graham-1@medctr.osu.edu
[4] 412-641-4203, fax 412-641-1132, e-mail mstadler@mail.magee.edu
[5] 313-966-7780, fax 313-745-9609, e-mail: sargentk@kci.wayne.edu

Cancer Genetics for the Clinician, edited by Shaw.
Kluwer Academic / Plenum Publishers, New York, 1999.

Familial Cancer Risk Counseling

Familial cancer risk counseling (FCRC) is a communication process between a health care professional and an individual concerning the occurrence, or risk of occurrence of cancer in the individual's family.[1,2] As such, FCRC addresses the genetic, medical, psychological, social, and ethical issues that arise in the context of cancer predisposition. The FCRC program may be established in a variety of settings to serve various different institutional and professional purposes. The program may be a free-standing clinical service, located in an academic medical center, an adjunct to general medical genetics, oncology practice, prenatal genetics service, high risk cancer clinic, or as an outgrowth of cancer registries, and genetic research protocols. There are both operational and programmatic aspects to developing such a clinical service. This chapter will emphasize the operational aspects of establishing such a program in the first section, with only brief mention of programmatic aspects of familial cancer risk counseling programs, as these are covered adequately elsewhere.

OPERATION OF A CANCER GENETICS PROGRAM

Program Justification

Those just beginning FCRC programs are often asked to justify the initial expenditure of resources. Table one outlines these. If 10–15% of patients with cancer have an underlying genetic mutation, there will be a significant number of individuals at your institution who will require specialized cancer management. The only way to identify this high-risk subset is through cancer risk assessment. Professional oncology societies such as American Society of Clinical Oncology (ASCO) have issued statements about the responsibilities of oncologists to take family histories that are adequate to ascertain families at risk for hereditary forms of cancer.[3] The FCRC program extends the oncology service to the at-risk relatives thus identified. The family history is the most cost-effective cancer prevention measure available.[4] While genetic counseling itself is not lucrative, families may remain loyal to medical centers that offer a complete package of oncology services. Spin-off services such as screening mammograms, colonoscopies, and laboratory testing can be profitable for the institution as a whole and may be used to subsidize the required genetic counseling and risk assessment. Relatives with average risk do not need to undergo unnecessary procedures. Finally, there is avoidance of negligence malpractice suits against physicians who fail to detect a hereditary cancer syndrome and to notify patients and family members of the medical implications of this diagnosis.

Table 1. Justifications for a Cancer Genetics Program

- Volume of potential families
- Professional standard of care
- Complete package of services
- Financial incentive
- Fear of lawsuits
- Wave of future practice

Adapted from Schneider, 1998, unpublished.

Missions and Models

The overall mission of an institution's oncology program may be to reduce mortality, increase quality of care, increase direct and indirect institutional revenues, improve cancer control, or conduct research.[1,5] Whatever the institutional mission, the FCRC program will facilitate its achievement.

Eeles[6] has provided a comprehensive list of functions of the FCRC. The most obvious objectives are to provide cancer risk assessment, to detect whether a family pattern of cancers is likely to be hereditary, and to diagnose rare cancer family syndromes. In countries with centralized healthcare systems, the clinic may provide accurate records archives and link familial data via registries. Often, clinical functions include genetic counseling and testing, if indicated, giving advice on early detection and preventive options, and conducting or participating in clinical trials. Also, the FCRC program is a training site for professionals, is available to guide, support, and consult for other clinical services. The genetics staff may also offer expert advice for purchasers and providers of cancer genetics services in the institution and regionally. For the forward-thinking oncologist, the FCRC can be the venue of a new generation of oncology practice in which an individual's genetic profile will figure into every phase of cancer prevention, diagnosis and treatment.

Different models have been developed for offering the FCRC services noted above.[1,2,6–11] Some FCRC services grow out of cancer registries,[12] international research collaborations[13] or translate epidemiological research into a family service.[14,15] Some centers will be primarily a single cancer type, e.g., breast or colorectal, and will be situated in a clinic dedicated to that disease, e.g., a Comprehensive Breast Center,[1,2] Digestive Disease Clinic[4,16] or Endocrine Clinic.[17] These models are useful in starting up FCRC programs because they provide focus and a clear set of guidelines for referral. However, the single disease programs are challenged by the nature of genetic susceptibility syndromes, which generally confer risk for more than one type of cancer, each requiring different combinations of medical specialty care. A variation of the single disease genetics clinic is forming an add-on service to already-existing services such as oncology practice, women's health center,[18] surgery consultation, or general medical genetics service.[19] There are also genetics programs affiliated with prevention clinics such as the Strang Breast Cancer Prevention Clinic (G. Rosenthal, personal communication, 1998). Some risk assessment is provided through behavioral science research protocols.[20–22] The prototype of the more comprehensive model is the Hereditary Cancer Prevention Clinic, which handles a variety of cancer types.[4,9,10,23]

While many FCRC programs are academically based, some are not. Kaiser Permanente is one of the first managed care organizations in the country to offer in-house genetic counseling on a routine basis, and, more recently, to initiate a systematic approach to handling FCRC and genetic cancer susceptibility testing. The Kaiser Permanente organization is also pioneering standardized clinical guidelines in regard to hereditary cancer.[24]

Increasingly, the importance of research in hereditary cancers is being recognized. As Ponder[25] (p. 734) argues, "there is hardly an aspect of familial cancer which does not require further research". Therefore, the FCRC clinic, while providing a service, should also be organized to promote research, or at the very least, collect data that could later contribute to research efforts.

Institutional Infrastructure and Resources

The decision as to whether FCRC will be provided onsite with institutional resources or through another mechanism is critical. If a program is established within an institution, one resource-saving strategy is to distribute costs of staff and resources among several departments. Other strategies involve forming collaborative groups within a city or region[19] or establishing a satellite network of affiliated clinics. Another alternative to establishing a local program is contracting with local geneticists or genetic counselors at a nearby institution to provide the FCRC service, or referral of cases to another institution. Finally, some commercial genetic diagnostic laboratories help to coordinate genetic counseling referrals for patients considering genetic susceptibility testing.

Infrastructure: Space, Human Resources, Budgets, Billing

Counseling and Office Space. The clinical consultation space should be quiet, private, comfortable, and large enough for lengthy discussions with multiple family members who may attend FCRC together. The traditional hospital setting and medical examination room are often sterile, cluttered, and an unwelcomed reminder of medical visits of ill relatives, and should be avoided whenever possible. A consultation space or small conference room is preferable. Access to an examination room is optimal for those patients who will require a physical examination, e.g., to evaluate dermatologic stigmata of Cowden's disease or Muir-Torre syndrome, or look for dysplastic nevi associated with hereditary melanoma. Empirical evidence from Stadler & Mulvihill[26,27] confirms the importance to families of these recommendations about the appearance of the clinical space.

In addition to clinic space, staff members will require office space for paperwork, telephone contact, and data management. Often this is a different location than the consultation room. If not, then table and chairs placed in the office should be arranged to separate the work area from the consultation space.

The outreach clinic, where clients are seen at a site separate from the administrative institution, is an alternative to the centralized cancer genetics clinic. Offering service at alternate sites may create more difficult logistics for the FCRC team, but may be very convenient and beneficial to the client. It also has the advantage of promoting professional networking and referral patterns with local providers.

Team Structures, Functions, Individual Roles

Adopting a multi-disciplinary approach to cancer genetics is of paramount importance in achieving an effective cancer genetics program. Assessing familial cancers involves coordination of complex sets of activities that require input from a variety of specialists from different disciplines.[8,11,14,19,25,28–34] The complementary expertise of oncologists, genetic counselors, medical geneticists, pathologists, molecular laboratory scientists, nurses, social workers, and/or psychologists is usually required. Each professional provides a unique perspective and information pertinent to their specialty.

One of the subtle challenges of setting up programs is to blend the distinct professional cultures of clinical genetics and medical oncology (Robin Clark, USC-CSU Northridge Cancer Genetics Conference, 1996). For example, the nature of diagnosis differs dramatically in these two specialties. Oncologists use a combination of clinical examination, medical imaging, and pathology findings to make a definitive diagnosis of a malignancy or metastases in an individual who is then treated according to somewhat standardized guidelines. In contrast, geneticists rarely diagnose a cancer; rather, they are trained to make syndrome diagnoses based on recognizing constellations of physical characteristics and family history of certain associated cancers. Cancer etiology is not of primary concern to the oncologist in the fundamental way that it is to the geneticist, whose business it is to determine the relative contributions of heredity and environment. Only in the past few years has molecular genetic testing been able to augment the genetic diagnosis. Whereas an oncology diagnosis is definitive and leads to specific treatment, a genetic diagnosis is often uncertain and may not lead directly to treatment recommendations. An interesting study suggests the possibility of personality differences as well; e.g. geneticists often have a greater personal tolerance for ambivalence than other medical professionals.[35] While the oncologist is often seen as the general who aggressively "wages war on cancer", the genetics professional will often use softer images of "learning to live with" the consequences of genetic disease. There is also an important difference in the definition of who is the patient. The oncologist takes the more traditional medical view of evaluating, diagnosing, treating, and hopefully curing a person with cancer, whereas the geneticist may view the whole family as the patient. These differences may have an impact on how professionals choose to form interdisciplinary teams, the goals they establish for the local cancer genetics program, and their marketing strategies to generate referral patterns.

The genetic counselor may act as clinic or program coordinator, research team leader, psychosocial crisis interventionist, or genetics expert. In the capacity of genetic counselor, he or she can help evaluate familial clusters of cancer. This might include presenting referrals to the core group; retrieving, reviewing, and summarizing medical records and relevant medical literature; and other information pertinent to the reason for referral. Genetic counselors and clinical geneticists have primary responsibility for constructing and interpreting pedigrees, recognizing known hereditary cancer susceptibility syndromes, calculating risk assessments, and communicating these to clients. The genetics team can also offer education about risk factors for cancer, the basic concepts of inheritance, and the significance of one's unique family history. The genetic counselor may also delineate and work with family dynamics, social, and ethical concerns. The medical oncologist has primary responsibility for medical management. The psychologist, nurse, social worker, and genetic counselor raise issues relevant to both pre-symptomatic testing, cancer diagnosis and management.[36] In some programs, a clinical psychologist or social worker is also on staff to be available to families or individuals with specific psychotherapeutic needs. Together the team develops differential diagnoses and, if possible, determines cancer risk estimates, the likelihood of the family having a specific mutation in a particular cancer susceptibility gene, the appropriateness of offering DNA testing, and cancer prevention and screening recommendations.

There are significant differences in offering cancer risk assessment and testing in research settings. The translation and integration of clinically relevant research efforts into the clinical setting is also promoted through the multi-disciplinary approach.[11,32]

Human Resources. There have been a number of commentaries on the need for primary care physicians, oncologists, and nurses to become knowledgeable about genetics.[3,37–41] However, we are presently far from this ideal situation; hence, cancer

Table 2. Components of Genetic Counseling

The genetic counseling process helps families to:
- comprehend the medical facts of the condition, including the diagnosis, probable course of the disorder and available management;
- appreciate the hereditary contribution and recurrence risk for the disorder in specific relatives;
- understand their options for dealing with the risk of recurrence in terms of medical care, reproduction, testing, etc.
- choose which of the options, including doing nothing, is appropriate for them at this point in time in view of their risk, disease burden, and family goals and values; and
- make the best possible adjustment to the condition in oneself and/or one's loved ones and/or to the risk of recurrence of the disorder.

Definition adapted from the ASHG Ad Hoc Committee on Genetic Counseling, 1975.

genetics programs should always include genetics professionals. While genetic counselors and medical geneticists are well known and utilized in perinatology, obstetrics, neonatology, and pediatrics, they have been less visible in oncology, internal medicine, and primary care. Thus, it might be helpful to briefly describe the genetic counselor and medical geneticist.

Genetic Counseling. Who does genetic counseling? The majority of genetic counseling is performed by certified genetic counselors, medical geneticists, or advanced practice nurses with graduate genetics training.

One of the first formal definitions of genetic counseling was offered by Clarke Fraser in 1974, when he stated that genetic counseling is "a communication process which deals with the human problems associated with the occurrence, or risk of occurrence, of a genetic disorder in a family. This process involves an attempt by one or more appropriately trained persons to help the individual or family . . ."[42] (p. 637). A year later, in 1975, an Ad Hoc Committee of the American Society of Human Genetics accepted this definition[43] and further defined the basic components of the genetic counseling process listed in Table 2.

Through the genetic counseling process, the family can learn about the features, natural history, and variability of a disorder, as well as possible genetic contribution to its occurrence; surveillance, diagnostic testing, treatment, and other medical management options, and reproductive options. The goals are to help the family feel competent in coping with the risk and impact of the genetic condition, diminish guilt or blame and restore self-esteem, make decisions about testing, treatment, and/or reproduction; anticipate and deal with medical and/or learning problems associated with the condition; and identify and utilize resources for psychological, social, and financial support.

As a distinct profession, genetic counseling has its own code of ethics,[44,45] nationally accredited master's level training programs and clinical internships. A national certification process leading to the privilege of using the "certified genetic counselor" (CGC) designation has been established by the American Board of Genetic Counseling. In the U.S., most genetic counselors belong to the professional society known as the National Society of Genetic Counseling (NSGC) and most attend an annual national education conference. Publications include the peer reviewed *Journal of Genetic Counseling*, and a newsletter, *Perspectives in Genetic Counseling*, as well as various informational materials.

Some health professionals think there is a lack of trained genetic counselors, leading them to offer risk assessment and genetic testing without adequate and qualified genetic counseling. This is a grave error. Schneider, a well-respected cancer genetics researcher has stated, "If and when there is a greater demand for cancer genetic counselors, the training programs will almost certainly respond accordingly by increasing the number of individuals trained"[36] (p. 97). Currently, in addition to more than one thousand genetic counselors working in prenatal and pediatric settings who can handle the rudiments of cancer genetics, there are at least several hundred genetic counselors in North America who are members of the NSGC Cancer Genetics Special Interest Group (CA-SIG). The NSGC CA-SIG provides genetic counselor members with starter packets of basic ingredients for starting FCRC programs, discussion via an active e-mail listserve and newsletter, and multiple continuing education and collaborative research opportunities.

Hiring, Job Descriptions, Support. Hiring new staff (professional, administrative, and clerical) for the FCRC program will require development of job descriptions and responsibilities, recruitment, training, and supervision. Cancer genetics is currently a highly competitive field appealing to both new and experienced counselors. New genetic counseling graduates have had cancer genetics coursework and training experience with hereditary and familial cancers. More experienced genetic counselors have had continuing education opportunities and bring essential clinical and administrative experience and judgement to the FCRC program and promote smooth day-to-day operations.

All health professionals need adequate time and resources to learn and remain current with new developments in the rapidly expanding field of cancer genetics. To do so, they will require resources for purchasing reference books and doing adequate library and electronic literature searches prior to consultations with patients with hereditary cancer diagnoses. It is essential to access genetic testing databases to locate and compare genetic testing laboratories, which usually differ from one another in cost, service, and type of test being offered. Designated resources should also include membership in appropriate genetics and oncology societies, travel expenses, and continuing education at appropriate genetics, oncologist, and behavioral medicine conferences.

Having support staff allows the FCRC program to optimize professional time and expertise. Nursing, database, computer, statistical staff along with administrative and clerical personnel should be considered essential to the efficient and thriving program.

Budgets

The development of operational and capital budgets should be accomplished prior to the initiation of the clinical service. Operational budgets generally include a one-year projection of estimated expenses for the following categories: salaries, medical, and non-medical supplies, postage, duplication, publications, and minor equipment, including software under $500. Additional budgetary projections to consider are the extensive telephone consultations, travel, consultant, or physician services, professional memberships and certifications, reference books and periodicals, and seminar/conference/training expenses. It may be helpful to model your first operational budget after a similar sized program with a comparable mission.

While the operational budget can be thought of as the day-to-day expenses, the capital budget generally encompasses the large items, which have a longer shelf-life or are sold as a system. Items such as expensive software, office furniture, and computers are considered capital expenses. The capital budget can be defined very differently from institution to institution so it is extremely important that one know the rules before making budget requests.

Both operational and capital budgets need justification for when, how, and why the funds are needed for a particular item or service. After the initial year of operation, budget increases often need to be justified using the same criteria.

Billing and Reimbursement

There are a variety of ways to handle billing for FCRC. Some programs bundle clinic costs together (e.g., oncology, genetics, psychology, nutrition). Others itemize the costs for each provider separately. Universally, this bill does not include the cost of DNA testing, which can range from $200–$2500 per person in the current market. Reimbursement often depends on receiving pre-approval for the FCRC service and testing from the patient's insurance carrier. Because of concerns about confidentiality and possible discrimination, many patients prefer to pay out-of-pocket for the consultation and/or genetic testing.

Often, institutions classify services provided by a specific practice group into "cost centers", complete with unique institutional account number. These cost centers make it possible to track revenues and expenses. If the program bills for services rendered, then the cost center is considered to be "revenue generating". Even if the FCRC program is provided as service or research only, without charge to the patient, establishing a cost center may be advantageous for tracking indirect costs and revenues from related services, e.g., the amount that the radiology cost center recovers from providing mammograms for patients and their relatives referred by the FCRC program.

FCRC programs are funded by a variety of mechanisms including private donors, institutional foundation funds, one-time start-up grants, support from one or more departments, direct service billing, public moneys, and research granting mechanisms. Standards have not yet been developed for billing for FCRC. A national survey was conducted in 1996 of 110 GC members of the NSGC Cancer Special Interest Group about their current billing and record keeping practices.[46] These genetic counselors saw families in clinical service clinics, research studies, or in settings where clinical care and research are undertaken, most often at a comprehensive cancer center or research institute.

About one third of genetic counselors billed for FCRC in 1996. There was a wide range of billing codes and fees summarized in Tables 3 and 4. Over 80% billed under a supervising or participating physician's name, according to who was present and the level of service, based on the amount of time, type, and complexity of service. When seeing multiple family members, half charged a flat family fee. The ICD-9 codes varied depending on who was seen, e.g., most counselors billed using the "V" ICD-9 codes for family history of cancer for unaffected individuals and cancer diagnosis for persons with cancer. Many programs were not able to obtain exact reimbursement rates from their institutions.[46]

Billing and reimbursement experiences with genetic testing also varied widely. In 1996, the majority of counselees were at risk for hereditary breast cancer and were seen in a research setting, reflecting the state of test availability in 1995–6. Estimated rates of testing uptake among eligible persons varied from 0–75%, with an average of

Table 3. Familial Cancer Risk Counseling and Testing Billing
and Reimbursement

Billing Method	Revenue To	Sources of Support
Group fee/superbill	Unique cost center	Patient billing, institutional support, grant funds
Fee for each service	Each cost center providing service	Patient billing, institutional support, grants
No bill	None	Grant funding, donations

30–40% of patients who were offered testing deciding to pursue it. The percentages of patients whose insurance company covered testing at that time depended on the disease being tested as well as national, state, and local insurance laws and the differing policies of specific insurance companies. Many genetic counselors had patients who chose not involve their insurance company and to pay for a visit, and/or testing, out of pocket.[46]

There remain many potential barriers to successful billing and reimbursement in the current healthcare environment. These include:

- lack of a specific billing code(s) for genetic counseling, necessitating need to bill as physician consultation, out-patient office visit, or preventive care;
- no licensure for genetic counselors;
- the time-consuming nature of FCRC;
- the perception by third-party payers that genetic counseling falls into a category of prevention or education;
- specific billing idiosyncracies through different practice plans; and
- confusing billing mechanisms, e.g., for facility fees.

Other issues may also be addressed, including creating superbills inclusive of the team, using stacking codes, and choosing CPT/ICD-9 codes with highest reimbursement potential and favorable division of revenues.

Information Management

Patient Records. It has been a longstanding practice within the genetic counseling field to maintain within the genetics department "shadow files" on patients and families seen in genetics clinics. Genetic testing results should be treated as extremely

Table 4. Familial Cancer Risk Counseling Billing Types and
Fees

Type of Billing Code	Charges
Consultation codes	$50–$340
Outpatient visit	$30–$226
Preventive Medicine	$25–$225
Other/Unsure	various

Adapted from Bernhardt, Peshkin, Yemel, 1997.

private, and every effort should be made to guarantee confidentiality within the medical care and health insurance systems. Generally, limited portions of the genetics file are entered into the institutional medical record. However, the exact type and extent of cross-documentation varies widely. In their 1996 survey of genetic counselors, Bernhardt et al.[46] found that in FCRC, shadow charts are universal; however, only 20% send a complete consultation to the patient's institutional medical record. Even when a consultation summary is sent to the medical records department, references to testing decisions and genetic test results are often omitted. Incomplete charting can further complicate billing practices, as well as confuse efforts at achieving coordinated care. However, many feel that these steps are justified in order to protect the client's privacy, confidentiality, and minimize opportunities for employment or insurance discrimination. Others take the approach of fully documenting genetic assessment and testing in notes to the referring physician, but clearly mark these as being exempt from being copied or sent to other parties (Wendy Rubinstein, 1998, personal communication). Typically, results are released to a referring physician, other health professionals, insurers, or even family members only with a patient's written authorization.[46] The patient needs to be told and fully comprehend the implications of the fact that even in the most secure situations, complete protection can never be guaranteed.

Access/Privacy. There are different practices for research and clinical record-keeping in the U.S.[47] At a minimum, the privacy of clinical FCRC records should be as private as any medical records. It is best to keep records in locked files and secured computer databases, with access limited to members of the department who have a specific reason to read or handle them. Computer databases should have access limited by security codes. It is best that data sent to common databases be stripped of identifying information, whenever possible.

When FCRC occurs in the research setting, charts, records, and test results can be protected by certificates of confidentiality.[48] These are government issued documents that protect research files from release to third parties, except under specific legal conditions. However, once test results are given to the patient for medical management decisions, the certificate can no longer protect the genetic information from further disclosure in the healthcare system. Also, one family member may disclose information about another. Thus, genetic research also is not without risk of discrimination.

Referral and Scheduling Mechanisms and Processes

Generally, two types of clients will be referred to the FCRC: those with a personal cancer history and those with a family history of cancer. Specific relatives may be at average or at increased risk for certain cancers based on their family history and other risk factors.

The marketing and advertising strategies of the FCRC will determine how individuals become aware of, and are referred for, consultation (see Table 5). Mass marketing of the FCRC services through local and regional print and broadcast media could trigger a substantial number of inquiry calls that result in referrals. For example, Stadler and Mulvihill,[27] held a press conference with local TV and radio stations to announce the newly formed Cancer Genetics Program, a joint undertaking between the University of Pittsburgh Medical Center and Magee-Womens Hospital. In addition, a letter introducing the services of the program was mailed to more than 5000 physicians of different specialties. During the two weeks following the announcement, over

Table 5. Marketing and Advertising the Familial Cancer Risk
Counseling Program

- Direct mailing to current and previous patients
- Direct mailing to professionals
- Brochures and fact sheets in clinical areas
- Cancer Information Services
- Direct advertisement in newsletters, media
- Mail materials in response to inquiries
- Presentations at local, national, international meetings
- Lecture to private lay and community health organizations

250 calls were received and 60 persons were scheduled for appointments. Over the next three years, the number of calls to the program monthly has been influenced by what marketing efforts were undertaken at that time (Stadler, personal communication, 1998).

Given the current environment of healthcare and the prevalence of managed care, most clients are referred by their physician. Patients under certain types of insurance plans need an authorization to be seen if they intend to submit the cost of consultation for reimbursement. It is also important to note that if a patient is physician referred, the CPT code for billing purposes allows one to bill at a higher rate as a consultation (vs. an out-patient visit) provided that other evaluation and management requirements are met.

Referrals to the FCRC originate from many different sources (see Table 6). They can be straightforward, such as a client calling to schedule an individual appointment based on physician recommendation or self-motivation. Referrals may also result from screening questionnaires that the FCRC program supplies to various specialty cancer clinics and private physicians' offices. No matter how the referral was made, an efficient scheduling mechanism is essential to the success of the clinic.

Clearly, the FCRC must have a clinical supervisor or program coordinator to oversee the daily operations and ensure a smoothly running service. Sometimes the coordination functions are divided between two individuals, one clinically oriented, and the other with administrative or operations expertise (Peters, personal communica-

Table 6. Sources of Referrals for Familial Cancer Risk
Counseling Program

- Genetics clinics
- Oncology service
- Direct self-referral
- Cancer Information Service
- NCI/PDQ Cancer Genetics Directory
- Radiology and mammography
- Surgery, general, oncological, and reconstructive
- Gynecology/Obstetrics
- Gastroenterology clinics
- Managed care systems
- Cancer support groups
- Public health agencies
- Professional organizations/networks
- Clinical diagnostic laboratories

tion). Preferably, the clinical coordinator will be a genetic counselor with a strong clinical background and experience in cancer risk consultation who can triage referrals, respond to professional inquiries, and provide clinical services. Generally calls come via a designated scheduling telephone line or information hotline to a central scheduling desk. At the time of referral, the scheduler records demographic information along with the reason for referral. Referral information should be entered into a computerized database so that a permanent and searchable record of all calls is available. It is important to record these referrals for compiling program statistical summaries, and for future reference. Sometimes, intake forms, questionnaires, and/or medical record requests for diagnosis documentation will be sent out at the time of scheduling so that the consultation time may be utilized efficiently.

Quality Assurance, Quality Control, Evaluation, Satisfaction

Quality assurance (QA) is obtaining an acceptable measurable level of performance; quality improvement (QI) is the incremental increase in level of performance; and total quality management (TQM) is the whole process which includes quality assurance and improvement.[49] The issue of quality medical care is a concern not only in the US but internationally. The World Health Organization definition[50] of quality assurance (QA) in healthcare was established in 1989:

> ... to assure that each patient receives such a mix of diagnostic and therapeutic health services as is most likely to produce the optimal achievable health care outcome for that patient, consistent with the state of the art of medical science, and with biological factors such as the patient's age, illness, concomitant secondary diagnoses, compliance with the treatment regimen, and other related factors; with the minimal expenditure of resources necessary to accomplish this result; and with maximal patient satisfaction with the process of care, his/her interaction with the healthcare system, and the results obtained.

On the national level, the NSGC held a workshop in 1992 to begin addressing QA efforts at the institutional, state, and regional levels.[51] A 1996 survey by the QA sub-committee of the NSGC found that the most common QA measurements across different types of institutions are patient surveys or letter/chart review.[49] Few centers collect follow-up or outcome information. Fewer centers utilize a QA committee, peer review practices, survey referring physicians, hold case conferences or participate in a formal QA program. Efforts are under deliberation by the American College of Medical Genetics, the American Society of Human Genetics, NSGC and various regional genetics networks to describe and document the value of genetic services.

Evaluation of genetic counseling has been approached in a number of ways, depending on the aspects of genetic counseling which one most highly prizes. Some of these are similar to quality measures used in hospitals to satisfy state and federal regulators of healthcare. These types of measures may include assessments of professional competence, counting of clinic visits or contributions to lessening decreased morbidity and mortality due to genetic conditions. Decreased burden of disease is often difficult to demonstrate in health systems where quarterly or annual accounting are the norm; in contrast, genetic conditions may take decades or generations to develop. Despite these limitations, effectiveness of genetic counseling programs, which identify rare genetic disorders in individuals at risk, make it possible to use the knowledge of the natural history of the condition to design appropriate surveillance protocols to maximize the likelihood of desired health outcomes.[52] For example, reductions in screening costs and disease morbidity have been demonstrated in von Hippel-Lindau syndrome,[53] MEN2;[54,55] and HNPCC.[56] Genetic counselors are also actively involved in formulating meaningful, outcome-oriented guidelines for practice and developing methods to evaluate the effectiveness of genetic counseling.[52]

With regard to the genetic educational and counseling aspects of genetics, there have been studies of patient knowledge, information retention, emotional reactions to genetic information or judgements regarding the influence of genetic counseling on risk perception, decision-making, and reproductive intentions. Some have criticized these approaches as shallow and irrelevant.[57]

Uniform counseling guidelines for specific situations, self-assessment tools, elements required in genetics centers, standardized letters and glossary paragraphs to enable continued improvement, quality of care indicators, staff functions, and minimal standards of care are all in various stages of development. Additional methods include looking at formalized peer review of genetic counseling skills and consumer involvement in the development of genetic counseling materials.[52] Several concrete issues to consider in establishing FCRC programs of high quality are addressed below.

Board Certification. The theory, practice, and professional development of genetic counseling has evolved over these past 25 years as advances in genetics have produced applications which require increasingly complicated healthcare decisions. In order for the purchaser and/or consumer of FCRC services to know that the professional has adequate training in genetics, it is useful to examine professional qualifications. Since 1996, genetic counselors have adopted practice-based competencies for accreditation of and training in graduate programs in genetic counseling.[58] The four domains of competency are communication skills, critical-thinking (including calculation of genetic risks), interpersonal counseling and psychosocial assessment, and professional ethics and values. Professionals offering genetic counseling are trained at the M.D., Ph.D., or M.S. level and are usually certified by the American Board of Genetic Counseling (ABGC) and/or the American Board of Medical Genetics (ABMG). Board certified genetic counselors are recognized by the CGC initials; medical geneticists are certified by the American Board of Medical Genetics, and may use the FACMG designation, referring to membership in the American College of Medical Genetics. Genetic counselors who specialize in cancer genetics can be identified by membership in the Cancer Genetics Special Interest Group (CA-SIG) of the NSGC.

Patient Satisfaction. While the flurry of genetics research has increased the possibilities for cancer genetic counseling and susceptibility testing, there has been little attention given to satisfaction with such services. Stadler & Mulvihill[27] argue that "periodic self-inspection and evaluation of nascent programs are needed to ensure that cancer genetics programs are meeting the needs of the physicians and patients they are intended to serve". Therefore, after one year of operation of a FCRC program, they surveyed participants about how the cancer genetics services were perceived and how much information was retained about the consultations in order to modify and enhance the counseling service.

Overall, Stadler & Mulvihill[26,27] found that their clinical service met the needs and expectations of most counselees seen in the first year, 1995. They found that patient satisfaction was high with regard to the length of the consultation; along with the summary letter and attached pedigree, it was worth the expended time and money, and met client expectations. Clients reported the best parts of the experience were having personalized information, learning that cancer risk was lower than thought, allowing cleansing of one's conscience of burdensome guilty feelings, realizing that one had been justified in suspecting the inheritance of cancer in one's family, and just having a chance to talk about cancer.

The satisfaction survey also allowed for feedback to improve the FCRC service. For example, clients placed a great emphasis on the size and appearance of office space, prompting the program to move to a larger counseling room. Other issues that clients mentioned were frustration about wanting DNA testing without having to involve certain family members, and collecting all family records before the appointment. Several found it difficult to revisit unresolved psychosocial and family issues around the family history of cancer. Many worried about possible insurance discrimination.

Solutions to some of these concerns are possible, others will require deeper systemic changes. Perhaps an enriched psychotherapeutic component might help to transform some of the unresolved emotional issues. In response to frustration about family records, the program relaxed the criteria as to which records were truly needed prior to consultation and focused efforts on reviewing records for ambiguous or crucial histories or key relatives. Staff also helped participants secure essential records. Other concerns about fair access to services, privacy and confidentiality of medical information, and the specter of discrimination will require economic and political solutions.

Other forms of outcome studies will also be needed to test the worth of FCRC programs. For example, while there are many studies on the amount of information that patients can remember following counseling, simple recall fails to assess the additional dimensions of interpretation, i.e., how patients make sense of medical information; and commitment, i.e., how patients evaluate the providers' ideas in the context of their own explanatory models and how they plan in using this information to guide their subsequent behaviors.[57,59] Lea and colleagues[52] have gone a step further in incorporating consumers in design of patient-oriented materials.

PROGRAMMATIC ASPECTS OF A CANCER GENETICS PROGRAM

While the call for genetic counseling for familial cancers has sounded for decades,[60-62] widespread establishment of FCRC clinics is just beginning. In fact, even within NCI-funded comprehensive cancer centers, deficiencies and inconsistencies in cancer genetics services have been identified.[39]

Coordinating a successful FCRC program is analogous to irresistible cooking. Just as the successful chef requires ingredients of good quality, has the proper cooking appliances, a tested recipe, a sense of what flavors complement each other, and creative improvisation to create the many courses of a gourmet meal, so too the successful FCRC program director collects the essential ingredients mentioned in the operational section, identifies a proven recipe from other successful programs, adds a sense of what will work at the local institution, and exercises the creativity to craft a comprehensive program that satisfies creator and consumer alike. Next we shall consider the components of such a program (see Fig. 1).

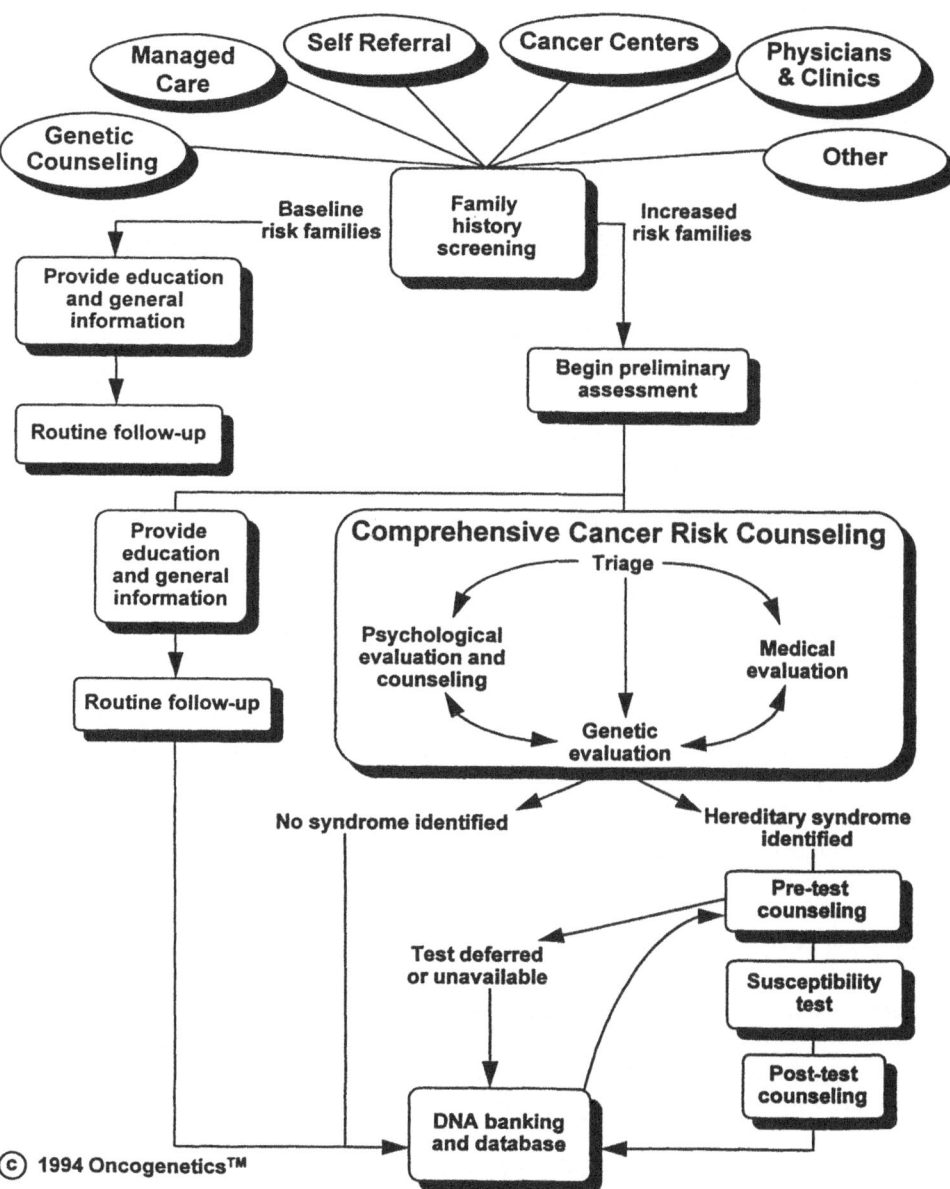

Figure 1. Cancer risk assessment and counseling protocol.

Ascertainment, Screening, and Triage

It has been estimated repeatedly that about 5–10% of most of the common cancers have strong hereditary components due inherited germline mutations.[4] In addition to the public health import, this figure represents a significant number of families for any oncology practice. This places significant burden on the oncologist to correctly identify and treat these cases accordingly. One way to meet the challenge is by developing a useful family history screening tool to consistently monitor one's clinical population. The screening tool can range from a single sheet that asks patients to list relatives and cancers[25a] (Mulvihill & Stadler, 1996), to sophisticated, computerized systems that can generate pedigrees and stratify the population by risk category.[63]

The preliminary report highlights this point about the use of family history screening. Mulvihill & Stadler[26] reviewed 187 gynecological and family planning charts and found that 47% had no family history of any kind noted, and 26% noted a family history limited to cancer. To correct this deficiency, they devised a two page self-administered family history questionnaire, which was completed by 266 out of the 269 patients approached in a six-week period. The forms took about five minutes for patients to complete. On review, 14% of completed questionnaires gave evidence of possible increased risk for cancer. This study suggests that self-administered cancer family history questionnaires can provide a quick and efficient way to aid identification of families for genetics referral.

The purpose of this preliminary screening is NOT to make a definitive genetic diagnosis, but rather, to identify those who have potentially increased cancer risk and merit further evaluation. In families with cancer clusters, it is customary to take a genetic pedigree, and further evaluate the family. Because there is evidence that self-reported family history may be inaccurate at certain cancer sites, the clinician, nurse, or geneticist should document cancer diagnoses.[64]

Increasingly, there will be molecular means of screening tumors for specific genetic markers that may indicate the presence of an underlying genetic cancer susceptibility. One example is the microsatellite instability (MSI) seen in some colon, endometrial, and other cancers. Some (but not all) cases of high levels of MSI can be associated with Hereditary Non-Polyposis Colorectal Cancer (HNPCC).[65] While the yield of this genetic screening seems low at present, one could foresee a day when additional markers may be available to improve the sensitivity of molecular screening of tumors to enhance the oncologists' ability to understand biological responses, tailor treatment choices, and improve clinical outcomes.[66,67]

Cancer Risk Assessment

Cancer risk assessment refers to the process of quantifying the statistical probability of an individual's developing cancer due to the presence of variables such as family history, cancer susceptibility genes, lifestyle, environmental exposures, and chance.[68] Most modeling of familial clusters of cancer has been done in relation to breast cancer.[23,69-75] These methods are best suited to women who do not have a recognized hereditary cancer susceptibility syndrome; hence, these models are not reliable for a truly high risk woman carrying a germline mutation. In hereditary cancer families, women may be at significantly higher risk for more than one type of cancer, e.g., ovarian cancer in persons carrying *BRCA1* mutations or thyroid disease or cancer in those with *PTEN* mutations causing Cowden disease. Further, risk assessment should be offered in the context of genetic counseling, where the implications of risk notification can be explored and risk reduction discussions can occur.

Medical Management of Genetic Risk

Medical management of cancer is on the verge of a revolution. For example, in the traditional model, a colon cancer patient would be treated with standard therapy determined by the size and stage of tumor. At-risk relatives might be identified through family history and offered screening. The advent of genetic testing changes the equation. Now genetic testing offers the prospect of customizing treatment for the cancer patient and identifying more accurately which relatives would benefit from enhanced cancer surveillance and prevention and which could be spared these costly and anxiety-producing strategies since they are not at increased cancer risk. Furthermore, those who know *prior to* developing cancer that they bear a deleterious, cancer-predisposing gene mutation could be prepared at the time of diagnosis to incorporate this genetic information into their treatment decision-making.

Medical management will vary with the situation and answers to questions such as the following. Does the proband have present or past cancer? Is the proband an unaffected relative at risk? Is the person a relative with cancer who is coming for genetic testing only for the sake of another relative, but who does not want to use genetic information personally for deciding medical management?

Clients seen in current FCRC programs usually assume that they are at high risk for developing cancer and are interested in what they can do about it. Many people seek cancer risk assessment, with or without testing, to pinpoint their cancer risk, get reassurance, and/or to help them decide what medical surveillance or preventive strategy to pursue. Often, people in families with many affected individuals may already be engaged in heightened surveillance; however, they may seek reassurance about the appropriateness of this strategy. Others with negative DNA test results may have difficulty abandoning their habits of heightened surveillance. While the medical management benefits of knowing genetic mutational status are clear-cut in some cancer predisposing disorders such as MEN2 or VHL, definite benefits have yet to be established in others, e.g. most notably, in hereditary breast or breast-ovarian cancer syndrome and HNPCC.[76,77] Genetic testing is also an opportunity to deal with the emotional and relational aspects of coping with inherited cancer risk. The FCRC program should have current medical management options available at the time of counseling as well as referrals to colleagues in other specialty areas for ready referrals.

One venue where genetic screening can make a significant impact is in the multi-disciplinary case conference or the treatment planning conference.[78,79] Cases being presented for consideration of treatment options should have very detailed family histories taken and evaluated to identify sub-groups at significantly increased risk for developing second primary cancers or malignancies at different organ sites due to a hereditary germline mutation. We predict that genetic information will increasingly be integrated into every aspect of clinical care.[66,67] While the testing for genetic mutations in breast cancer susceptibility genes is still expensive, cumbersome, and too slow for making immediate clinical treatment decisions at present, genetic testing is already augmenting biochemical and imaging strategies for management of other cancers. For example, DNA testing for mutations in the *RET* gene in medullary thyroid cancer, for *VHL* mutations causing von Hippel-Lindau disease, and for protein-truncating alterations of the *APC* gene for classical Familial Adenomatous Polyposis (FAP) are being successfully integrated with medical screening into clinical care of patients within affected kindreds. Thus, having a cancer genetics program can potentially reduce medical liability of failing to recognize genetic diagnoses which could alter medical management.

Genetic Susceptibility Testing for Hereditary Cancer

Genetic testing is not like other tests where test batteries are ordered with minimal discussion between physician and patient and, subsequently, only abnormal results discussed. Therefore, the Task Force was created by the National Institutes of Health (NIH)-Department of Energy (DOE) Working Group on Ethical, Legal, and Social Implications (ELSI) of Human Genome Research to review genetic testing in the US and to make recommendations to ensure the development of safe and effective genetic tests. The Task Force's final report has expanded the discussions of safety and effectiveness from a narrow definition of validity and utility to include also genetic test delivery in laboratories of assured quality and their appropriate use by health care providers and consumers.[80]

Genetic counseling should both precede and follow genetic testing.[36,68,80-84] For this reason, genetic testing should be considered a multi-step process, first assessing risk and determining likelihood of positive results, then choosing a particular test and laboratory and discussing details of a specific test, disclosing test results, discussing implications, and dealing with reactions and medical management.

Patients should be told at the outset that genetic testing is not for everyone. Testing is most typically helpful in families likely to have a deleterious mutation. Each center should set its own policy establishing statistical and psychosocial threshholds for when testing will be offered. Before widespread genetic screening is undertaken in the general population, many scientific and ethical issues must be addressed. Questions remain regarding the role of genetic, nutritional, and environmental factors in modifying the expression of cancer susceptibility gene mutations, as well as the frequency and penetrance of these mutations in the population at large. We also need to know the safety and effectiveness of genetic screening and establish mechanisms to ensure high quality control of test laboratories, and for adequate genetic education and informed consent processes for every person considering testing.[83] Furthermore, improvements in prevention and treatment of inherited cancers are needed before the genetic tests can truly make large differences in disease rates and outcomes.

Genetic counseling plays a crucial role in the genetic susceptibility testing process.[4,16,31,36,68,81] Genetic counseling in conjunction with quantitative risk assessment should be offered to evaluate the appropriateness of testing, and incorporated into pre-test and post-test discussions with the patient of the costs, risk, benefits, limitations, and implications of testing. It is especially important to discuss the worth of the test result for the individual and the family.

Pre-test Genetic Counseling and Informed Consent. Genetic discussions are woven into the informed consent process.[3,37,82] Informed consent in genetic testing must accurately and completely describe the information necessary for individuals to make fully informed decisions regarding whether or not to partake in predisposition testing.[84] Informed consent often involves transmitting extensive information about the description of test procedures, specificity and sensitivity of a given laboratory method, possible test results, implications of results to the patient and relatives, and risks, benefits, and limitations of currently available tests. Counselees should understand that DNA testing is voluntary, and that there are viable alternatives to testing at present, e.g., medical screening or tissue storage for DNA testing at a future date when test characteristics and cost are likely to improve. The possible test outcomes typically are not a clear all-or-nothing answer to questions about risk, but rather, they imply a relative increase or decrease in the probability for developing one or more neoplasms. The possibility of an inconclusive test result (either false positive or false negative) should be thoroughly discussed with counselees prior to testing in order to minimize later misunderstandings, disappointments, or outright errors in interpreting test results, as has already been demonstrated in APC screening for FAP.[85]

Genetic Test Disclosure. Most people are nervous as they await test results, generally becoming more so as the disclosure date approaches. In cases of newly developed DNA tests, results may take months or even years to become available, while others are commercially available in a few weeks. For this reason, it may be necessary to maintain contact by telephone and/or to repeat some of the pre-test counseling and update the family or personal medical history when results are given. However, in all cases, genetic test results, whether positive or negative, should be disclosed in person to the individual tested in straightforward language and with a compassionate manner. Consultands are encouraged to bring a support person with them to provide emotional support, to ask questions that the consultand may not raise, and to help recall the details of the discussion afterwards. At disclosure of test results, individuals generally focus on their personal cancer risk, medical management options, and the testing of other at-risk relatives, including children. It is important that the counselor be attentive to subtle emotional reactions, and undercurrents of awkwardness, secrecy, avoidance, resentment or guilt in the family dynamics.

Follow-up to Genetic Counseling and Testing. The effects of genetic counseling and DNA testing have been demonstrated to be long-lasting in other genetic conditions,[86,87] and we assume that hereditary cancers will be similar. Therefore, FCRC programs should make provisions for the availability of follow-up services for consultands and relatives for at least one year following testing. This follow-up should be offered to those with negative and inconclusive test results, as well as those with positive results, since adverse and unexpected effects have also been seen in those receiving decreased genetic risk.[88]

Psychosocial Aspects of Genetic Counseling

As was mentioned in the genetic counseling section, the goals of genetic counseling go beyond medical goals of reducing disease incidence, morbidity, and mortality. Genetic counseling is also concerned with the adjustment of the individual and the family to the condition. Even the goals of education and medical decision-making are deeply influenced by psychological factors. For example, it has been long argued that counselees may not be able to hear, understand, remember, or assimilate information if they are having an emotional response to what is being presented.[15,42,89,90] Despite this recognition, genetic counseling is often confused with genetic education, perhaps because the counseling aspect is more difficult to describe accurately. However, there is a slowly accumulating body of literature by social scientists who use participant observation, interviews, transcript analysis, and other qualitative methods to enrich our understanding of genetic counseling interactions.[59,91,92]

Although genetic education is vital to ensuring informed consent for genetic testing, the psychosocial issues go far beyond the education process. Lerman and Croyle[20] emphasize that psychological processes permeate nearly all aspects of clinical risk identification and reduction programs. To work successfully with patients and their relatives about genetic risk in meaningful ways, genetic counseling should be considered a process that deals simultaneously with informational content and psychological implications.

Lerman and Croyle[20] identified program components that can help prevent and manage adverse reactions to the disclosure of genetic status. These components include: providing pre-disclosure education and informed consent, bolstering coping skills, facilitating decision-making, identifying the need for referrals, and protecting patient privacy. Several of these issues will be discussed below.

Familial Cancer Psychosocial Assessment. Psychosocial evaluation within genetic counseling can be brief or comprehensive depending on the setting, reason for referral, the family needs, and the training and expertise of the genetic counselor, nurse, psychologist, or social worker. Assessment strategies should encompass individual, family, religious, and cultural considerations. This evaluation includes an assessment of the motivation for seeking genetic evaluation, the expectations of what would be gained from a genetics consultation, and the experiences, beliefs and attitudes about the condition in the family as well as standardized psychosocial information. It is important to get a sense of language usage, background knowledge, and level of medical sophistication in order to blend one's counseling style with their views and vocabulary. The psychosocial history also includes inquiry regarding previous emotional problems, current levels of functioning, and perception of one's own risk, as well as the responses to that risk on emotional state and daily function, general worldview of optimism or pessimism, and coping style and strategies.

In genetic conditions, the family is the patient. Because genetic conditions affect whole families, the spouse or family members may be invited to the counseling session. The genetic counselor, nurse, or social worker will often form a gestalt of family beliefs and attitudes, communication patterns, and family constellation and dynamics around information-sharing, secrecy, power distribution, and support systems. The counselor asks explicitly about employment, insurance status, native language, ethnicity, and educational level. The personal experience of genetic risk may be influenced by the closeness of relationship to affected individuals, psychological identification with affected individual, impact of disease on affected individuals, and one's developmental issues.

Testing for cancer susceptibility usually proceeds without undue psychosocial distress (Lerman, et al., 1996). However, there may be subsets of persons at emotional risk who exhibit fragility in the face of significant stressors. For example, Croyle, et al.[93] found that *BRCA1* gene mutation carriers manifested significantly higher levels of test-related psychological distress compared with non-carrier relatives; the highest levels were observed among mutation carriers with no personal history of cancer or cancer-related surgery. Recognizing persons who are psychologically vulnerable to becoming distressed through the counseling or testing processes is of paramount importance, since these are persons most helped by psychosocial interventions.[94] There should be psychiatric referral protocols and resources in place, prior to the need for them to handle unexpected crises. Providers should be prepared to defer the drawing blood for testing or providing test results if the person seems seriously depressed, suicidal, or unusually anxious, lacks all social support, or is dealing with intense grief reactions or other stressful life events. A consideration in the establishment of the FCRC is inviting a mental health professional to play a key role on the inter-disciplinary team, both on an ongoing basis, and as needed for crisis referrals.

Genetic Counseling Psychosocial Interventions. While the literature about psychological implications is growing, there is not yet a clear connection between psychosocial characteristics and interventions. Some believe that there is therapeutic value in the cancer genetic counseling experience, regardless of whether or not a person is considering having genetic testing.[1,2,68] For instance, genetic counseling can be an opportunity for the individual to untangle confusions and misunderstanding about genetic risk for cancer and to face up to and make meaning of past history of cancer in oneself or one's family.[27] Some individuals appreciate the chance to talk openly about cancer, while others find this aspect of cancer risk assessment unpleasant or threatening. Positive test results may lead to increased feelings of control, relief from uncertainly, and greater motivation to pursue cancer monitoring. On the other hand, knowledge that one carries a mutation in a cancer susceptibility gene could result in closer identification with affected relatives and greater fear of cancer[82] while negative results may engender relief and joy, and lessen depression, anxiety and cancer worry.[20–22,36]

There are also family benefits from undergoing genetic evaluation and supportive counseling. "Testing is performed on an individual basis, yet each result has implications for other family members"[36] (p. 95). The FCRC program needs sufficient structure so that individuals and families know what to expect, yet be flexible enough to proceed differently with different families depending on their unique needs and preferences. For example, some families operate in secrecy about testing, while others prefer to attend counseling together, and openly share test results. As a general rule, the family members should be the ones to disseminate information through the family rather than the FCRC staff. Having adequate family systems assessment of family communication and decision-making patterns can help in planning a strategy that will be most likely to work well in a given family.

One of the most important ways that the genetic counselor may be helpful is identifying and working to remove psychological barriers to recommended medical screening. Kash et al.[95] have shown that women attending a high-risk breast cancer prevention program had impaired follow-through with cancer screening recommendation in inverse proportion to their anxiety levels. Addressing this observation, they found that a short, psycho-educational support group including genetic counseling helped to alleviate the anxiety and improve medical screening.

SUMMARY

Genetic counselors are uniquely prepared to offer FCRC service due to specialized education, counseling expertise, and technical understanding of genetic disease. In our experience, the following recommendations are most helpful in beginning a cancer genetics program.

- Establish a multi-disciplinary team with strong leadership, stable administration, collegial exchange, and close coordination of family services to handle the diverse needs of families with hereditary cancers.
- Set realistic goals. A FCRC program cannot be established quickly, or become an overnight success, but rather, should be considered a cornerstone for future oncology practice.
- Consider the mission statement the first step and develop the program around the mission.

- Shadow other programs of compatible size, resources, and goals to find the right recipe for your institution.
- Insist on program excellence.
- Plan ahead both for program success and growth and also for the increasing incorporation of genetic advances into all phases of cancer prevention, screening, diagnosis, and treatment.

RESOURCES

A timely and focused summary of other internet oncology resources is available.[96] For additional information about genetic counseling and cancer genetics, visit the following web sites:

- National Society of Genetic Counselors—http://www.nsgc.org
- Genetics Professional Societies—http://www.faseb.org
- American Cancer Society—http://www.cancer.org/index_4up.html
- Alliance of Genetic Support Groups—http://www.geneticalliance.org
- National Human Genome Research Institute (NHGRI)—http://www.nhgri.nih.gov
- National Cancer Institute (NCI) CancerNet—http://cancernet.nci.nih.gov
- OncoLink, University of Pennsylvania—http://www.oncolink.upenn.edu
- Genetic Education Center—http://www.kumc.edu/gec
- National Action Plan on Breast Cancer (NAPBC)—http://www.napbc.org

ACKNOWLEDGMENTS

This manuscript began with an invitation to offer a workshop offered at the Cancer Genetics for the Clinician Conference on how to set up cancer genetics clinics. It was expanded through the compilation of the collective experience of the authors along with other colleagues who have described the experiences of establishing cancer genetics clinics. The authors would especially like to thank members of the NSGC CA-SIG who generously shared materials and information that have become part of the NSGC Cancer Clinic Starter packs. We are also grateful to Dr. John Mulvihill who shared his publications, personal experiences, and editing skills to enrich the manuscript.

REFERENCES

1. Peters JA: Familial cancer risk, Part I: Impact on today's oncology practice. Journal Oncology Management 3:18–30, 1994
2. Peters JA: Familial cancer risk, Part II: Breast cancer risk counseling and genetic susceptibility testing. Journal Oncology Management 3:14–22, 1994
3. ASCO: Statement of American Society of Clinical Oncology (ASCO): Genetic testing for cancer susceptibility. Journal of Clinical Oncology 14:1730–1736, 1996
4. Lynch HT, Lynch JF: Genetic counseling for hereditary cancer. Oncology 10:27–34, 1996
5. Ponder BA: Familial cancer: Opportunities for clinical practice and research. European Journal Surgical Oncology 13, 1997

6. Eeles RA, Murday VA: The cancer family clinic., in Eeles RA, Ponder BAJ, Easton DF, et al (eds): Genetic Predisposition to Cancer. London, UK, Chapman & Hall, 1996
7. Egan C: Models for cancer genetic risk assessment programs. Oncology Issues 12:14–17, 1997
8. Evans DGR, Cuzick J, Howell A: Cancer genetics clinics. European Journal Cancer 32A:391–392, 1993
9. Lemon SJ, Tinley ST, Fusaro RM, et al: Cancer risk assessment in a hereditary cancer prevention clinic and its first year's experience. Cancer 80:606–613, 1997
10. Lynch HT, Fitzsimmons MS, Lynch J, et al: A hereditary cancer consultation clinic. New England Journal Medicine 74:351–359, 1989
11. McKinnon WC, Guttmacher AE, Greenblatt MS, et al: The familial cancer program of the Vermont Cancer Clinic: Development of a cancer genetics program in a rural area. Journal Genetic Counseling 6:131–145, 1997
12. Vasen HFA, Griffoen G, Offerhaus GJA: The value of screening and central registration of families with familial adenomatous polyposis. A study of 82 families in the Netherlands. Diseases Colon Rectum 33:227–230, 1990
13. Vasen HFA, Mecklin J-P, Meera Khan, P: The international collaborative group on hereditary non-polyposis colorectal cancer (ICG-HNPCC). Diseases Colon Rectum 34:424–425, 1991
14. Lynch HT, Lynch JF, Cristofaro G: Genetic epidemiology of colon cancer, in Lynch HT, Hirayama T (eds): Genetic Epidemiology of Cancer. Boca Raton, FL, CRC Press, Inc., 1989
15. Kelly PT: Breast cancer risk analysis: A genetic epidemiology service for families. Journal Genetic Counseling 1:155–168, 1992
16. Menko FH, Whijnen JTH, H.F.A. V, et al: Genetic counseling in hereditary nonpolyposis colorectal cancer. Oncology 10, 1996
17. Grosfeld FJM, Lips CJM, Ten Kroode HFJ, et al: Psychosocial consequences of DNA analysis for MEN type 2. Oncology 10:141–145, 1996
18. Burke W, Press N, Pinsky L: Breast carcinoma genetics from a primary care perspective. Cancer 80:621–626, 1997
19. Stadler MP, Mulvihill JJ: Establishing a cancer genetics program in an academic medical center. American Journal Human Genetics 57:A348, 1995
20. Lerman C, Croyle R: Emotional and behavioral responses to genetic testing for susceptibility to cancer. Oncology 10:191–195, 1996
21. Lerman C, Narod S, Schulman K, et al: BRCA1 testing in families with hereditary breast-ovarian cancer: A prospective study of patient decision making outcomes. JAMA 275:1885–1892, 1996
22. Lerman C, Schwartz MD, Miller SM, et al: A randomized trial of breast cancr risk counseling: interactiong effects of counseling, educational level, and coping style. Health Psychology 15:75–83, 1996
23. Offit K: Clinical Cancer Genetics. New York: Wiley and Sons, 1998
24. Bachman RP, Bass HN, Bergoffen J, et al: An evidence-based BRCA1 testing guideline. American Journal of Human Genetics 59:56A, 1996
25. Ponder BAJ: Setting up and running a familial cancer clinic. British Medical Bulletin 50:732–745, 1994
25a. Mulvihill JJM, Stadler MP: Cancer family history: Baseline collection vs. self-reporting in a gynecology clinic. American Journal of Human Genetics 59:A76, 1996
26. Stadler MP, Mulvihill JJ: After cancer risk counseling: Consultands' satisfaction and subsequent behavior. American Journal Human Genetics 59:A7, 1996
27. Stadler MP, Mulvihill JJ: Cancer risk assessment and genetic counseling in an academic medical center: Consultants' satisfaction, knowledge, and behavior in the first year. Journal Genetic Counseling 7(3):279–297, 1998
28. Josten DM, Evans AM, Love RR: The cancer prevention clinic: A service program for cancer-prone families. Journal Psychosocial Oncology 3:5–20, 1985
29. Hoskins IA: Genetic counseling for cancer patients. Oncology 3:84–98, 1989
30. Peters JA, Stopfer JE: Role of the genetic counselor in familial cancer. Oncology 10:160–166, 1996
31. Petersen G, Brensinger J: Genetic testing and counseling in familial adenomatous polyposis. Oncology 10:89–94, 1996
32. Baty BJ, Venne VL, McDonald J, et al: BRCA1 testing: Genetic counseling protocol development and counseling issues. Journal of Genetic Counseling 6:223–244, 1997
33. Calzone KA, Stopfer JE, Blackwood A, et al: Establishing a cancer risk evaluation program. Cancer Practice 5:228–233, 1997
34. Graham J, Sargent K: How to set up a cancer genetics clinic. Workshop, in Peshkin B, Matloff E (eds): NSGC Cancer Genetics Shortcourse. Baltimore, MD, NSGC, 1997

35. Geller G, Tambor ES, Chase GA, et al: Measuring physicians'tolerance for ambiguity and its relationship to their reported practices regarding genetic testing. Medical Care 31:989–1001, 1993
36. Schneider KA: Genetic counseling for BRCA1/BRCA2 testing. Genetic Testing 1:91–98, 1998
37. Collins FS, Kahn MJE, Calzone KA, et al: Hereditary susceptibility testing for breast cancer, National Action Plan on Breast Cancer (NAPBC), Position Paper. National Action Plan on Breast Cancer, 1996
38. Collins FS: Preparing health professionals for the genetic revolution. JAMA 278:1285–1286, 1997
39. Thompson JA, Wiesner GL, Sellers TA, et al: Genetic services for familial cancer patients: A survey of National Cancer Institute cancer centers. Journal National Cancer Institute 87:1446–1455, 1995
40. Touchette N, Holtzman NA, Davis JG, et al: Toward the 21st Century: Incorporating Genetics into Primary Health Care. Cold Spring Harbor, NY, Cold Spring Harbor Laboratory Press, 1997
41. Dimond E, Calzone K, Davis J, et al: The role of the nurse in cancer genetics. Cancer Nursing, 1997
42. Frazier FC: Genetic counseling. American Journal Human Genetics 26:636–659, 1974
43. ASHG (Ad hoc committee of the ASHG): Genetic counseling definition. American Journal Human Genetics 27:240–242, 1975
44. Benkendorf JS, Callanan NP, Grobstein R, et al: An explication of the National Society of Genetic Counselors (NSGC) Code of Ethics. Journal of Genetic Counseling 1:31–40, 1992
45. NSGC: National Society of Genetic Counselors (NSGC) Code of Ethics. Journal Genetic Counseling 1:41–44, 1992
46. Bernhardt B, Peshkin B, Yemel Y: Billing and record keeping for familial cancer risk counseling: A national survey. Journal of Genetic Counseling 6:491, 1997
47. Mark HFL, Annas G, Ricker R, et al: Clinical and resarch issues in breast cancer genetics. Annals Clinical Laboratory Science 26:396–408, 1996
48. Early CL, Strong LC: Certificates of confidentiality: A valuable tool for protecting genetic data. American Journal Human Genetics 57:727–731, 1995
49. Connerton-Moyer K, Doyle DL: Total quality management in genetic services. Perspectives in Genetic Counseling 19:12, 1997
50. Vuori H: World Health Organization (WHO) and quality assurance. Quality Assurance in Health Care 1, 1989
51. Greendale K, Knutson C, Pauker SP, et al: Quality assurance in the clinical genetics setting—Report of a workshop. Journal Genetic Counseling 3:169–185, 1994
52. Lea DH: Emerging quality improvement measures in genetic counseling. Journal Genetic Counseling 5:123–137, 1996
53. Green J: Health care evaluation and cost analysis of clinical and genetic screening for von Hippel-Lindau disease in Newfoundland. American Journal Human Genetics 57:A295, 1996
54. Lips CJM, Landsvater RM, Hoppener JWM, et al: Clinical screening as compared with DNA analysis in families with multiple endocrine neoplasia type 2A. New England Journal Medicine 331:828–835, 1994
55. Wells SA, Chi DD, Toshima: Predictive DNA testing and prophylactic thyroidectomy in patients at risk for multiple endocrine neoplasia type 2A. Annals Surgery 3:237–250, 1994
56. Vasen H, van Ballegoijen M, Buskiens E, et al: Cost-effectiveness analysis of colorectal cancer screening in HNPCC, ICG-HNPCC Eighth Annual Meeting. Buffalo, NY, 1996
57. Michie S, Marteau T: Genetic counseling: some issues of theory and practice, in Marteau T, Richards M (eds): The troubled helix. Cambridge, UK, Cambridge University Press, pp 104–139, 1996
58. Fine BA, Baker DL, Fiddler MB: Practice-based competencies for accreditation of and training in graduate programs in genetic counseling. Journal Genetic Counseling 5:113–122, 1996
59. Hallowell N, Statham H, Murton F, et al: "Talking about chance": The presentation of risk information during genetic counseling for breast and ovarian cancer. Journal Genetic Counseling 6:269–286, 1997
60. Lynch HT: Dynamic Genetic Counseling for Clinicians. Springfield, MA, C.C. Thomas, 1969
61. Parry DM, Mulvihill JJ, Miller RW, et al: Strategies for controlling cancer through genetics. Cancer Research 47:6814–6817, 1987
62. Mulvihill JJ: Genetic counseling of the cancer patient., in DeVita FT, Jr, Hellman S, Rosenberg SA (eds): Cancer Principles and Practices of Oncology (ed 4th). Philadelphia, Lippincott, pp 2529–2537, 1993
63. Hampel H, Kuhn T, Markowitz A, et al: The use of optically scannable forms and computerized algorithms for mass family history cancer risk assessment. American Journal Human Genetics 59:A56, 1996

64. Aitken J, Bain C, Ward M, et al: How accurate is self-reported family history of colorectal cancer? American Journal of Epidemiology 141:863–871, 1995
65. Rodgriguez-Bigas MA, Boland CR, Hamilton SR, et al: A National Cancer Institute workshop on hereditary non polyposis colorectal cancer syndrome: Meeting highlights and Bethesda guidelines. Journal Nationa Cancer Institute 89:1758–1762, 1997
66. Peters JA: Applications of genetic technologies to cancer screening, preventiona, diagnosis, prognosis, and treatment. Seminars Oncology Nursing 13:74–81, 1997
67. Peters JA, Dimond E, Jenkins J: Genetic technologies in cancer care. Cancer Nursing 20:359–377, 1997
68. Peters JA, Biesecker BB: Genetic counseling and hereditary cancer. Cancer 80:576–586, 1997
69. Benichou J, Gail MH, Mulvihill JJ: Graphs to estimate an individualized risk of breast cancer. Journal of Clinical Oncology 14:103–110, 1996
70. Berry DA, Parmigiani G, Sanchez J, et al: Probability of carrying a mutation of breast-ovarian cancer gene BRCA1 based on family history. Journal of the National Cancer Institute 89:227–237, 1997
71. Claus EB, Risch N, Thompson WD: Genetic analysis of breast cancer in the cancer and steroid hormone study. American Journal Human Genetics 48:232–242, 1991
72. Claus EB, Risch N, Thompson WD: Autosomal dominant inheritance of early-onset breast cancer: Implications for risk prediction. Cancer 73:643–651, 1994
73. Gail MH, Brinton LA, Byar DP: Projecting individualized probabilities of developing breast cancer for white females who are being examined annually. Journal National Cancer Institute 81:1879–1886, 1989
74. Hoskins KF, Stopfer JE, Calzone KA, et al: Assessment and counseling for women with a family history of breast cancer: A guide for clinicians. JAMA 273, 1995
75. Offit K, Brown K: Quantitative risk counseling for familial cancer: A resource for clinical oncologists. Journal Clinical Oncology 12:1724–1736, 1994
76. Burke W, Petersen G, Lynch P, et al: Recommendations for follow-up care of individuals with an inherited predisposition to cancer. I. Hereditary nonpolyposis colon cancer. Cancer Genetics Studies Consortium. JAMA 277:915–919, 1997
77. Burke W, Daly M, Garber J, et al: Recommendations for follow-up care of individuals with an inherited predisposition to cancer. II. BRCA1 and BRCA2. JAMA 277:997–1003, 1997
78. Lee CZ, Coleman C, Link J: Developing comprehensive breast centers—Part one: Introduction and overview. Journal Oncology Management 1:20–23, 1992
79. Lee CZ, Coleman C, Link J: Developing comprehensive breast centers—Part two: Critical success factors. Journal Oncology Management 1:20–26, 1992
80. Holtzman NA, Watson MS: Task force on genetic testing of the National Institute of Health working group on ethical, legal, and social implications of human genome research: Promoting safe and effective genetic testing in the United States. Final Report, Bethesda, MD, National Institutes of Health, 1997
81. Biesecker BB, Boenke M, Calzone K, et al: Genetic counseling for families with inherited susceptibility to breast and ovarian cancer. JAMA 269:1970–1974, 1993
82. Geller G, Botkin JR, Green MJ, et al: Genetic testing for susceptibility to breast and ovarian cancer. JAMA 277:1467–1474, 1997
83. Holtzman NA: Are we ready to screen for inherited susceptibility to cancer? Oncology 10:57–64, 1996
84. MacDonald DJ: Informed consent in cancer predispostion testing-Implications for genetic cousnelors. Journal Genetic Counseling 6:457–458, 1997
85. Giardello FM, Brensinger JD, Petersen GM, et al: The use and interpretation of commercial APC gene testing for familial adenomatous polyposis. New England Journal Medicine 336:823–827, 1997
86. Wiggins S, Whyte P, Huggins M: The psychological consequences of predictive testing for Huntington's disease. New England Journal Medicine 327:1401–1405, 1992
87. Bloch M, Adam S, Wiggins S: Predictive testing for Huntington disease in Canada: The experience of those receiving an increased risk. American Journal Medical Genetics 42:499–507, 1992
88. Huggins M, Bloch M, Wiggins S: Predictive testing for Huntington disease in Canada: Adverse effects and unexpected results in those receiving a decreased risk. American Journal Medical Genetics 42:508–515, 1992
89. Kessler S: Genetic Counseling: Psychological Dimensions. New York, NY, Academic Press/Harcourt, Brace, Jovanovich, 1979
90. Hallowell N, Richards MPM: Understanding life's lottery. Journal Health Psychology 2:31–43, 1997
91. Beeson D: Nuance, complexity, and context: Qualitative methods in genetic counseling research. Journal of Genetic Counseling 6:21–44, 1997

92. Green J, Richards M, Murton F, et al: Family communication and genetic counseling: The case of hereditary breast and ovarian cancer. Journal Genetic Counseling 6:45–60, 1997
93. Croyle RT, Smith KR, Botkin JR, et al: Psychological responses to BRCA1 mutation testing: Preliminary findings. Health Psychology 16:63–72, 1997
94. Baum A, Friedman AL, Zakowski SG: Stress and genetic testing for disease risk. Health Psychology 16:8–19, 1997
95. Kash KM, Holland JC, Halper MS, et al: Psychological distress and surveillance behavior of women with a family history of breast cancer. Journal National Cancer Institute 84, 1992
96. Sikorsky R, Peters R: Oncology on the Internet: Where to find reliable cancer information on the internet. JAMA 277:1431–1432, 1997

2

GENETIC COUNSELING FOR THE INDIVIDUAL WITH INHERITED CANCER SUSCEPTIBILITY

Barbara Bowles Biesecker

Genetic Counselor and Co-Director
Genetic Counseling Research and Training Program
Medical Genetics Branch/NHGRI/NIH
Bldg. 10, Room 10C101
10 Center Drive MSC 1852
Bethesda, MD 20892-1852

I. INTRODUCTION

Molecular discoveries into common diseases are occurring at an astounding rate. Cancer is no exception. There are now a number of genes that, when mutated, confer a significantly increased risk of cancer. Additional genes that confer a more modest risk of cancer are also being discovered. Together with improved understandings of environmental risk factors, increasingly accurate predictions of individual cancer risk will become available. Further, improved treatments will result from better understanding of the underlying cause(s) and contributions to cancer development. Yet, with the promise of these new discoveries comes the current introduction of new clinical tools that are not yet well understood. For oncology providers, it is challenging to determine which patients are most likely to have a cancer predisposing gene mutation. Those patients deemed eligible for genetic testing must consider risks and benefits of testing, as well as the limitations. Genetic counseling is the process by which patients can explore their interest in genetic testing and make informed decisions. As more genetic tests become available, aspects of the genetic counseling process will need to be increasingly provided by oncologists and oncology nurses. Research that identifies innovative and effective approaches to support patients and facilitate test decision-making will improve and expand genetic counseling services in the future.

Telephone: (301) 496-3979

Cancer Genetics for the Clinician, edited by Shaw.
Kluwer Academic / Plenum Publishers, New York, 1999.

II. GENE DISCOVERY

The discovery of cancer susceptibility genes has outpaced development of improved treatments. These discoveries have lead to the development of genetic tests that can be used to improve the accuracy of cancer risk prediction for certain high risk individuals. However, more accurate risk predictions by way of genetic testing may be available for many years prior to having evidence that cancer detection or intervention strategies are successful. This time gap leaves patients to struggle with the decision whether to avail themselves of new genetic tests. For those who do and are found to be at increased risk, there are uncertainties in deciding how to act on the results. The lack of known outcomes of testing and medical recommendations make genetic testing a personal medical decision. Some patients may find the test result information useful while others may not. Genetic counseling helps patients determine whether they may benefit from cancer gene testing. This chapter discusses cancer risk assessment, the role of cancer gene testing, and genetic counseling for cancer risk.

III. CANCER RISK ASSESSMENT

When a patient identifies herself/himself as concerned about a personal risk for developing cancer based on family history, it behooves the provider to assess the risks and offer appropriate counseling. The counseling may focus on understanding the cancer-related concern, discussion of any differences between perceived and actual risk, a surveillance or prevention plan, and/or on the role genetic testing may play in accurately assessing cancer risks.[1] Genetic testing is currently infrequently used as a tool for assessing an individual's cancer risks. The responsibility to assess who may benefit most from genetic testing falls to the provider. Determining the likelihood that a gene mutation has contributed to the cause of the cancer in the family is an important first step. Ultimately, this will lead to identification of patients most likely to have inherited a susceptibility to cancer.

Although cancer can cluster in families, this does not necessarily imply that there is an inherited cancer predisposition. When taking the family history, the provider needs to determine whether: multiple people are affected in different generations; the ages of onset are remarkably young; and the pattern of cancers present in the family are consistent with a recognizable syndrome or association. This is done by taking a thorough multiple generation family history; verifying the types of cancer reported in the family; documenting ages of onset; assessing non-genetic (environmental) risk factors; and evaluating the pattern of cancer occurrence. Unfortunately, there is no absolute definition of a hereditary cancer family that makes this effort straightforward (see chapter by Hoskins). If there is reasonable suspicion of an inherited predisposition, then the provider should further consider whether the patient is interested in genetic testing and is likely to personally benefit from the information gleaned from testing. Risk assessment may lead to referral for genetic counseling in order to assist the patient in exploring the role of cancer gene testing.

IV. WHAT'S DIFFERENT ABOUT GENETIC TESTING?

Determining who is most likely to harbor a cancer gene mutation is important not only to maximize the utility of testing, but also to put genetic testing into context for the patient. Cancer gene testing as it is currently offered is relevant to only a small proportion of families and individuals afflicted with cancer. For instance, of all cases of breast cancer in the United States, perhaps 5% are due to an inherited single gene susceptibility.[2] The vast majority of breast cancer is sporadic, however it occurs frequently enough in the general population (12% lifetime risk) that having a family history is very common. Further, genetic testing differs from other tools in medicine. The very nature of genetic tests with their inherent limitations and implications suggest the importance of individual testing decisions and the role of genetic counseling.

Genetic testing for cancer is predictive, but not diagnostic. Identifying a cancer gene mutation in an individual does not mean he or she certainly will develop cancer. Further, for any individual with a gene mutation the timing and severity of cancer development cannot be accurately predicted. Most current recommendations for early detection strategies following a "positive" cancer gene test are based on expert medical opinion rather than on medical evidence.[3] It will require decades of longitudinal research on mutation carriers to gather sufficient data to make sound recommendations for medical follow-up.

When potential risks and benefits of cancer gene testing are presented to a member of a hereditary breast and ovarian cancer family for instance, it should be made clear to the patient that while she may choose to learn more precisely whether she faces a high risk for cancer there is limited evidence that taking certain medical action(s) will result in increased longevity or quality of life. This is complicated when patients assume test results will be motivating to them but the guidelines for surveillance and early detection may not lead to reduced morbidity and mortality. Thus, discussions of potential benefits must focus on the potential inherent value of the information. If a patient is anxious about living with continued uncertainty of whether she inherited a cancer gene mutation from her father and finds herself distressed and obsessing about her risk of cancer, learning her status, one way or the other, may be emotionally beneficial to her. It may not alter her surveillance activities (other than to reduce them in the event that she learns she did not inherit the mutation present in the family) nor may the information prevent her from developing breast cancer. But the psychological relief from the uncertainty may make it worthwhile in her case. Further, it clarifies the risks to her children. If she inherited the mutation, there is a 50% chance she has passed it on to each of her children. If she did not inherit it, she does not have it to pass on to her children or to her grandchildren. The psychological benefits of knowing this information may be as important as the benefits of using the information to alter behaviors.

Genetic test results are also considered by many to be personal and private.[4] This may be due partly to the socially stigmatizing aspects of carrying an aberrant gene, but also due to concerns about insurance discrimination.[5] The personal aspect of testing is paradoxical given that by their very nature, genetic test results provide information about an entire family. An individual who carries a cancer gene mutation reveals that his/her first degree relatives (parents, children, and sibling) have up to a fifty percent chance of carrying the same gene mutation. As well as genetic, there are emotional and financial ramifications for the family when a person's results predict that they are at increased risk to develop cancer. Together, these descriptors of genetic testing, coupled with a paucity of data on the interpretation of certain laboratory results and medical recommendations for follow-up, suggest cancer gene testing should be offered only to those who understand the potential risks and limitations and are most likely to benefit from the results. Upholding personal choice is of utmost importance in offering cancer gene testing and is considered a basic tenant of genetic counseling.[6]

V. GENETIC COUNSELING FOR INHERITED CANCER RISK

The process of genetic counseling can assist patients in making informed decisions about cancer gene testing. However, the introduction of cancer gene testing presents interesting challenges to traditional genetic counseling. Most genetic testing offered to date has been performed for uncommon disorders. The intent of testing has been to make a diagnosis of a genetic condition or to determine whether someone carries a gene mutation that predisposes their child to a genetic condition. Thus, use of the information has focused primarily on reproductive decision-making. Rarely have adults faced the option of learning their own risk status based on genetic testing. In this case, risks to children are also a concern but test results are used mainly to understand ones own health status. Other than state-mandated newborn screening, most genetic testing has been offered within the context of clinical genetics services coupled with genetic counseling. Testing has been done primarily for rare disorders (for diagnosis of an affected family member or for reproductive planning) and the needs of patients have been (more or less) met by the relatively small number of genetic counselors and medical geneticists operating specialty genetics services.

Cancer gene testing, while currently relevant to a small number of cancer cases, will become useful for a much larger target population in the future. As testing becomes more accurate and recommendations more sound, the frequency of genetic testing will undoubtedly rise. As cancer is far more common than most genetic conditions, the number of patients likely to need genetic counseling services will increase. Also, the nature of the tests for individual risk prediction differs from testing for diagnostic purposes and introduces significant ambiguities into the test decision-making process.

Traditional genetic counseling has emphasized the importance of upholding personal, autonomous decision-making, particularly in the arena of prenatal diagnosis and decisions on whether or not to continue pregnancies when the fetus is affected with certain conditions. Non-directiveness describes the practice in which clients are encouraged and supported in their own decision-making without explicit influence from the counselor. This counseling approach of educating, exploring, facilitating, and supporting is both time and labor intensive. Given a much larger population considering testing, certain aspects of counseling will need to be made more widely available. There is a need for other medical professionals to be trained to address aspects of genetic testing. Providers will need to appreciate the importance of individual decision-making and personal choice due to the ambiguities and limitations of test results.

VI. GENETIC COUNSELING MYTHS OR MISUNDERSTANDINGS

In an effort to suggest how these new challenges to genetic counseling ought to be met, I present for consideration misconceptions about genetic counseling as it is currently practiced. For one, genetic counseling has been described as a service to provide recurrence risk information.[7] This suggests that a pedigree analysis is done, a risk calculated and information presented to the patient. While patients often seek genetic counseling with questions about recurrence, the process of counseling goes far beyond the provision of information. Genetic counseling might be better described as a dual process of education coupled with exploration of the emotional impact of the information.[8] This process can be described as a client-centered counseling approach that assists patients in assimilating genetic information, exploring its meaning, making decisions, and living contentedly with the outcomes of those decisions. In the case of cancer risk counseling, while it may be important to review the factual information about the genes involved and the risk of cancer, the counseling specifically addresses how the patient might use the information and how it fits with other health-related decisions made in the past.

Another common misconception of genetic counseling is that patients understand risk information provided, retain it, and use it in their childbearing (or other health-related) decisions. Outcomes research in genetic counseling, although sparse, suggests that patients often do not retain much of the information provided and may not find what is viewed by the counselor to be important as most useful in making their decisions.[9-11] The relative importance to the clients of the information provided in genetic counseling depends on the timing of the session in the patients life and their receptivity. They may be more prepared to understand information about inheritance if they've had time to adapt to their circumstances. Further, life planning decisions are often far more complex than simply applying information learned in genetic counseling. While clients often come seeking answers to specific questions about inheritance, it is the importance placed on that information (such as how they perceive the burden of the condition) in their particular life circumstances (such as one of limited resources) that is likely to be more relevant to their decisions. Thus, the emotional and social context in which the information is presented contributes significantly to how it is assimilated and used to make decisions. Overall, genetic counseling strives to provide personally tailored education and client-centered counseling addressing the decision whether or not to undergo genetic testing.

VII. EDUCATIONAL CHALLENGES IN PROVIDING GENETIC COUNSELING

During counseling, genetic and cancer information must be effectively transmitted to the patient, recognizing the importance of exploring its personal meaning and relevance. The process involves discussion of abstract concepts such as probabilities or likelihood. The manner in which the information is conveyed can help to maximize patient comprehension of such abstractions. Further, there are many uncertainties or unknowns in cancer genetics that are also difficult for patients to appreciate. One example is the lack of precise understanding of the penetrance (the chance for developing cancer) of many mutations. Analogies may be employed to illustrate such concepts. Terms used to teach both genetics and cancer stem from biological and medical sciences. When patients have no background in these scientific vocabularies, familiar concepts and terms of conversational speech must be adopted.

An important goal of genetics education is to convey the information in an accurate and balanced way. For instance, if the hazards of test results are overemphasized that may lead patients to choose not to undergo testing when they otherwise would like to know their risk status. On the other hand, if the promise of cancer surveillance activities is stressed perhaps those who would rather not know their risk status choose to undergo testing. The counselor must take great care not to convey personal opinions about testing that are not based on evidence. Similarly, they must strive to provide information in a balanced way that accurately reflects the current state of knowledge. Although personal decision-making is stressed, the counselor may directly influence a patient's choice about testing based on how the information is presented and what information is included. An important role of genetic counseling is to ensure patient comprehension based on a balanced view of the information.

Within the educational goals of counseling is the risk of overloading patients with information. While there are many bits of relevant information that counselors may believe patients need to know to make their test decisions, too much information may be counterproductive. Patients may become overwhelmed with the details and have a difficult time prioritizing information or determining relevance to their own decision-making. Further, it is important for the counselor to learn what information the patient perceives to be most useful and relevant. The tailoring of information is critical to facilitating decision-making and assumes that not all patients need precisely the same information. If left to the judgment of the counselor alone, aspects of testing outcomes critical to the patient may not be included.

VIII. PSYCHOLOGICAL CONTEXT OF GENETIC INFORMATION

The context in which an individual faces a choice about genetic testing influences the decision and the long-term outcomes. Importantly, genetic counseling considers psychological factors that may play a role. This is not to imply that individuals who may choose to undergo genetic testing are psychologically weak or mentally ill but rather that the information itself is potent. Some describe it as life-altering. Others cannot believe that anyone at high risk would choose not to know their test results. Once someone does choose to know their results, there is no turning back if the results are not what was desired. Thus, one objective of the counseling process is to help patients be prepared for either outcome and to make "good" decisions for themselves.

Insufficient research has been conducted to anticipate with certainty the psychological outcomes of cancer gene testing. Several studies have suggested that certain psychological parameters, such as cancer-related distress, are correlated with the decision to undergo testing.[12] Test decisions in our studies of members of hereditary cancer families seem to be related to marital status, age, and family cohesion (based on preliminary analysis of 188 family members). Several studies have followed individuals who chose to be tested to better understand the impact of test results. Those who, at a variety of ages, learn that they harbor a BRCA1 mutation have significantly less depressive symptoms six months after receiving test results than those who choose not to undergo testing.[13] It is expected that further research will indicate that individuals' reactions to test information will be related to personality traits (such as optimism), how they cope with stress-provoking information, the perceived personal threat of the information, and the control they perceive themselves to have over their own health. While additional research is needed to understand whether there are significant toxic psychological harms of cancer gene test information, preliminary evidence suggests there are not.[5,13,14]

Research into psychological outcomes of other genetic tests and of genetic counseling can be used to inform our predictions for cancer gene testing. For instance, the perceived burden of a genetic condition being tested for has been one of the strongest predictors of use of genetic test results.[10] It is not unexpected that an elevated cancer burden or worry coupled with a high perceived risk may predict interest in the use of cancer gene test results.[15] Further, health behavioral research and clinical "hunches" based on counseling hereditary cancer families can lead to additional informed hypotheses.[16,17] For instance, individuals with a greater tolerance for ambiguity or uncertainty may be less likely to undergo cancer gene testing.[18] Those who are optimists or more hopeful may be more likely to choose to undergo testing. They may be more tolerant of the potential results of genetic testing. Those who fear cancer may be highly motivated to pursue testing yet also sufficiently scared of the results to avoid testing. Fear or distress has been shown in the past to be both a motivator of health-related behavior as well as an obstacle.[19,20] Thus, these character traits and feeling states need to be investigated over time in order to make more accurate predictions about how they will effect testing decisions and outcomes.

These personality traits and emotions become more complex when considered alongside various cultural values and beliefs of patients. Cancer itself is viewed, discussed, and treated in a variety of ways in differing cultures. For instance, until recently, in Japanese culture a cancer diagnosis has not been discussed directly with the patient.[21] Further, if one's belief about the cause(s) of cancer have no grounding in scientific thought but are based on spiritual beliefs or forces, then genetic status may be irrelevant to the client. Future studies must include patient populations from a variety of ethnic and religious backgrounds in order to gather at least preliminary data on the correlation of certain beliefs with testing outcomes.

Genetic counselors often address feelings of patient guilt and shame in their clinical work. Despite the lack of control we have over our genetic destiny and (for the most part) our children's, there are often strong feelings of responsibility expressed by patients in counseling interactions. In cancer genetic counseling this has been described by our group and others as survivor guilt.[18,22] Those that have been spared the family's genetic "destiny" may express grave concern over why they have been so fortunate. Some voice a preference that they "trade places" with those less fortunate (and often younger) in the family. Smith and associates have investigated the issue of survivor guilt and report that it is not uniform between members of one large extended family.[23] For instance, sisters seem to be less distressed by differing test results than noncarrier brothers who have carrier sisters.

As in any therapeutic relationship, there are also practical issues that counselors face in meeting the psychological needs of their patients. If the patient has a topic agenda that conflicts with that of the counselor, meeting the needs of both patient and counselor (in serving that patient) may be quite challenging. Patients at times have agendas that are hidden or not apparent to the counselor, making patient satisfaction even more of an abstraction. Effective clinical skills are needed to assess patient concerns, needs, abilities, and expectations in order to deliver effective counseling services and facilitate cancer gene test decisions.

IX. ALTERNATIVE MODELS FOR GENETICS EDUCATION AND COUNSELING

Current challenges to genetic counseling practice and future anticipated changes to the field suggest a need for new efficient but effective approaches to genetic counseling. Perhaps it is easiest to begin by standardizing the informational aspects of counseling. For instance, a well-developed videotape may present patients with thoroughly balanced information about cancer gene testing. It can even include vignettes that model different decision-making processes and outcomes.[24] The use of videotapes removes the burden from the counselor to present lots of factual information and frees him or her up to spend the counseling session helping the patient to process and apply the information gleaned from the tape. It ensures that patients making decisions about testing are provided similar information upon which to base their decisions. A further advantage of a videotape is the use of graphics to illustrate complex concepts. While this tool needs to be investigated in terms of it effectiveness and appeal to patients, it may be one option to address the time consuming nature of genetic counseling services. Use of videotapes for education also introduces a risk that tapes will be regarded as inexpensive alternatives to professional genetic counseling services. Other providers may assume that they offer an alternative to personal counseling. Effective tools for genetics education offer no substitute for the processing of the information provided by a professional counselor. A client may be able to successfully recite facts about cancer gene testing following the viewing of a videotape and yet be no further along in her own test decision-making.

Another educational tool worthy of investigation for cancer gene testing is interactive computer programs.[25] This tool offers similar advantages to videotapes but can also be individualized by the patient. In other words, the patient can customize the information he or she wants to learn and can review any topics chosen. It remains to be determined whether patients enjoy learning from a computer and whether it is successful; but interactive computer programs may be one of the most promising tools for future models of genetics education. Again, education via the computer should be followed by personal counseling and should be regarded as a potential adjunct rather than a replacement of genetic counseling services. Both videotapes and computer programs offer opportunities to foster the effectiveness of the short-term genetic counselor.

An information age is upon us and the surge in rapidly accessible information via the internet cannot be ignored. Patients currently attend genetic counseling visits armed with far more information than ever before. This revolution will continue to unfold and provide an increasingly large sector of the population with rapid access to information. Further, the use of e-mail listserves or chat boxes provides opportunities for patients to interact and learn from one another. For instance, members of the hereditary cancer families that participate in our NIH research are initiating a support group via the internet and postal service. There will be more channels for patients to compare information they have uncovered and to process it with one another. In my opinion, this type of peer education and counseling should be encouraged. There are many advantages to patients receiving information and support through non-providers and those familiar with living in a hereditary cancer family. Of course there are risks to it as well, such as receiving and believing incorrect or irrelevant information. But we don't and can't control what our patients are exposed to or choose to adopt. We can work with peer counselors and support group leaders to help ensure accuracy and completeness of information but this is a daunting task.

Access to information via the internet and its impact on gene testing decisions is difficult to investigate and represents a moving target. However its increasing presence cannot be ignored. How successful it will be in increasing the overall knowledge base of patients prior to genetic counseling is unknown. It does serve to remind us that a more important role of genetic counselors is that of a psychological counselor, rather than a genetics educator. No matter how educated the patient-population becomes they may be no further along in evaluating the various ways cancer gene testing may or may not be appropriate for themselves.

In addition to new models for genetics education, there may be a need for new models of short-term decision-making or problem-solving types of counseling. Such approaches are used in other areas of health behavior counseling and may offer useful structure for genetic counseling. Currently no practice standards exist even for prenatal genetic counseling, which might adapt to standardization more readily than other arenas in which genetic counseling is practiced.[26] Most prenatal patients participate in genetic counseling to make a decision (or to review a prior decision) to undergo prenatal testing (amniocentesis or chorionic villus sampling). They are involved in a decision-making process that applies the information they have been given to their interest in learning more about their developing baby's chromosomes. That interest may be greater if the risks are high, if the burden of the conditions tested for is perceived to be great, and if there is an interest in pursuing an abortion if the fetus is found to be abnormal. Such a prediction is not intended to ignore patients who choose to undergo testing simply for the perceived value of the information given low risks, low perceived burden and/or no interest in abortion. It simply rehearses reported clinical experience with prenatal decisions. This is a subspecialty of genetic counseling where decision-making models have been proposed.[27] It remains one where the application of a clinical decision-making tool may prove to be an effective model for genetic counseling following education, perhaps by a videotape or interactive computer program. While cancer gene testing is a new and burgeoning field and for that reason less amenable to standardization, most patients are facing test decisions. Decision-making tools have been applied to decisions about cancer surveillance, for instance, and may serve as useful models for investigation of gene testing.[28] In a similar light, some authors have proposed the application of values self-awareness exercises for patients undergoing genetic counseling.[29] Helping patients to clarify their personal values about cancer risk, cancer worries, and early detection methods, for instance, may be useful within psychological counseling. Yet it remains only one piece of a larger decision-making process. Information, values and beliefs are all important to test decision-making but so are emotions: how patients may feel about, and therefore act on, test results.

Another short-term counseling model that we are currently investigating is a problem-solving model.[30] This model is based on cognitive-behavioral psychotherapy and offers a brief intervention that focuses on the patient's approaches to coping with stress-inducing circumstances such as facing an elevated cancer risk. It teaches patients how to identify a problem (such as how to make a decision whether or not to undergo cancer gene testing) and to brainstorm and prioritize solutions. The exercise continues with exploration of the potential consequences of the identified solutions including the potential long-term benefits of certain choices. Overall, it provides patients with the structure in which to contemplate outcomes of their test decisions. It also provides a model for future decision-making. This may prove particularly useful in cancer genetics since those choosing to be tested who are found to have a mutation, may face additional complex cancer risk-related decisions in the future. Arming patients with a technique they might employ again in the future could turn out to be even more valuable than a one-time interaction.

X. RESEARCH NEEDS

Throughout this paper, the need for research has been reiterated. Genetic counseling is a young profession and one that has evolved from clinical care.[6,31] In an effort to better understand patient needs and effective interventions, there is a need for clinical investigation and behavioral studies particularly as they apply within new subspecialties of genetic counseling and in the integration of new technologies. Cancer gene testing is an important arena in which to investigate patient education needs, effective counseling strategies and the test decision-making process. Barriers to services and other access issues can be investigated. Patients from a variety of ethnocultural backgrounds may be included in order to gain insights into the effects of their beliefs and values on counseling for cancer gene testing. The need for balanced and effective educational tools has been presented along with new models for short-term counseling decision-making strategies. Important research into various genetic counseling approaches will not only improve the effectiveness of specialty services, but will also help to clarify what aspects of the cancer genetics education and counseling oncologists and hem/onc nurses will play in the future.

Much of cancer gene testing is currently offered by genetic counselors working within teams of high risk oncology providers. Those being offered testing have been determined to be highly likely to carry a gene mutation. As testing becomes increasingly widespread oncology patients will be educated and offered testing more often without the assistance of a genetic counselor. It will remain critical to patient care that when they receive "positive" gene test results they are referred for follow-up counseling to a genetic counselor in order to review the impact of the information and for assistance in making future cancer-risk related health care decisions. Services of other subspecialists such as radiologists, surgeons, and ob/gyns will also be imperative in the comprehensive follow-up care of patients.

REFERENCES

1. Peters J, Stopfer JE: Role of the genetic counselor in familial cancer. Oncology 10:159–182, 1996
2. Easton DF: The inherited component of cancer. Br Med Bull 50:527–535, 1997
3. Burke W, Daly M, Garber J, et al: Recommendations for follow-up care of individuals with inherited predisposition to cancer. II.BRCA1 and BRCA2. Cancer Genetics Studies Consortium. JAMA 277:997–1003, 1997
4. Fanos JH, Johnson JP: Barriers to carrier testing for adult cystic fibrosis sibs: The importance of not knowing. Am J Med Genet 59:85–91, 1995
5. Lerman C, Narod S, Sculman K, et al: BRCA1 testing in families with hereditary breast-ovarian cancer: A prospective study of patient decision-making and outcomes. JAMA 275:1885–1892, 1996
6. Biesecker B: Future directions for the genetic counseling profession: Practical and ethical considerations. Kennedy Institute of Ethics Journal, 8:145–160, 1998
7. Shiloh S, Saxe L: Perception of risk in genetic counseling. Psychol Health 3:45–61, 1989
8. Kessler S: Psychological aspects of genetic counseling. IX. Teaching and counseling. J Genet Counsel 6:287–296, 1997
9. Sorenson JR, Swazy JP, Scotch NA: Medical genetics and genetic counseling in Reproductive Pasts Reproductive Futures: Genetic Counseling and Its Effectiveness. Birth Defects: Original Article Series, XVII (4). New York, NY, Allan R. Liss, pp 131–144, 1981
10. Lippman-Hand A, Fraser FC: Genetic counseling: Provision and reception of information. Am J Med Genet 3:113–127, 1979
11. Michie S, McDonald V, Marteau TM: Genetic counseling: Information given, recall, and satisfaction. Patient Educa Counsel 32:101–106, 1997

12. Lerman C, Croyle R: Psychological issues in genetic testing for breast cancer susceptibility. Arch Int Med 154:609–616, 1994
13. Lerman C, Hughes C, Lemon S, et al: What you don't know can hurt you: Adverse psychologic effects in members of BRCA1-linked and BRCA2-linked families who decline genetic testing. J Clin Oncol 16:1650–1654, 1998
14. Croyle RT, Smith KR, Botkin JR, et al: Psychological responses to BRCA1 mutation testing: Preliminary findings. Health Psych 16:63–72, 1997
15. Struewing JP, Lerman C, Kase RG, et al: Anticipated uptake and impact of genetic testing in hereditary breast and ovarian cancer families. Cancer Epidemiol Biomarkers Prev 4:169–173, 1995
16. Lerman C, Glanz K: Stress, Coping, and Health Behavior, in Glanz K, Lewis FM, Rimer B (eds). Health Behavior and Health Education: Theory, Research, and Practice. San Francisco, CA, Jossey-Bass Publishers, pp 113–138, 1997
17. Biesecker BB, Boehnke M, Calzone K, et al: Genetic counseling for families with inherited susceptibility to breast and ovarian cancer. JAMA 269:1970–1974, 1993
18. Lippman-Hand A, Fraser FC: Genetic counseling–The postcounseling period: I. Parents' perceptions of uncertainty. Am J Med Genet 4:51–71, 1979
19. Becker MH (ed): The Health Belief Model and Personal Health Behavior. Thorofare, NJ: Charles B. Slack, Inc, 1974
20. Lerman C, Lustbader E, Rimer B, et al: Effects of individualized breast cancer risk counseling: A randomized trial. J Natl Cancer Inst 87:286–292, 1995
21. Strazar MD, Fisher NL: Traditional Japanese Culture, in Fisher NL(ed): Cultural and Ethnic Diversity: A Guide for Genetics Professionals. Baltimore, MD, The Johns Hopkins University Press, p 109, 1996
22. Krell R: Holocaust Families: The survivors and their children. Com Psychiatry 20:560–568, 1979
23. Smith KR, West J, Croyle R, et al: Familial context of genetic testing for cancer susceptibility: the moderating effect of siblings' test results on psychological distress following BRCA1 mutation testing. Cancer Epidemiol Biomarkers Prev 8:385–392, 1999
24. Magyari T, Smith ACM, Wholey K, Gold RS: Evaluation of the effecticeness of multimedia decision-support materials vs. traditional genetic counseling for CF carreir screening (Abstract). J Genet Counsel 3(4):318–319, 1994
25. Green MJ, Fost N: Who should provide genetic education prior to gene testing? Computers and other methods for inproving patient understanding. Genet Test 1:131–136, 1997
26. Matloff ET: Practice variability in prenatal genetic counseling. J Genet Counsel 3:215–232, 1994
27. Degner LF, Beaton JI: Life-Death Decisions in Health Care. New York, NY, Hemisphere Publishing Corp., 1987
28. Salazar MK, deMoor C: An evaluation of mammography beliefs using a decision model. Health Educat Quarterly 22:110–126, 1995
29. Doukas D: personal communication within the Univeristy of Michigan Human Genome Ethics Committee, 1992 (see related article: Doukas DJ, Giorenflo DW, Venkateswaran R: Understanding patients' values. J Clin Ethics 4(2):199–200, 1993)
30. D'Zurilla TJ: Problem-Solving Therapy: A Socl Competence Approach to Clinical Intervention. New York, NY, Springer, 1988
31. Kenen, Regina H, Smith Ann CM: Genetic counseling for the next 25 years: Models for the future. J Genet Counsel 4:115–124, 1995

3

ESTIMATING INDIVIDUALIZED RISK OF BREAST CANCER

Mitchell H. Gail[1] and Jacques Benichou[2]

[1]Biostatistics Branch, Division of Cancer Epidemiology and Genetics
National Cancer Institute
6130 Executive Blvd., Room EPN 431
Rockville, MD 20892
[2]University of Rouen Medical School
Biostatistics Unit 1, rue de Germont
76031 Rouen Cedex, France

1. INTRODUCTION

It is estimated[1] that 179,000 women in the United States will be diagnosed with breast cancer in 1998 and that 44,000 will die from it. About one in eight women will develop breast cancer sometime in her life.[2] Many women are therefore concerned about the risk of developing breast cancer, especially women with known risk factors such as a history of breast cancer in close relatives. The purpose of this paper is to review and compare two models for projecting the individualized risk of developing breast cancer over defined age ranges. One model,[3] based on data from the Breast Cancer Detection Demonstration Project (BCDDP), uses information on family history, age at menarche, age at first live birth, number of biopsies, and the presence of atypical hyperplasia. A second model by Claus, Risch, and Thompson,[4] which we refer to as the "Claus model", relies on detailed family history information, including age at breast cancer onset in affected relatives. Published tables[5] based on that model cover individuals with at least one affected relative.

1.1. Absolute Risk versus Relative Risk

It is important to distinguish absolute risk from relative risk. Most studies of risk factors for breast cancer estimate relative risk. Relative risk is the ratio of the age-specific incidence rate among women with specific risk factors to the incidence rate among women without risk factors. For example, using the BCDDP model,[3] one can estimate that a forty-year-old nulliparous woman who began menstruating at age 14,

Cancer Genetics for the Clinician, edited by Shaw.
Kluwer Academic / Plenum Publishers, New York, 1999.

39

who has had no breast biopsies, and whose mother had breast cancer has a relative risk of 2.76 compared to a forty-year-old woman with no risk factors. Although relative risk estimates are useful for identifying risk factors and for comparing the risk of one woman with that of another, they do not directly measure the chance that a woman will develop breast cancer over a defined age interval.

Absolute risk is the chance that a woman with defined risk factors will develop the disease of interest over a defined age interval. For example, one might want to know the chance that the forty-year-old woman described above would develop breast cancer between ages 40 and 70. From the BCDDP model,[3] one estimates this absolute risk as 0.116 or 11.6%.

Four elements influence the absolute risk of breast cancer. One is the age of the woman. For example, the absolute risk that a thirty-year-old woman who is otherwise like the forty-year-old woman described above would develop breast cancer in the next 30 years is 8.5%, rather than the 11.6% calculated previously. The duration of the age interval is also important. Shorter time periods yield smaller absolute risk. For example, the chance that the thirty-year-old woman above would develop breast cancer in the next ten years is 1.2%. The particular risk factors that a woman has also influence absolute risk. Thus a woman whose risk factors put her at high relative risk will have a higher absolute risk over a given age interval than a woman at lower relative risk. A fourth element that influences absolute risk is the chance of dying of some other disease before the disease of interest develops. These competing risks reduce the absolute risk of breast cancer and can have an appreciable impact in old age. The impact of these four factors is expressed quantitatively in equation (5) of Gail et al.[3] that takes current age, age interval, risk factors, and competing risks into account.

Absolute risk is directly relevant to counseling, because it allows a woman to evaluate the magnitude of the risk over various time periods. An appreciation of absolute risk can lead to a better understanding of the potential benefits of medical options and management strategies. For example, a woman with several risk factors and high relative risk may be reassured to learn that her absolute risk of developing breast cancer over the next ten years is small, and she may elect to follow a program of surveillance. Conversely, she may be very concerned about a large absolute risk over a period of 30 years, and she may decide to undergo prophylactic mastectomy. Such decisions are complicated and depend importantly on the particular concerns of the woman and on the medical options. However, an estimate of absolute risk is a useful ingredient in devising a sound management plan. Information on the range of uncertainty in the estimate of absolute risk is also useful to the woman and health care provider.

1.2. Outline

In Section 2, we review factors associated with increased breast cancer risk. We describe the BCDDP model,[3] easy ways of obtaining absolute risk estimates from this model, and validation studies in Section 3. We review the Claus model[4,5] in Section 4 and compare it to the BCDDP model. In the Discussion (Section 5), we consider how to apply these models in counseling and how to deal with special factors that affect risk, such as demonstration of a mutation in the breast cancer genes, BRCA1 or BRCA2.

Table 1. Selected Risk Factors for Breast Cancer Incidence

Factor	Comparison Group	Approximate Relative Risk	References
Age 60–64	Age 25–29	56	26
Western country	Japan	5	27
Family history of breast cancer			
One first-degree relative	No affected first-degree relative	1.4–3	3, 28
Two or more first-degree relatives		4–6	3
Early age of onset (30 yrs) in an affected relative	Age 50 at onset	2.6	4
BRCA1 or 2 mutation carrier risk (to age 70)	Non-carrier	5–15	6, 7
Age at menarche 11	Age 16	1.3	28
Age at first birth ≥30	Age <20	1.9	28
Age at menopause after 55	Age 45–55	1.5	28
Exposure to 100 rads	No exposure	3	28
Two alcoholic drinks/day	Nondrinker	1.7	28
Hormone replacement therapy ≥10 yrs	None	1.3	28
A breast biopsy	No biopsy or aspiration	1.3–1.7	3, 28
Proliferative disease on biopsy	No biopsy or aspiration	2	28
Atypical hyperplasia on biopsy	No biopsy or aspiration	4	29, 30
≥75% dense tissue on mammogram	No dense tissue	5	31
Contralateral breast cancer	None	5	28

2. RISK FACTORS

Epidemiologists have identified many factors associated with breast cancer risk. It is useful to divide these into factors that may induce cancer and features of the medical history, such as the presence of atypical hyperplasia on a biopsy, that serve as markers of increased risk but may not cause cancer. These two types of risk factors are grouped separately in Table 1.

Age is the most important risk factor; a woman age 70–74 has 56 times the risk of developing breast cancer in the next year as a woman age 25–29 (Table 1). As shown in the solid semi-logarithmic plot in Fig. 1, risk rises with age at a rapid exponential rate for young women and continues to rise exponentially, though at a slower rate, for women over 50 years old. Living in a western country is associated with a relative risk of 5 (Table 1). Women with two or more affected first degree relatives (e.g., mother, sister, or daughter) have high relative risks (4–6), and women known to carry mutations of the breast cancer genes BRCA1 or BRCA2 have cumulative relative risks to age 70 estimated to be between 5 (see Struewing et al.[6]) and 15 (see Whittemore et al.[7]). Relative risks are even higher at younger ages. Aspects of the reproductive history, such as age at menarche, age at first live birth, and age at menopause also affect risk, but the associated relative risks are moderate (Table 1). Recent evidence suggests an association with elevated alcohol intake and with prolonged hormone replacement therapy. Exposure to 100 rads of radiation is associated with a relative risk of 3.

Certain features of the medical history are prognostic, even though they may be markers of the disease process rather than causal agents. Having more than 75% dense tissue on a mammogram carries a relative risk of 5 compared to a woman with no dense

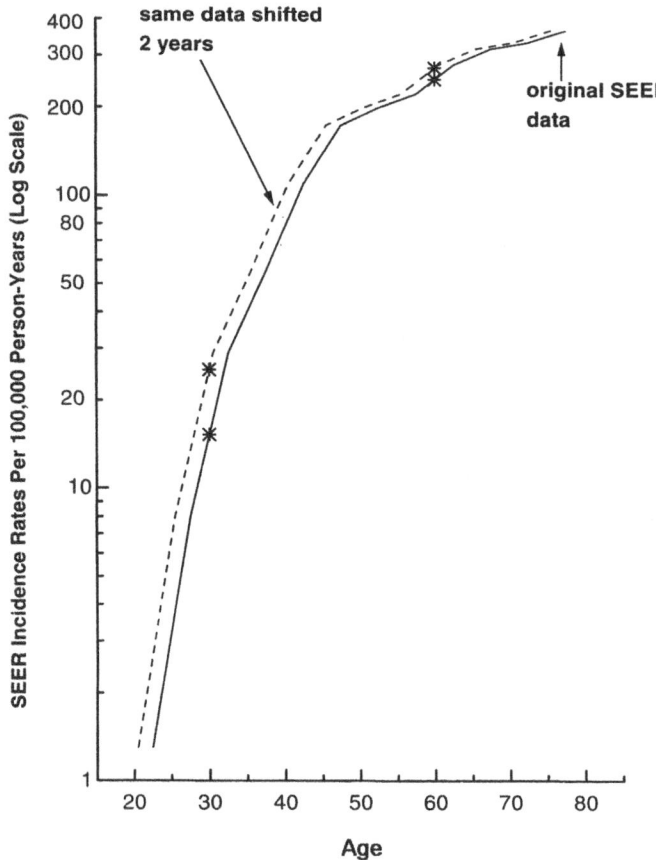

Figure 1. Age-specific breast cancer incidence rates from the Surveillance, Epidemiology, and End Results (SEER) program of the National Cancer Institute are shown by the solid curve. Taken from Gail and Benichou.[32] The dashed curve represents the effect of a two-year lead time from screening. Asterisks correspond to relative risks from screening of 1.67 and 1.12 for 30- and 60-year-old women, respectively.

tissue (Table 1). A history of contralateral breast cancer also increases the risk five fold. Demonstration of atypical hyperplasia or proliferative disease on biopsy is associated with elevated risk, and even a history of biopsies with non-proliferative disease is associated with a modest elevation in risk. Such features of the medical history may be useful in projecting risk, even though some of them, such as mammographic density, have not yet been incorporated into models for projecting risk.

It is clear that models for projecting breast cancer risk should at least account for age and family history. Both the BCDDP model[3] and the Claus model[4,5] do this, though the methods used differ.

3. BCDDP MODEL

3.1. Study Population and Modeling Approach

The BCDDP model[3] was based on a study of 243,221 white women who volunteered to be screened annually with mammography and physical exams for five years beginning in 1973–1975. Because the age-specific breast cancer incidence rates are higher in women in regular screening, Gail et al.[3] noted that "the risk projections from this model are probably most reliable for counseling women who plan to be examined about once a year."

Gail et al. used data from an embedded case-control study to empirically model relative risks from family history and aspects of reproductive and medical history. Although they did not posit a particular genetic model for breast cancer, genetic features are captured to some extent by empirical modeling of risks associated with family history. Gail et al. combined case-control information on relative risks with cohort information on age-specific breast cancer incidence rates to obtain estimates of absolute risk for women with particular risk factors.

3.2. Estimating Risk from the BCDDP Model

The BCDDP model first calculates a multivariate relative risk that takes age at menarche, age at first live birth, number of biopsies, atypical hyperplasia, and number of affected first-degree relatives (mothers or sisters) into account (Table 2). To compute a relative risk from Table 2, one multiplies the four relative risks corresponding to factors A, B, C, and D. For example, the forty-year-old woman considered previously began menstruating at age 14 (relative risk factor 1.00), had no breast biopsies (relative risk factor 1.00), was nulliparous and had an affected mother but no affected sisters (relative risk factor 2.76), and had no atypical hyperplasia (1.00). Thus the combined relative risk is $1.00 \times 1.00 \times 2.76 \times 1.00 = 2.76$. Now consider a 40-year old woman who began menstruating at age 12 (relative risk factor 1.10), and who had one breast biopsy (relative risk factor 1.70). Her first child was born when she was 31 years old, and her mother, but none of the sisters, had a diagnosis of breast cancer (relative risk factor 2.83). There is no information on atypical hyperplasia from the biopsy (relative risk factor 1.00). Her combined relative risk is therefore $1.10 \times 1.70 \times 2.83 \times 1.00 = 5.29$. If atypical hyperplasia had been present the relative risk estimate would be $1.10 \times 1.70 \times 2.83 \times 1.82 = 9.63$.

Gail et al.[3] showed how to convert relative risk estimates into absolute risk estimates using their Table 4 for various ages at counseling and years of follow-up. It is simpler and sufficiently accurate for clinical applications to read absolute risk estimates from the graphs of absolute risk versus relative risk prepared by Benichou, et al.[8] We have reproduced their graphs in Fig. 2 for 30 year risk projections. Panel A is for women with no biopsies, panels B and E for women with one biopsy, and panels C and F for women with more than one biopsy. Separate plots are given for 20-, 30-, 40-, and 50-year-old women. The thirty year risk for the forty-year-old woman with relative risk 2.76 and no breast biopsies can be estimated from Fig. 2A as 12%. From Fig. 2B, one estimates an absolute risk of 17% for the forty year old woman with one biopsy and no information on atypical hyperplasia. From Fig. 2E, the estimate of absolute risk is 28% for the forty year old woman with atypical hyperplasia on her biopsy.

Twenty- and ten-year projections can be obtained from Fig. 2 in Benichou et al.[8] (not shown here). To obtain projections for a 35 year-old woman, one can interpolate between projections for a 30-year-old woman and a 40-year-old woman. Benichou et at.[8] also provide a graph, reproduced as our Fig. 3, of upper and lower confidence level limits plotted against absolute risk. Figure 3 can be used to construct a confidence interval for the risk projection. For example, the woman with an estimated risk of 28% and atypical hyperplasia would have a confidence interval on the risk projection of (17%, 43%). Note from Fig. 3 that the width of the confidence interval increases with

Table 2. Relative Risk Computation for the BCDDP Model. Adapted from Gail et al.[3]

Risk Factor	No. of first-degree relatives with breast cancer	Relative Risk
A. Age at menarche, years		
≥14		1.00
12–13		1.10
<12		1.21
B. Number of breast biopsies		
Age at counseling < 50 years		
0		1.00
1		1.70
≥2		2.88
Age at counseling ≥ 50 years		
0		1.00
1		1.27
≥2		1.62
C. Age at first live birth, years		
<20	0	1.00
	1	2.61
	≥2	6.80
20–24	0	1.24
	1	2.68
	≥2	5.78
25–29 or nulliparous	0	1.55
	1	2.76
	2	4.91
≥30	0	1.93
	1	2.83
	≥2	4.17
D. Atypical hyperplasia (AH)		
No biopsies		1.00
At least one biopsy and no AH found on any biopsy		0.93
No AH found and AH status unknown for at least one biopsy		1.00
AH found on at least one biopsy		1.82

To compute overall relative risk, multiply four component risks from categories A, B, C, and D. For example, a 40-year-old nulliparous woman who began menstruating at age 14, who has had no biopsies, and whose mother had breast cancer has an overall relative risk of $1.00 \times 1.00 \times 2.76 \times 1.00 = 2.76$.

increasing estimated absolute risk, reflecting greater uncertainty with higher projected risks.

A simpler and more accurate approach is to use the computer program RISK written by Benichou.[9] This program calculates risk using formulas in Gail et al.,[3] and calculates confidence intervals based on Benichou and Gail[10] and Benichou.[11] Figure 4 depicts an interactive computer dialogue for the forty-year-old woman with atypical hyperplasia and relative risk 9.63. RISK calculates her risk as 29.7%, with 95% confidence interval (19.8%, 41.8%). The previous graphical estimates of 28% with confidence interval (17%, 43%) are close to the exact results from RISK.

3.3. Validation of the BCDDP Model

Several investigators have checked the relative risk calculations of the BCDDP model against other data sources. Because data on atypical hyperplasia are not consis-

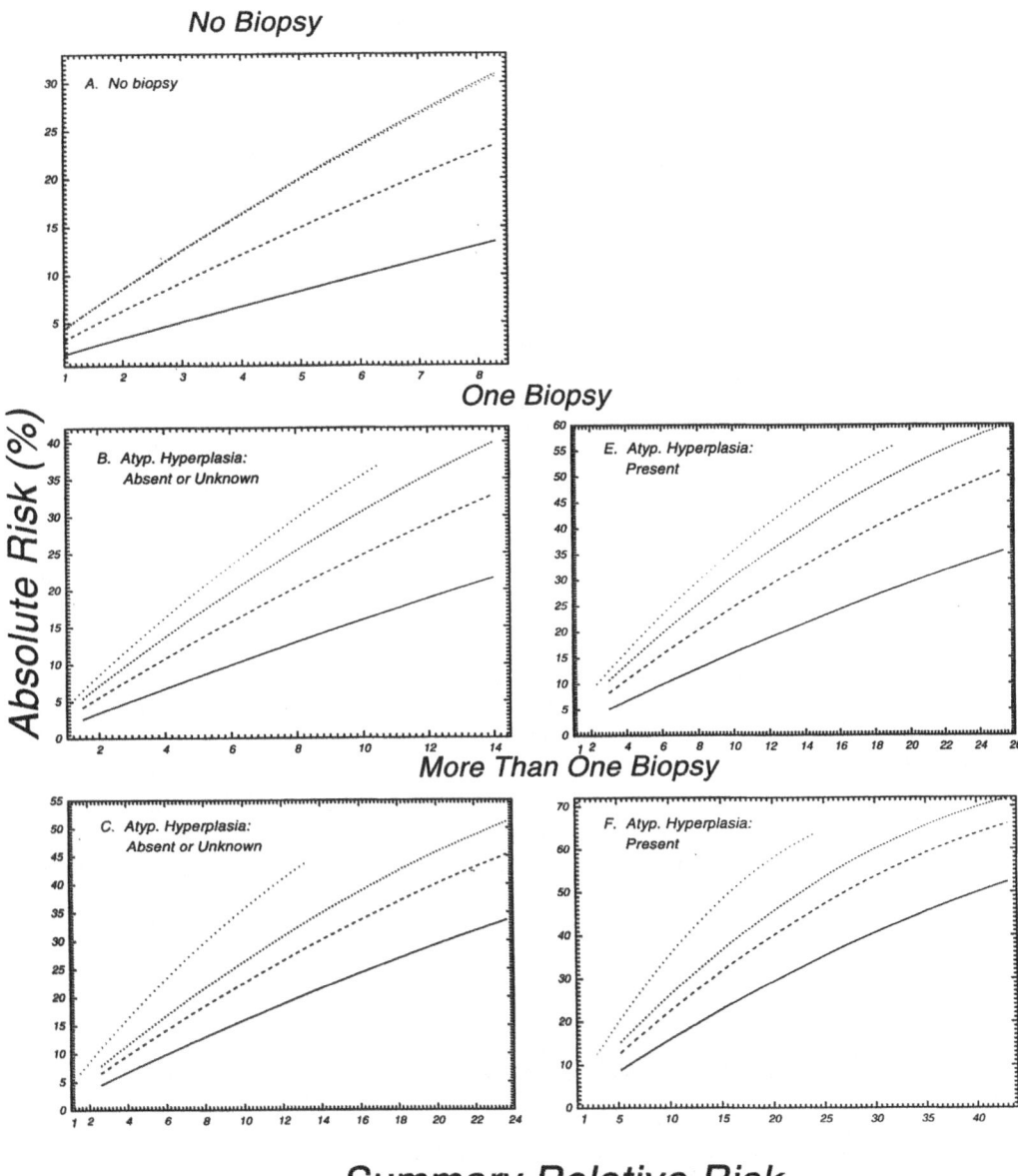

Figure 2. Plots from Benichou et al.[8] of the absolute risk of developing breast cancer in thirty years versus relative risk. Separate curves depict risk for women who are 20 (——), 30 (– – –), 40 (-----), and 50 (·······) years old at the time of counseling. Figure A corresponds to no biopsies, Figures B and E to one biopsy, and Figures C and F to two or more biopsies.

tently available, only the relative risks associated with age, age at menarche, number of biopsies, number of affected first degree relatives, and age at first live birth have been checked. Gail and Benichou[12] found very similar relative risks when fitting these factors to data from the Cancer and Steroid Hormone (CASH) study. CASH was a population-based case-control study of women between ages 20–54 from the general U.S. population. Cases and controls accrued between December 1, 1980 and Decem-

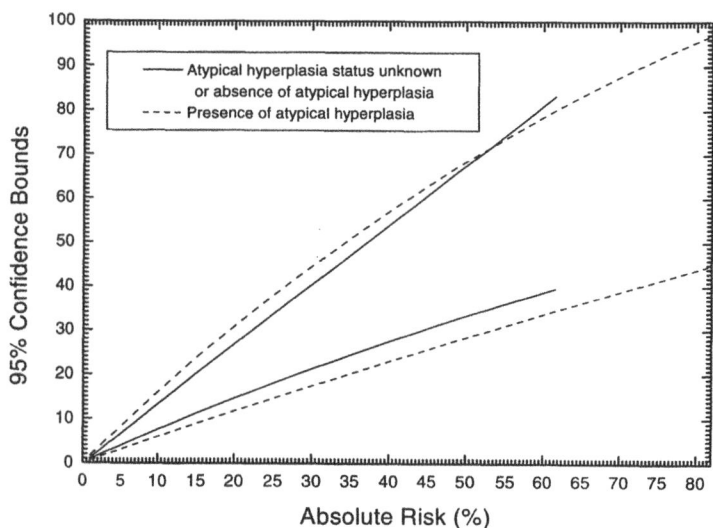

Figure 3. Lower and upper 95% confidence bounds versus estimated absolute risk. Dashed curves apply if atypical hyperplasia has been documented. Otherwise, use solid curves. Taken from Benichou et al.[8]

ber 31, 1982, when there was very little screening mammography. Spiegelman et al.[13] fitted the risk factors in the BCDDP model to data from the Nurses Health Study. Follow-up of this cohort of nurses began in 1976, when the nurses were between the ages of 30 and 55, and follow-up information was used through 1987. Spiegelman et al.[13] found good agreement between the relative risks of the BCDDP model and those obtained by refitting these risk factors to data from the Nurses Health Study, except that relative risks associated with having affected first-degree relatives were smaller.

```
A:\>risk

            Individualized Breast Cancer Risk Projections

    current age (20-80): 40
    upper age limit (20-80): 70

    age at menarche: 12
    age at first live birth (0 if no live birth): 31
    number of previous breast biopsies: 1
    at least one biopsy with hyperplasia
        (y:yes, n:no, u:unknown) ? y
    number of first-degree relatives
        (mother and/or sister(s)) with breast cancer: 1


            absolute risk = 29.7%

        95% CI = [ 19.8%, 41.8% ]

A:\>
```

Figure 4. Interactive output from RISK[9] for 40 year-old woman with risk profile shown and relative risk 9.63.

Bondy et al.[14] also found consistency between the relative risks from the BCDDP model and those obtained by fitting these risk factors to a cohort of women who participated in the Texas Breast Screening Project and were found to have at least one first-degree relative when screened initially in 1987. Thus, the relative risk portion of the BCDDP model has been shown to apply quite well in three independent groups of women.

The situation is more complicated for absolute risk projection. In their original report,[3] Gail et al. warned that the BCDDP model would overestimate risk in younger women who are not being screened annually. Gail and Benichou[12] noted that the breast cancer rate found in the BCDDP population below age 55 was about 1.62 times that in the general CASH population and that a higher prevalence of risk factors in the BCDDP population could only account for a ratio of 1.15. They concluded that the BCDDP model would overestimate risk in unscreened younger women, such as those in the CASH population, by about $\{1.62/1.15) - 1\} \times 100 = 41\%$.

Why should screening have such an impact on breast cancer rates for younger women but not older women? Mammographic screening allows one to look about 2 years into the future for a young woman. The amount by which one looks into the future is called the "lead time" of the screening test. Thus, a screened 30-year-old woman has the risk of a 32-year-old woman. Figure 1 illustrates the effect of this two-year lead time (see the dotted curve). Because this is a semi-logarithmic plot with a steep slope at younger ages, even a two-year shift increases risk sharply. For example the relative risk for a 30-year-old screened woman, compared to a 30-year-old unscreened woman, is 1.67. For a 60-year-old woman, the relative risk associated with a two-year lead time is only 1.12, because the slope of the age-specific log-incidence curve is much shallower in older women. Screening effects could easily explain much of the discrepancy that arises when the BCDDP model, which was derived from women in regular annual screening, is applied to unscreened or sporadically screened younger women.

Bondy et al.[14] found that the BCDDP model overestimated risk in younger but not older women in the cohort derived from the Texas Breast Screening Project. For women under age 60, the ratio of expected breast cancers under the BCDDP model to observed cancers was 30.58/12 = 2.55. For women age 60 and over, the ratio was 20.74/25 = 0.83. The overall ratio of expected to observed cancers was 1.32. When, however, the BCDDP model was applied to the subset of women who adhered to American Cancer Society screening guidelines, the overall ratio of expected to observed cancers was 0.89, with 95% confidence interval 0.62–1.33. Bondy et al. concluded: "Overall, the Gail et al. model accurately predicts risk in women with a family history of breast cancer and who adhere to American Cancer Society guidelines. The model should be used as it was intended, for women who receive annual mammograms."

Speigelman et al.[13] found expected to observed ratios of 1.48 for women under age 50 and 1.16 for women age 50 or more. The discrepancies were greatest in the years 1976–1981, during which mammographic screening was rarely performed, and less during 1982–1987, when there was sporadic screening in the Nurses Health Study cohort.

Another good opportunity to validate the BCDDP model will arise when data from the Breast Cancer Prevention Trial are fully analyzed. This study recently announced that tamoxifen reduced the incidence of breast cancer, compared to placebo, in women above age 59 or in younger women whose risk factors put them at a risk equivalent to that of an average 60-year-old woman.[15] Because women in this study are screened annually, the control arm will be useful for assessing predictions from the BCDDP model. Preliminary unpublished analyses indicate that the BCDDP model does, in fact, predict absolute risk well in this population.

To summarize, absolute predictions from the BCDDP model may very well be accurate for women in regular screening, but the BCDDP model overestimates risk in younger women who are not screened regularly. Relative risk estimates from the BCDDP model are applicable to screened and unscreened populations.

4. THE AUTOSOMAL DOMINANT MODEL OF CLAUS ET AL.[4]

4.1. The Claus Model

Claus et al.[4] performed segregation analyses on data from relatives of cases and controls in the CASH study. They concluded that an autosomal dominant model for a single breast cancer gene accounted for familial aggregation of disease better than other models. We now know that there are at least two important breast cancer genes, BRCA1 and BRCA2. Nonetheless, the simple autosomal model used by Claus et al.[4] captures much of the useful prognostic information in family history. Claus et al. assumed that carriers of a dominant breast cancer gene would have one age-specific breast cancer incidence rate function (or cumulative risk function) and non-carriers would have another lower age-specific breast cancer incidence rate function. Even though no genotyping was performed, Claus et al. were able to estimate the frequency of the mutant allele as 0.0033 and the cumulative risk functions for carriers and non-carriers. They estimated a cumulative risk to age 70 of 67% for carriers and 5% for non-carriers.

Claus et al. found that the relative risk of cancer comparing carriers with non-carriers is very large in young women (e.g., 43 for ages 30–39) but smaller in older women (e.g., 5 for ages 70–79). If a relative develops breast cancer while young, she is therefore more likely to be a mutation carrier, which increases the chance that the woman being counseled is a carrier. Thus Claus et al. use not only the number of affected relatives but their ages at disease onset.

Because the CASH study recruitment took place in 1980–1982, at which time family history was elicited, the data used to fit the Claus model represent an unscreened general population. It can be anticipated, therefore, that risk projections for younger women from the Claus model will often be lower than projections from the BCDDP model.

Claus et al.[5] present tables for projecting risk according to the age of the woman being counseled and the ages at onset in affected relatives. They give tables for one affected first-degree relative, one affected second-degree relative, two affected first-degree relatives, an affected mother and maternal aunt, an affected mother and paternal aunt, one affected maternal and one paternal second-degree relative, and two affected maternal or paternal second-degree relatives.

Consider again the 40-year-old woman who began menstruating at age 14, who had no breast biopsies, and whose mother developed breast cancer (see Section 3.2). Her 30 year risk was estimated from the BCDDP model as 11.6%. Table 3, which is taken from Table 2 in Claus et al.,[5] describes the cumulative probability of breast cancer for such a woman according to her age and the age at onset in a first-degree relative. Suppose the mother developed breast cancer at age 63. According to Table 3, the

Table 3. Predicted Cumulative Probability of Breast Cancer for a Woman Who Has One First-Degree Relative Affected With Breast Cancer, by Age of Onset of the Affected Relative Taken from Claus et al.[5]

Age of Woman (yr)	First-Degree Relative with Age of Onset (yr)					
	20–29	30–39	40–49	50–59	60–69	70–79
29	0.007	0.005	0.003	0.002	0.002	0.001
39	0.025	0.017	0.012	0.008	0.006	0.005
49	0.062	0.044	0.032	0.023	0.018	0.015
59	0.116	0.086	0.064	0.049	0.040	0.035
69	0.171	0.130	0.101	0.082	0.070	0.062
79	0.211	0.165	0.132	0.110	0.096	0.088

cumulative risk of breast cancer in the woman being counseled is 0.006 through age 39 and 0.070 through age 69. Therefore, the 30 year risk for this 40-year-old woman is (see the formula in Claus et al.[5]) $(0.070-0.006)/(1-0.006) = 0.064$. If the mother had developed breast cancer at age 28, the risk would be $(0.171-0.025)/(1-0.025) = 0.150$ or 15%.

No validation studies of the Claus model have been published. No confidence intervals have been presented for projections under this model. This model also does not take competing risks into account, but such risks would have only a small impact for projections to age 60. For projections to age 80, however, competing risks would tend to reduce absolute risk of breast cancer below the values in Table 3.

4.2. Comparison of BCDDP and Claus Models

As the previous example illustrates, it may be difficult to compare projections from the BCDDP and Claus models because they employ different risk factors. In particular, the Claus model does not include reproductive factors or information on biopsies, while the BCDDP model does not use data on age at onset in affected relatives. The BCDDP model incorporated family history information empirically based on logistic regression, and it was found that age at onset in affected relatives did not add useful information to logistic models that contained all the other factors in Table 2. This observation does not imply that age at onset is not useful for predicting risk in other models, such the Claus model.

The tables given by Claus et al.[5] only pertain to counselees with at least one affected relative, whereas the BCDDP model also makes projections for women without affected relatives.

Some comparisons may be drawn for women with given family histories by considering BCDDP projections in the absence of other risk factors and in the presence of all other risk factors except atypical hyperplasia (Table 4). Projections for the Claus model are made assuming that the relatives are affected either at age 50 or at age 20. No projections are available for the Claus model with no affected relatives (Table 4). For 1 affected relative, projections of risk for ages 30 to 60 range from 8% to 22% for the BCDDP model and from 5% to 11% for the Claus model. Although these projections overlap, the BCDDP projections tend to be higher. This probably reflects the lack of screening in the CASH population and the fact that the projections are for a 30-year-old woman. For a 60 year old woman, the corresponding 20 year risks are 3.0%

Table 4. Comparison of Estimated Absolute Risks from Age
30 to Age 60 from the BCDDP and Claus Models

	BCDDP		Claus Model	
Number of affected first-degree relatives	No other factors	All other factors[a]	Affected at age 50	Affected at age 20
0	3%	13%	NA	NA
1	8%	22%	5%	11%
2	20%	35%	13%	28%

[a]Assumes biopsy status for atypical hyperplasia is unknown.

and 25% for the BCDDP model and 6.4% and 10.7% for the Claus model. With two affected first degree relatives (Table 4), there is considerable overlap between projections under the two models, but again results from the BCDDP model tend to be higher.

McGuigan et al.[16] applied both models to 111 women with at least one affected relative in a high risk breast cancer clinic at the University of California at Los Angeles. They estimated the risk from the woman's current age to age 80. Most risks from the BCDDP model were under 20%, the highest risk was 51%, and a typical risk projection of 15% from the BCDDP model corresponded to a risk of about 10% for the Claus model. There were, however, 11 cases in which the Claus model yielded risks above 25% that were more than twice as large as the BCDDP model projections, presumably because these women had relatives with early-onset disease.

5. DISCUSSION

We have reviewed the BCDDP model and Claus model and indicated how to use them. McTiernan et al.[17] compared these methods with earlier life-table projections based on smaller cohorts of relatives of women with breast cancer[18,19] and with a method that classifies a woman into one of four relative risk categories but does not specify absolute risk.[20]

In using the BCDDP model, it is important to consider the nature of the counselee. Projections are likely to be most accurate if she is white, has just been screened and found to be free of disease, and plans to continue in a program of annual follow-up with screening mammography. As we have indicated, the BCDDP model overestimates risk in young women who do not receive annual mammography. The model was fitted to data on white women because there were too few black or Asian women in the BCDDP to obtain reliable estimates.

The data used to fit the Claus model derived from unscreened women. It is possible, therefore, that projections from this model underestimate risk when applied to younger women in regular follow-up, but no validation studies have been reported.

Neither of these models take certain special features into account, and the counselor has an indispensable role in determining the applicability of the model. For example, if the woman is a recent immigrant from rural Japan or China, her relative risk may be reduced by a factor of five (Table 1). If she has had a diagnosis of breast cancer in the contralateral breast, her relative risk is increased five fold. One may wish to modify risk projections to take such factors in Table 1 into account by multiplying the relative risk from the new factor times the relative risk calculated from Table 2 before using the graphs of Benichou et al.[8] to obtain modified BCDDP projections. The counselor must, at a minimum, interpret projections from the BCDDP model and the Claus model in light of information not included in these models that can have an important modifying influence.

A nice feature of the BCDDP model is that estimates of uncertainty are expressed in the form of confidence intervals. These confidence intervals tend to be wider for larger estimated risks (Fig. 3). Although these confidence intervals measure uncertainty from random variation due to limitations of sample size, they do not reflect systematic errors that could arise, for example, when applying the model to an unscreened population or to a woman with a previous history of breast cancer or previous exposure to radiation.

Exciting progress has been made in identifying the major breast cancer susceptibility genes, BRCA1 and BRCA2. Whittemore et al.[7] estimated the chance that a BRCA1 mutation carrier would develop breast cancer by age 70 at 69%, whereas Ford et al.[21] estimated 87%. Results in Claus et al.,[4] who implicitly studied BRCA1, BRCA2, and possibly other genes, yield cumulative risk to age 70 of 67% for such carriers. Struewing et al.[6] estimated 56% for carriers of three mutations in BRCA1 and BRCA2 among Ashkenazi Jews. To some extent, risks from BRCA1 or BRCA2 mutations are reflected in the family history data in the BCDDP model and Claus model. Nonetheless, if a woman is known to carry a cancer-causing mutation in BRCA1 or BRCA2, that information should be used to project risk. This information could become available through genotyping several members of a highly affected family. If women with breast cancer share the same mutation, that mutation is very likely to confer risk.

Very few women in the general population carry mutations of BRCA1 or BRCA2. Data in Claus et al.[4] suggest a carrier frequency of 0.7% for BRCA1 or BRCA2 mutations, and data for BRCA1 mutations alone suggest carrier frequencies ranging from 0.1 percent[22] to 0.3 percent.[7] Thus, only a very small fraction of women in the general population carry disease-conferring mutations of BRCA1 or BRCA2, although the carrier frequency may approach 2% in Ashkenazi Jews.[6] Even if a woman is found to carry a mutation in BRCA1 or BRCA2, it is not certain that the mutation confers increased risk unless it has been previously identified as a risk-producing allele or unless it is linked with disease in relatives.

Thus, models such as the BCDDP model and Claus model remain useful for the vast majority of women for whom no disease-causing mutation has been identified. Nonetheless the counselor will want to use available information on mutations of BRCA1 and BRCA2 and on other inherited syndromes that confer greatly increased breast cancer risk. The Li-Fraumeni cancer family syndrome, particularly when supported by evidence of a shared mutation in the p53 gene, is indicative of high breast cancer risk.[23] The Cowden multiple hamartoma syndrome is a rare autosomal dominant condition that also confers greatly increased breast cancer risk.[24] These syndromes are exceedingly rare, however.

Ongoing work by several investigators may lead to improved models. One line of research would incorporate additional strong risk factors, such as the presence of dense tissue on mammograms. Barry et al.[25] use family history to estimate the probability that a woman carries a mutation in BRCA1 or BRCA2; this approach may allow one to summarize complex family history data in risk models that also include other risk factors.

An estimate of absolute risk from these models is a useful tool in the counseling process, but it is only one element. The counselor must gather the best available prognostic information, including a careful personal and family history and results of histopathologic examinations, before using such models and must be alert to features not accounted for in the models. Most important, the counselor will need time to put risk estimates, and their uncertainties, into perspective for the counselee and to carefully explain management options in the context of estimated risks. Giving risk projections for several age intervals may be useful. Only by working closely with the counselee to convey information and support and to understand the counselee's preferences and reactions to such information, can the counselor use these models effectively.

REFERENCES

1. Landis SH, Murray T, Bolden S, et al: Cancer Statistics, 1998. CA-A Cancer Journal for Clinicians 48:6–29, 1998
2. Ries LAG, Kosary CL, Hankey BF, et al: SEER Cancer Statistics Review, 1973–1994 Bethesda, MD, National Cancer Institute, NIH Pub. No. 97-2789, page 131, 1997
3. Gail MH, Brinton LA, Byar DP, et al: Projecting individualized probabilities of developing breast cancer for white females who are being examined annually. J Natl Cancer Inst 81:1879–1886, 1989
4. Claus EB, Risch NJ, Thompson WD: Genetic analysis of breast cancer in the Cancer and Steroid Hormone Study. Am J Hum Genet 48:232–242, 1991
5. Claus EB, Risch N, Thompson WD: Autosomal dominant inheritance of early onset breast cancer: Implications for risk prediction. Cancer 73:643–651, 1994
6. Struewing JP, Hartge P, Wacholder S, et al: The risk of cancer associated with specific mutations of BRCA1 and BRCA2 among Ashkenazi Jews. N Engl J Med 336:1401–1408, 1997
7. Whittemore AS, Gong G, Itnyre J: Prevalence and contribution of BRCA1 mutations in breast cancer and ovarian cancer: Results from three U.S. population-based case-control studies of ovarian cancer. Am J Hum Genet 60:496–504, 1997
8. Benichou J, Gail MH, Mulvihill JJ: Graphs to estimate an individualized risk of breast cancer. J Clin Oncol 14:103–110, 1996
9. Benichou J: A computer program for estimating individualized probabilities of breast cancer. Comput Biomed Res 26:373–382, 1993
10. Benichou J, Gail MH: Methods of inference for estimates of absolute risk derived from population-based case-control studies. Biometrics 51:182–194, 1995
11. Benichou J: A complete analysis of variability for estimates of absolute risk from a population-based case-control study on breast cancer. Biometric J 37:3–24, 1995
12. Gail MH, Benichou J: Assessing the risk of breast cancer in individuals, in DeVita VT, Hellman S, Rosenberg SA (eds): Cancer Prevention. Philadelphia, PA, Lippincott, pp 1–15, 1992
13. Spiegelman D, Colditz GA, Hunter D, et al: Validation of the Gail et al. model for predicting individualized breast cancer risk. J Natl Cancer Inst 86:600–607, 1994
14. Bondy ML, Lustbader ED, Halabi S, et al: Validation of a breast cancer risk assessment model in women with a positive family history. J Natl Cancer Inst 86:600–607, 1994
15. Redmond CK, Costantino JP: Design and current status of the NSABP breast cancer prevention trial, in Senn HJ, Gelber RD, Goldhirsch A, Thurlimann B (eds): Recent Results in Cancer Research 140: Adjuvant Therapy of Breast Cancer. Berlin, Springer-Verlag, pp 309–317, 1996
16. McGuigan KA, Ganz PA, Breant C: Agreement between breast cancer risk estimation methods. J Natl Cancer Inst 88:1315–1317, 1996
17. McTiernan A, Gilligan MA, Redmond C: Asessing individual risk for breast cancer: Risky business. J Clin Epidemiol 50:547–556, 1997
18. Ottman R, Pike MC, King MC, et al: Practical guide for estimating risk for familial breast cancer. Lancet ii:556–558, 1983
19. Anderson DE, Badzioch MD: Risk of familial breast cancer. Cancer 56:383–387, 1985
20. Taplin S, Thompson RS, Schnitzer F, et al: Revisions in the risk-based breast cancer screening program at Group Health Cooperative. Cancer 66:812–818, 1990
21. Ford D, Easton DF, Bishop DT, et al: Risk of cancer in BRCA-1 mutation carriers. Lancet 343:692–695, 1994

22. Ford D, Easton DF, Peto J: Estimates of the gene frequency of BRCA1 and its contribution to breast and ovarian cancer incidence. Am J Hum Genet 57:1457–1462, 1995
23. Li F: Familial aggregation, in Schottenfeld D, Fraumeni JF, Jr (eds): Cancer Epidemiology and Prevention (ed 2). New York, Oxford University Press, pp 546–558, 1966
24. Hanssen AMN, Fryns JB: Cowden syndrome. J Med Genet 32:117–119, 1995
25. Berry DA, Parmigianni G, Sanchez J, Schildkraut J, Winer E: Probability of carrying a mutation of breast-ovarian cancer gene BRCA1 based on family history. J Natl Cancer Inst 89:227–228, 1997
26. Miller BA, Ries LAG, Hankey BF, et al: Cancer statistics review: 1973–1989. Natl Cancer Inst. NIH Publ. No. 92-2789, Washington, DC, US Government Printing Office, 1992
27. Kelsey JL: A review of the epidemiology of breast cancer. Epidemiol Rev 1:74–109, 1979
28. Harris JR, Lippman ME, Veronesi U, et al: Breast cancer. N Engl J Med 327:319–328, 1992
29. Dupont WD, Page DL: Risk factors for breast cancer in women with proliferative disease. N Engl J Med 312:146–151, 1985
30. Carter CL, Corle DK, Micozzi MS, et al: A prospective study of breast cancer in 16,692 women with benign breast disease. Am J Epidemiol 128:467–477, 1988
31. Byrne C, Schairer C, Wolfe J, et al: Mammographic features and breast cancer risk: Effects with time, age, and menopause status. J Natl Cancer Inst 87:1622–1629, 1995
32. Gail MH, Benichou J: Validation studies on a model for breast cancer risk. J Natl Cancer Inst 86:573–575, 1994 (editorial)

4

GENETICS OF BREAST AND OVARIAN CANCER

A Continuum of Risk

Wylie Burke

Department of Medicine
University of Washington
Seattle, WA 98105

INTRODUCTION

Genetics contributes to the risk of breast and ovarian cancer to a variable degree. Rare families show dramatic clustering of breast and ovarian cancer, with cancers occurring at an early age.[1] Most such families carry genetic alterations (or mutations) conferring an inherited predisposition to cancer. These families are often referred to as cancer-prone or high risk families; women from these families, if they inherit the cancer predisposition, may face a lifetime probability of cancer as high as 85–90%.[1]

The majority of women with a family history of breast or ovarian cancer, however, are from families that are far less dramatic. About 5–10% of women have a first degree relative (a mother, sister, or daughter) with breast cancer, but fewer than 1% have two first degree relatives with breast cancer.[2] Yet even one affected relative may cause a woman to perceive herself at high risk.[3]

Many women over-estimate their risk of breast cancer.[3,4] Anxiety about breast cancer may be fueled by over-estimates of breast cancer mortality. In a 1995 Gallup survey, women respondents estimated that 40% of female deaths are due to breast cancer,[5] although actual mortality data indicate the figure was only 4%.[6] Breast cancer has been the subject of much media attention, with advocates expressing anger at the slow progress of efforts to cure or prevent breast cancer.[7] For many women, this cov-

Department of Medicine Box 354765, University of Washington, 4245 Roosevelt Way NE, Seattle, WA, 98105. Phone: (206) 598-8779; Fax: (206) 598-8957

Cancer Genetics for the Clinician, edited by Shaw.
Kluwer Academic / Plenum Publishers, New York, 1999.

erage may contribute to a pervasive sense of risk, amplified by personal knowledge of women with breast cancer. "Sadly, all of us know a woman who has had breast cancer. With one in nine American women predicted to get the disease at some point over the course of her lifetime, it's hard to imagine being spared the anguish of seeing a relative, friend or acquaintance suffer. And of course, what woman doesn't fear being stricken herself?"[8] As new knowledge about cancer genetics emerges, clinicians will challenged to identify and help those at high risk, without contributing further to unnecessary breast cancer worry.

SIGNIFICANCE OF A FAMILY HISTORY OF BREAST OR OVARIAN CANCER

Five to 10% of women have a first degree relative with breast cancer, and about twice that many have either a first or a second degree relative with breast cancer.[2,9,10] The risk conferred by a family history of breast cancer varies with the age at which the affected relative was diagnosed: the younger the age of the affected relative, the greater the risk posed to relatives.[9-12] A woman whose mother or sister had breast cancer in her thirties has a relative risk of breast cancer of 2 to 3, compared to a woman with no family history of breast cancer.[9-11] However, the risk is lower if her mother or sister was affected at an older age,[9-11] and may approach that of the average women if her relative was affected beyond age 60.[12]

The number of affected relatives and their biologic relationship to the person whose risk is being considered are also important factors.[9-12] In general, the greater the number of affected relatives and the closer the biologic relationship, the greater the risk.[9-12] In assessing family history for these factors, one must take into account family size and constitution. In the case of breast and ovarian cancer, the number of female relatives in the family influences both informativeness and significance of the family history. In families with few women, it may be difficult to identify a genetic susceptibility to cancer, even if one is present. If there are many female family members, the proportion of affected to unaffected may be an important indicator of risk: one affected sister among six is less suggestive of genetic risk than one affected sister among two.

A recent study of family history of breast cancer used statistical methods to account for both family size and age of cancer onset in affected relatives.[2] In this analysis, the observed breast cancer status for each family member was compared to the risk expected for that relative from cancer incidence rates in the population. The result was a family history score, with the numerical value of the score increasing as the number of breast cancer cases in the family increased above the number expected from population rates. Using data from a prospective mortality study, the authors were able to show that a third of women with a family history of breast cancer (those with the lowest family history scores) were at no higher risk for breast cancer than women who lacked a family history of the disease.[2]

Less is known about a family history of ovarian cancer, but in general, the family characteristics that influence risk are the same as for breast cancer, ie, number of affected relatives, age of onset of disease, and closeness of the biologic relationship.[13-15] The relative risk of ovarian cancer is 2–4 for women with an affected first degree relative, compared to those with no family history of ovarian cancer.[13] Unlike breast

Table 1. Breast and/or Ovarian Cancer Risk Associated with Genetic Mutations

Gene(s) in Which Mutation Occurs	Breast Cancer Risk	Ovarian Cancer Risk	Risk for Other Cancer(s)
BRCA1[1,19,20]	Yes	Yes	Prostate, Colon?
BRCA2[1,29,20]	Yes	Yes	Prostate, Pancreatic?, Other?
HNPCC⁻ Associated[21,22]	Uncertain	Yes	Colorectal, Endometrial, Ureteral
p53[23,24] (LiFraumeni)	Yes	No	Sarcoma, Leukemia, Brain, Adrenal Gland
PTEN[25] (Cowden)	Yes	No	Thyroid

cancer, the risk appears to be significantly greater when cancer occurs in a sister than when it occurs in the mother.[13-15] As with breast cancer, the risk is greater if two first degree relatives are affected and smaller when a second degree relative is affected.[13,14]

Studies of the effect of family history also suggest an interaction between breast and ovarian cancer. A family history of ovarian cancer is a weak risk factor for breast cancer and vice versa.[1,13,14] The presence of both cancers in a family increases the likelihood that a cancer-predisposing mutations is present.[16,17]

INHERITED PREDISPOSITION TO BREAST AND OVARIAN CANCER

Several genes associated with breast or ovarian cancer risk have been identified; some are associated with significant risk for other cancers as well (Table 1). Such mutations are rare, even among women with cancer, and probably account for fewer than 5% of breast cancer cases overall.[26,27] All mutations known to cause a predisposition to breast or ovarian cancer are inherited as autosomal dominant (AD) traits. Thus the family characteristics that suggest AD inheritance of cancer predisposition are important indicators of high risk and of the presence of a cancer-predisposing mutation. These include the following:

Vertical Transmission of Cancer Risk

Vertical transmission refers to a genetic trait being passed from one generation to the next; a person must inherit the cancer predisposition from a parent who also had it.

Both Males and Females Can Inherit the Cancer Predisposition

The mutation producing the cancer predisposition can be passed on to both male and female children. In the case of breast and ovarian cancer, cancers occur predominantly in women (though some male carriers develop breast cancer, and male carriers may also have other cancer risks). Thus a male who inherits the cancer predisposition may show no evidence of it, but can still pass the predisposition on to his sons and daughters.

Inheritance Risk of 50%

When a parent carries a cancer-predisposing mutation, each child has a 50% chance of inheriting the mutation.

Other Clinical Characteristics

Cancers in people from high risk families typically occur at an earlier age than in sporadic cases. The mean age of breast cancer associated with BRCA1, for example, is in the early 40s.[19] In addition, two or more primary cancers may occur in a single individual. These could be multiple primary cancers of the same type (e.g., bilateral breast cancer) or primary cancer of different types (e.g., breast and ovarian cancer in the same individual).

Difficulties in Identifying an AD Inheritance of Breast or Ovarian Cancer Risk

The family history reported by a patient is not always accurate. When accuracy of family histories of breast and ovarian cancer was assessed, by comparing self-reported family history with data from medical records or cancer registries, the accuracy of reported breast cancers was high—in the range of 80–95%—but a history of ovarian cancer was less reliable.[28,29] In addition, small family sizes and premature deaths may limit the information obtained from a family history. In the case of breast and ovarian cancer, a history of cancer on the paternal side of the family may be missed if not actively sought.[30]

BRCA1 AND BRCA2

Families in which BRCA1 or BRCA2 mutations have been found demonstrate either a "site-specific" pattern of breast or ovarian cancer—ie, affected family members as a rule have only one type of cancer—or a predisposition to both breast and ovarian cancer.[1] Ovarian cancer is more frequently associated with BRCA1 than with BRCA2,[19] but mutations in both genes have been identified in breast/ovarian families.[19] The explanation for these differing clinical patterns remains to be determined. Clinical variation could result from differing clinical effects of different mutations—hundreds of different mutations have been documented in both genes[31]—or could be due to other environmental or genetic modifiers of risk, or to a combination of these factors.

Estimates of the proportion of high risk families who carry BRCA1 or BRCA2 mutations have varied. In initial gene mapping studies, BRCA1 mutations accounted for about half of such families, and BRCA2 mutations for an additional 20–30%.[19,32] However, in clinical series, mutations are identified less frequently.[16,17] This difference probably reflects the fact that families seen in the course of clinical care are more heterogeneous than those enrolled in research studies, and may include some families in which cancer aggregation has occurred by chance or as the result of an interaction between milder genetic variants and environmental modifiers. A very small percentage of high risk families carry other known mutations, such as P53 and PTEN (Table 1).[1,23,24] Some families with pedigrees suggesting high risk may carry mutations in other genes yet to be discovered.

CANCER RISK ASSOCIATED WITH BRCA1 AND BRCA2 MUTATIONS

The lifetime cancer risk of women carrying BRCA1 and BRCA2 mutations appears to be variable. The breast cancer risk associated with BRCA1 mutations has been estimated to range between 50 and 85%,[32-34] and appears to be similar for BRCA2 mutations.[19,20] Lifetime risk of ovarian cancer is estimated to be between 16 and 66% for BRCA1 mutation carriers and 27% for BRCA2 mutation carriers.[19,32] Men who carry BRCA1 or BRCA2 mutations appear to have a small increased risk of prostate cancer, and BRCA1 carriers of both genders may have an increased risk of colon cancer.[1,19,32] In families with BRCA2 mutations, a variety of cancers other than breast and ovarian have occurred, including include prostate, pancreatic, laryngeal, esophageal, colon, and hematopoietic cancers.[20] Whether these cancers are part of the cancer risk associated with BRCA2 mutations is not yet known. A number of family studies have shown male breast cancer associated with BRCA2 mutations;[19,35] male breast cancer also occurs rarely in families carrying BRCA1 mutations.[19] These data indicate a complex relationship between cancer-predisposing mutations and risk of specific cancers.

BRCA1 AND BRCA2 MUTATIONS IN ETHNIC POPULATIONS

Most BRCA1 and BRCA2 mutations are rare; many have been observed in only a single family.[31] However, relatively common mutations have been identified in Icelandic and Ashkenazi Jewish populations. Studies of these mutations provide additional information about the variability in cancer risk seen with BRCA1 and BRCA2 mutations.

Among Icelandic individuals, a single BRCA2 mutation, termed 999del5, occurs with a prevalence of 0.6%, and is found in 8% of female and 40% of male Icelandic breast cancer patients.[35,36] In individuals of Ashkenazi Jewish descent, two mutations, the 185delAG mutation in BRCA1 and the 6174delT mutation in BRCA2, each occur with a prevalence of about 1%.[33,37] In both Icelandic and Jewish populations, the mutations are more common in people with a family history of cancer and in women with early breast cancer. However, they have also been found in people with late-onset cancer or little or no family history.[35,36,38-40] The 185delAG and 6174delT mutations appear to account for a substantial proportion of sporadic ovarian cancer cases among Jewish women.[38,40] These observations support the idea that the cancer risk associated with a given BRCA1 or BRCA2 mutation is variable and therefore likely to be influenced by environmental or other modifiers.

OTHER GENES ASSOCIATED WITH BREAST OR OVARIAN CANCER

Cowden Syndrome

Cowden syndrome is a rare autosomal dominant cancer syndrome that includes breast cancer, thyroid cancer, and meningiomas.[25] Diagnosis is established through identification of characteristic skin lesions (acral keratosis, facial trichilemmomas, and oral papules). Benign neoplasms of the breast and thyroid gland and hamartomatous polyps of the gastrointestinal tract are also seen. A candidate gene, designated PTEN or MMAC1, has been identified.[25]

Li-Fraumeni Syndrome

Li-Fraumeni syndrome is a rare autosomal dominant cancer syndrome that includes sarcomas, leukemia, and cancers of the brain, adrenal gland, and breast.[41] Approximately 50% of patients with Li-Fraumeni syndrome have identifiable mutations in the p53 gene.[42] In addition, p53 mutations have been detected in individuals with multiple primary cancers and in individuals with a strong family history of cancer who do not meet the diagnostic criteria for Li-Fraumeni syndrome.[24] P53 mutations account for less than 1% of early breast cancer cases.[23]

Hereditary Non-polyposis Colon Cancer (HNPCC)

HNPCC is an AD disorder conferring a high lifetime risk of colorectal cancer.[43,44] HNPCC is genetically heterogeneous, with mutations from at least four genes so far identified in different HNPCC families: hMSH2,, hMLH1, hPMS1, and hPMS2.[45] The risk of colorectal cancer in HNPCC is estimated to be 68–75% by age 65.[44] Endometrial cancer is the second most common cancer seen in HNPCC families, with a cumulative risk in female mutations carriers of 30–39%.[44,46] Women with HNPCC are also at increased risk for ovarian cancer. Watson and Lynch[22] reported ovarian cancer risk in HNPCC families to be 3.5 times higher than average. In a series of 116 unselected ovarian cancer cases, 2 of the affected women carried HNPCC-associated mutations (as compared with 10 who carried BRCA1 mutations).[21] Other cancers seen in HNPCC families include small bowel, stomach, and transitional cell carcinoma of the ureters.[43,44]

Metabolic Polymorphisms

Many additional genetic traits are being described as a result of rapid advances in genetic research. A number of normal variants, affecting metabolic processes such as drug detoxification and hormone metabolism, have been identified and found in some studies to be associated with cancer risk.[47] In the future, such genetic traits may be identified as an important contributor to population risks for breast and ovarian cancer.

CLINICAL FOLLOW-UP

There are no interventions of proven benefit for individuals with a genetic susceptibility to breast or ovarian cancer. Based on current information about risk and about the efficacy of screening procedures in the general population, recommendations for the care of people with BRCA1 and BRCA2 mutations have been made (Table 2).[48]

No studies have evaluated the outcome of early breast cancer screening in women with BRCA1 or BRCA2 mutations (or women from high risk families). The recommendations are based on expert opinion concerning presumptive benefit, given the early onset of breast cancer documented in high risk families.[48] Men with BRCA2

Table 2. Cancer Screening for Women with an Autosomal
Dominant Predisposition to Breast Cancer and Ovarian
Cancer[48]

Breast Cancer Screening
Evidence: expert opinion
Proof of efficacy: none
Monthly breast self-examination
Annual or semi-annual clinical breast examination beginning at age 25–35 years
Annual mammography beginning at age 25–35 years

Ovarian Cancer Screening
Evidence: expert opinion
Proof of efficacy: none
Annual or biannual pelvic examination, beginning at age 25–35
Annual or biannual transvaginal ultrasound examination with color Doppler, beginning at age 25–35
Annual serum CA-125 levels beginning at age 25–35 years

mutations also appear to be at increased risk for breast cancer, and evaluation of any breast mass or change is advisable, but no formal program of surveillance has been recommended.[48]

Ovarian cancer screening may also be considered, for women with an inherited disposition to ovarian cancer (Table 2).[48] However, the screening measures currently available have limited sensitivity and specificity, and have not been proven to reduce ovarian cancer mortality; they are not recommended for women of average risk.

Prophylactic surgeries (mastectomy and oophorectomy) have also been proposed as a means to reduce cancer risk in people with genetic susceptibility to breast and ovarian cancer. Evidence concerning the efficacy of these procedures is limited and incomplete.[48] Cancers have been observed after both procedures. A retrospective cohort study of women receiving a prophylactic mastectomy at the Mayo Clinic estimated a 90% reduction in risk from the procedure; a third of the women in the study were considered to have a strong family history of cancer, and experienced a risk reduction similar to that of the whole cohort[49] An observational study of women from high risk ovarian cancer families found no difference in the rate of peritoneal carcinomatosis or ovarian cancer after oophorectomy among women who had had an oophorectomy compared to those who had not.[50] In addition to providing incomplete protection, these procedures have personal and social implications, and are unacceptable to some.

No chemoprevention has yet been recommended as a treatment for high risk women. However, a randomized clinical trial of treatment with tamoxifen (a partial estrogen antagonist) in women with increased breast cancer risk (based on assessment of genetic and other risk factors) has provided evidence that the treatment reduces breast cancer risk.[51] Significant adverse consequences of tamoxifen treatment occurred in the trial, including excess cases of endometrial cancer, pulmonary embolism and other thromboembolic events. The study is promising, in that it has confirmed the risk-reducing effect of an estrogen-antagonist, but more information is needed about the risks and benefits of treatment before the use of this approach to prevention can be recommended.

Studies in the general population suggest that long-term estrogen therapy may increase breast cancer risk, but that short-term use to treat menopausal symptoms does not. Similarly, general population studies indicate that the use of oral contraceptives decreases ovarian cancer risk. No studies have evaluated hormone therapy in women carrying cancer-predisposing mutations.[48]

Where family history or genetic data indicate the risk for other cancers, additional screening needs to be considered. In women with HNPCC-associated mutations, for example, the risks for colon cancer and endometrial cancer are higher than the risk for ovarian cancer, and screening for these other cancer is recommended.[52] For male carriers of BRCA1 and BRCA2 mutations, prostate cancer screening may be of benefit, although this issue has not yet been studied. Further, the full spectrum of cancer risks associated with BRCA1 and BRCA2 mutations may not be known for some time. Preliminary data suggest that BRCA2 mutations may be associated with diverse cancer risks, some of which may be amenable to screening.

AFTERWORD

With the advent of molecular genetics, it is becoming possible to identify and define the multiple genetic mechanisms contributing to breast and ovarian cancer risk. This research effort is still in an early stage, but has already revealed a complex relationship between genetic traits and cancer risk. Continued research will undoubtedly contribute to a better understanding of the biology of breast and ovarian cancer, and hopefully will lead to new strategies for cancer treatment and prevention. In the near term, the primary outcome of genetic research will be the increasing ability to identify people who may have a genetic susceptibility to cancer. Clinicians face the formidable task of determining when such information is clinically useful.

REFERENCES

1. Ford D, Easton DF: The genetics of breast and ovarian cancer. Br J Cancer 1995;72:805–812
2. Yang Q, Khoury MJ, Rodriguez C, Calle EE, Tatham LM, Flanders WD. Family history score as a predictor of breast mortality: prospective data from the cancer prevention study II, United States, 1982–1991. Am J Epidem 147:652–659, 1998
3. Wellisch DK, Gritz ER, Schain W, et al: Psychological functioning of daughters of breast cancer patients. Part 1: Daughters and comparison subjects. Psychomatics 32:324–336, 1991
4. Alexander NE, Ross J, Sumner W, Nease RF, Littenberg B. The effect of an educational intervention on the perceived risk of breast cancer. J Gen Intern Med 11:92–97, 1995
5. Gallup Survey 1995, cited in Mortality vital statistics report, Medical Tribune, Jan 25, p 17, 1996
6. Parker SL, Tong T, Bolden S, Wingo PA: Cancer Statistics 1996. CA Cancer J Clin 46:5–27, 1996
7. Ferrar S. The anguished politics of breast cancer. NY Times Magazine 1993; Aug 15:24–27, 58–61
8. Shannon J: Portraints of breast cancer. Woman's Day 1993; Oct 21:85,88–90, 94, 95
9. Colditz GA, Willett WC, Hunter DJ, Stampfer MJ, Manson JE, et al: Family history, age, and risk of breast cancer. JAMA 270:338–343, 1993
10. Slattery ML, Kerber RA: A comprehensive evaluation of family history and breast cancer risk: the Utah population database. JAMA 270:1563–1568, 1993
11. Pharoah PDP, Day NE, et al: Family history and the risk of breast cancer: A systematic review and meta-analysis. Int J Cancer 71:800–809, 1997
12. Claus EB, Risch N, Thompson WB: Autosomal dominant inheritance of early onset breast cancer: Implications for risk prediction. Cancer 73:643–651, 1994
13. Kerber RA, Slattery ML: The impact of family history on ovarian cancer risk: the utah population database. Arch Intern Med 155:905–912, 1995
14. Easton DF, mathews FE, Ford D, Swerdlow AJ, Peto J: Cancer mortality in relatives of women with ovarian cancer: the OPCS study. Int J Cancer 65:284–294, 1996

15. Auranem A, Pukkala E, Makinen J, Samkila R, Grenman S, Salmi T: Cancer incidence in the first-degree relatives of ovarian cancer patients. Brit J Cancer 74:280–284, 1996
16. Couch FJ, DeShano ML, Blackwood MA, et al: BRCA1 mutations in women attending clinics that evaluate the risk of breast cancer. N Engl J Med 336:1409–1415, 1997
17. Shattuck-Eidens D, Oliphant A, McClure M, et al: BRCA1 sequence analysis in women at high risk for susceptibility mutations. JAMA 278:1242–1250, 1997
18. Wellisch DK, Gritz ER, Schain W, et al: Psychological functioning of daughters of breast cancer patients. Part 1: Daughters and comparison subjects. Psychomatics 32:324–336, 1991
19. Ford D, Eastin DF, Stratton M, et al: Genetic heterogeity and penetrance analysis of the BRCA1 and BRCA2 genes in breast cancer families. Am J Hum Genet 62:676–689, 1998
20. Easton DF, Steele L, Fields P, et al: Cancer risks in two large breast cancer families linked to BRCA2 on chromosome 13q 12–13. Amer J Hum Genei 61:120–128, 1997
21. Rubin SC, Blackwood MA, Bandera C, et al: BRCA1, BRCA2 and hereditary non-polyposis colorectal cancer gene mutations in an unselected ovarian cancer population: relationship to family hisotry and implications for genetic testing. Am J Ob Gynecol 178:670–677, 1998
22. Watson P, Lynch HT: Extracolonic cancer in hereditary nonpolyposis colorectal cancer. Cancer 71:677–685, 1993
23. Sidransky D, Tokino T, Helzlsouer K, et al: Inherited p53 gene mutations in breast cancer. Cancer Res 52:2984–2986, 1992
24. Malkin D, Li FP, Strong LC, et al: Germ line p53 mutations in a familial syndrome of breast cancer, sarcomas, and other neoplasms. Science 250:1233–1238, 1990
25. Liaw D, Marsh DJ, Li J, et al: Germline mutations of the PTEN gene in Cowden disease, an inherited breast and thyroid cancer syndrome. Nat Genet. 16:64–67, 1997
26. Malone KE, Daling JR, Thompson JD, et al: BRCA1 mutations and breast cancer in the general population: analyses in women before age 35 years and in women before age 45 years with first-degree family history. JAMA 279:922–929, 1998
27. Newman B, Mu H, Butler LM, et al: Frequency of breast cancer attributable to BRCA1 in a population-based series of American women. JAMA 279:915–921, 1998
28. Kerber RA, Slattery ML: Comparison of self-reported and database-linked family history of cancer data in a case-control study. Am J Epidem 146:244–248, 1997
29. Parent M-E, Ghadrian PV, Lacroix A, Perret C: The reliability of recollections of family history: implications for the medical provider. J Cancer Ed 12:114–120, 1997
30. Burke W, Press N, Pinsky L: Breast carcinoma genetics from a primary care perspective. Cancer 80(Suppl):621–626, 1997
31. Szabo C, King M-C: Population Genetics of BRCA1 and BRCA2. Am J Hum Genet 60:1013–1020, 1997
32. Narod SA, Ford D, Devilee P, et al: An evaluation of genetic heterogeneity in 145 breast ovarian cancer families. Am J Hum Genet 56:254–264, 1995
33. Struewing JP, Hartge P, Wacholder S, et al: The risk of cancer associated with specific mutations of BRCA1 and BRCA2 among Ashkenazi Jews. N Engl J Med 336:1401–1408, 1997
34. Whittemore AS, Gong G, Itnyre J: Prevalence and contribution of BRCA1 mutations in breast cancer and ovarian cancer: Results from three U.S. population-based case-control studies of ovarian cancer. Am J Hum Genet 60:496–504, 1997
35. Thorlacius S, Olafsdottir G, Tryggvadottir L, et al: A single BRCA2 mutation in male and female breast cancer families from Iceland with varied cancer phenotypes. Nat Genet 13:117–119, 1996
36. Thorlacius S, Sigurdsson S, Bjarnadottir H, et al: Study of a single BRCA2 mutation with high carrier frequency in a small population. Am J Hum Genet 60:1079–1084, 1997
37. Roa BB, Boyd AA, Volcik K, et al: Ashkenazi Jewish population frequencies for common mutations in BRCA1 and BRCA2. Nat Genet 14:185–187, 1996
38. Levy-Lahad E, Catane R, Eisenberg S, et al: Founder BRCA1 and BRCA2 mutations in Ashkenazi Jews in Israel: frequency and differential penetrance in ovarian cancer and in breast-ovarian cancer families. Am J Hum Genet 60:1059–1067, 1997
39. Richards CS, Ward PA, Roa BB, et al: Screening for 185delAG in the Ashkenazim. Am J Hum Genet 60:1085–1098, 1997
40. Abeliovich D, Kaduri L, Lerer I, et al: The founder mutations 185delAG and 5382insC in BRCA1 and 6174delT in BRCA2 appear in 60% of ovarian cancer and 30% of early-onset breast cancer patients among Ashkenazi women. Am J Hum Genet 60:505–514, 1997
41. Li FP, Fraumeni JF, Jr, Mulvihill JJ, et al: A cancer family syndrome in twenty-four kindreds. Cancer Res 48:5358–5362, 1988

42. Frebourg T, Barbier N, Yan YX, et al: Germ-line p53 mutations in 15 families with Li-Fraumeni syndrome. Am J Hum Genet 56:608–615, 1995
43. Marra G, Boland CR: Hereditary nonpolyposis colorectal cancer: the syndrome, the genes, and historical perspectives. J Natl Cancer Inst 87:1114–1125, 1995
44. Aarnio M, Mecklin J-P, Aaltonen LA, Nystrom-Lahti M, Jarvinen HJ, Willett WC: Life-time risk of different cancers in hereditary non-polyposis colorectal cancer (HNPCC) syndrome. Int J Cancer. 64:430–433, 1995
45. Rhyu MS: Molecular mechanisms underlying hereditary nonpolyposis colorectal carcinoma. J Natl Cancer Inst 88:240–251, 1996
46. Watson P, Vasen HFA, Mecklin JD, et al: The risk of endometrial cancer in hereditary on polyposis colorectal cancer. Am J Med 96:516–520, 1994
47. D'Errico A, Taioli E, Chen X, Vineis P: Genetic metabolic polymorphisms and the risk of cancer: a review of the literature. Biomarkers 1:149–173, 1996
48. Burke W, Daly M, Garber J, et al: Recommendations for follow-up care of individuals with an inherited predisposition to cancer II. BRCA1 and BRCA2. JAMA 277:997–1003, 1997
49. Hartmann LC, Schaid DJ, Woods JE, et al: Efficacy of bilateral prophylactic mastectomy in women with a history of breast cancer. N Eng J Med 340(2):77–84, 1999
50. Struewing JP, et al: Prophylactic oophorectomy in inherited breast/ovarian cancer families. J Natl Cancer Inst Monograph 17:33–35, 1995
51. Fisher B, Costantino JP, Wickerham DL, et al: Tamoxifen for prevention of breast cancer: Report of the National Surgical Adjuvant Breast and Bowel Project P-1 Study. J Natl Cancer Inst 90(18): 1371–1388, 1998
52. Burke W, Petersen G, Lynch P, Daly M, Garber JE, Botkin J, Kahn MJE, McTiernan A, Offit K, Thomson E, Varricchio C. Recommendations for follow-up care of individuals with an inherited predisposition to cancer. 1. Hereditary nonpolyposis colon cancer JAMA 277:915–919, 1997

5

TESTING FOR BREAST CANCER RISK IN THE ASHKENAZIM

Carole Oddoux,* Elsa Reich, and Harry Ostrer

NYU Medical Center
Human Genetics Program
Department of Pediatrics
550 First Avenue
New York, NY 10016

1. INTRODUCTION

Breast cancer is the most common gender-specific malignancy among women. In the United States, over 180,000 women are diagnosed with breast cancer each year, and 46,000 die of the disease.[1,2] One out of eight, or 12.6%, of all women can expect to develop breast cancer at some time during her lifetime and for 1 in 30 women, breast cancer will be the cause of death.[3] Although breast cancer may also affect men, the frequency among males is quite small, approximately 1% of the total number of breast cancers.[1]

Knowledge about genes that predispose to the development of breast cancer has exploded in recent years, but there is clearly much still to be learned. Two major breast cancer predisposition genes are currently known, BRCA1 and BRCA2. Although information about the number and frequency of mutations in these genes remains unclear, and the probability that carriers will develop breast cancer is incompletely defined, risk assessment can still be provided and may contribute to decisions about medical care for the patient and her family members. Molecular analysis of genes predisposing to breast cancer is an option that may provide further risk modification in selected families and/or individuals. Genetic testing and risk assessment should be carried out within the framework of a recommended genetic counseling protocol to assure informed and autonomous patient decision-making.

---

*To whom correspondence should be addressed: 212-263-7621, FAX: 212-562-2642, email: oddouc01@mcrcr6.med.nyu.edu

Cancer Genetics for the Clinician, edited by Shaw.
Kluwer Academic / Plenum Publishers, New York, 1999.

Mutations in cancer predisposition genes, including BRCA1 and BRCA2, are relatively common. It is estimated that the frequency of carriers in the general population is between 1 in 800 and 1 in 400, with a significantly higher frequency in selected populations.[4] Approximately 1 in 200 women develops breast cancer due to the inheritance of a high-risk gene and such genes account for 5–10% of all breast and ovarian cancers.[5] This implies that between 9000 and 18,000 of the women diagnosed each year in the United States have a heritable form of breast cancer and that more than 600,000 individuals in the U.S. are carriers of a mutant allele. For women of Ashkenazi Jewish ancestry, 2.4% are carriers of one of three common BRCA1 and BRCA2 mutations, a rate at least 8-fold greater than that of other populations. The cases that arise from the inherited mutations are thought to account for the excess of breast cancer among Ashkenazi Jewish women.[6]

Although new developments in molecular genetics enhance our ability to perform risk analysis, the task is complicated by several factors: 1) the discovery of a wide variety of different mutations causing common hereditary cancers; 2) incomplete ascertainment of all predisposing genes and mutations; and 3) incomplete knowledge of genotype-phenotype correlations, including penetrance estimates. The task is further complicated by the potential misuse of genetic information.

This chapter will review current information regarding the risk of developing breast cancer based on family history of breast and/or ovarian cancer, the role of genetic testing for modifying that risk, the potential benefits, drawbacks, and/or limitations of testing, and specific recommendations for follow-up care for people who are identified as "high risk". Although we expect explosive developments to continue in the field of cancer genetics, these protocols will provide a framework for the integration of the new information.

2. FOUNDER EFFECTS

2.1. Definition

Mutations that occur in members of small populations that remain isolated and expand dramatically in numbers can reach high frequencies. This effect, called genetic drift, does not require that the mutations confer any selective advantage. Such mutations are referred to as founder mutations and are frequently found in homogeneous endogamous populations.

2.2. Breast Cancer Genes and Founder Mutations

Two genes, BRCA1 and BRCA2, are known to be major causes of hereditary predisposition to breast cancer; current testing and surveillance focuses on these two genes. The BRCA1 gene was mapped in 1990 to 17q12 and cloned in 1994.[7,8] Shortly thereafter, the BRCA2 gene was mapped to chromosome 13q12–13 in 1994 and cloned in 1995.[9,10]

The contribution of mutations in BRCA1 and BRCA2 to hereditary breast cancer remains uncertain. Among the high-risk families selected for mapping studies and subsequently utilized for mutation analysis, these genes were thought to account for approximately 90% of all hereditary breast cancer. BRCA1 accounted for 40–50%

of hereditary breast cancer and BRCA2 approximately 35–45%.[9–11] More recent studies have suggested that the role of these genes in heritable site-specific breast cancer families may be less than the original estimates.[11–17] The distribution and frequency of mutations differ in diverse ethnic populations and do not contribute as expected among affected individuals. The frequency of mutations also appears to be age-dependent with a lower than expected contribution of BRCA2 mutations in early-onset breast cancer.[13] Mutations in BRCA1 remain the major etiologic factor in breast/ovarian and site-specific ovarian families.[15,18] Likewise, families in which there is an individual with both breast and ovarian cancer are far more likely to harbor mutations in BRCA1.[19] Mutations in BRCA2 contribute to an increased risk of breast cancer in males and may account for almost 15% of the total cases of male breast cancers.[11]

An inherited predisposition to the development of breast cancer is also associated with germline mutations in p53 and may be seen in families with an aggregation of other soft tissue tumors.[20] Heterozygotes for the mutant allele causing ataxia telangiectasia, a recessively inherited syndrome predisposing to cancer, have been observed to have an increased risk of developing breast cancer, but these genes contribute only marginally to the total number of cases.[21–23] In rare cases of male breast cancer, mutations in the androgen receptor gene may be contributory.[24] In addition, there is an unknown number of other predisposition genes that have yet to be identified.[16] Evidence also exists for genes which modify the expression of cancer predisposition genes. For example, a polymorphism in the Hras gene will increase the likelihood that BRCA1 mutations will be associated with ovarian cancer.[25]

2.2.1. Ashkenazi Jews. Both BRCA1 and BRCA2 are large genes. More than 130 unique mutations have been found in BRCA1 and more than 75 distinct mutations in BRCA2, many of which occur in single affected families. More than 85% of mutations in BRCA1 and 90% of mutations in BRCA2 result in truncation of the encoded protein.[26–28] Some mutations have been seen repeatedly, particularly among certain ethnic groups, indicating an historical progenitor or "founder". Among individuals of Ashkenazi Jewish origin, there are three recurrent common mutations: 185delAG and 5382insC in BRCA1 and 6174delT in BRCA2. Because 5382insC is common in other Eastern European groups, the 185delAG mutation and the 5382insC are the most frequently observed mutations in BRCA1 and account for 11.7% and 10.2% of the total mutations, respectively.[26] The three mutations are responsible for approximately 50% of all mutations in Ashkenazi breast cancer families, but a greater percentage, up to 90%, of breast/ovarian families.[15,18]

2.2.2. Other Populations. There are other populations in which founder mutations occur in breast cancer predisposing genes. In Iceland, a single BRCA2 mutation, 999del5, accounts for all heritable cancer in the country.[17] Founder mutations have been found in other countries as well, including Russia, Sweden, Finland, The Netherlands, Belgium, and France.[29–32] There are also founder mutations among individuals of African origin.[33] This list is not exhaustive. Awareness of these founder mutations may facilitate testing; targeted mutation analysis may provide a more efficient approach to testing for a given individual with a known ethnic origin. Many lessons learned in the development of testing and followup strategies for individuals of Ashkenazi Jewish ancestry will apply to individuals from other homogeneous populations.

3. PENETRANCE AND GENOTYPE/PHENOTYPE CORRELATIONS

3.1. Penetrance

BRCA1 and BRCA2 are transmitted as autosomal dominant traits. Any carrier, female or male, has a 50% chance to transmit the mutation to her/his offspring. The phenotype of the carrier is, however, gender-dependent and variable, and penetrance for both breast and ovarian tumors is less than 100%.

Having a dominantly inherited breast cancer predisposition gene therefore is not sufficient to cause the development of breast cancer. Data obtained from the original families recruited for the mapping studies demonstrated that the penetrance of breast and ovarian cancer among mutation carriers of BRCA1 and BRCA2 was high. These families were specifically selected because they were large, had multiple affected family members and thus had considerable bias of ascertainment. Penetrance of breast cancer in BRCA1 carriers in these high risk families was 51% by age 50 and 85% by age 80.[34] The penetrance of ovarian cancer in these same families was lower, 23% by age 50 and 63% by age 70. Comparable risks applied to the occurrence of a second tumor in the same individual. Penetrance estimates for breast cancer among BRCA2 carriers is also high (87%), but the penetrance of ovarian cancer was considerably lower, approximately 6–10%.

Among individuals with breast cancer, the frequency of founder mutations is higher, especially among women diagnosed at an earlier age. Among Jewish women diagnosed before 40, 21% have the recurrent 185delAG mutation.[35] In contrast, a population of young women unselected for their ethnic origin had a predisposition gene with a frequency of approximately 10%.[36] Among the Jewish founder mutations, it has been noted that despite the frequency of the BRCA2 6174delT mutation in the general population, its frequency in breast cancer families is lower than expected, about 1/3 that of the frequency of the BRCA1 185delAG mutation in affected families. This suggests that the penetrance of the BRCA2 mutation is less than that of the BRCA1 mutation.[37–39] Additional studies demonstrated that the median age of onset of breast cancer in carriers of BRCA2 mutations is higher than that of BRCA1 carriers.[16]

The penetrance values obtained from the high-risk families may not be appropriate to all carriers. Recent studies have demonstrated that penetrance of breast and ovarian cancer among carriers may be significantly lower in some families. In particular, in one recent study of Ashkenazi Jews, the penetrance of breast cancer was 56% and of ovarian cancer 16% by age 70 in carriers of BRCA1 mutations.[14] Families with the 185delAG mutation may also show interfamilial variability in penetrance of both breast and ovarian cancer.[40] In addition, two non-Jewish families were reported with identical mutations in which penetrances differed, one complete penetrance, one incomplete.

3.2. Genotype/Phenotype Correlations

Some studies have suggested that there is a correlation between the presence of specific mutations and expression of the phenotype. For example, some investigators have demonstrated that individuals carrying mutations in the first two-thirds of the gene have a higher frequency of ovarian cancer than those carrying mutations in the terminal one-third.[41] They have also reported that the occurrence of ovarian cancer is increased in BRCA2 carriers in whom the mutation is found in exon 11.[29] Others have found no correlation.[19]

3.3. Other Cancers

Mutations in BRCA1 and BRCA2 also have other effects in addition to pre-disposing women to breast and ovarian cancer. Although not as prevalent as breast and ovarian cancer in women, these additional effects are not gender specific and as a result have important implications for male BRCA1 and BRCA2 mutation carriers. The presence of a mutation in BRCA2 predisposes to the development of breast cancer in male carriers, whereas BRCA1 mutations do not.[11] The penetrance of breast cancer in male carriers of BRCA2 mutations may be as high as 14%.[11] In addition, the frequency of colon and prostate cancer is also increased in carriers of BRCA1 mutations whereas the frequency of colon, prostate, and pancreatic cancer is increased among carriers of BRCA2 mutations.[40,42,43] One study of Ashkenazi Jews carrying BRCA1 mutations suggests that the risk of prostate cancer in such individuals may be as high as 16% by age 70 and 39% by age 80.[14] The frequency of other malignancies remains to be defined.

4. PRIOR RISK

4.1. Moderate versus High Risk

Women who present for breast cancer risk assessment may generally be divided into two groups, those at moderate risk and those at high risk.[44] Women at moderate risk have fewer affected family members, absence of a family history of ovarian cancer and relatives with an older age at the time of diagnosis. The molecular basis of disease among such women may *not* be the result of inheritance of a single dominant susceptibility gene. For women at moderate risk, the likelihood of developing disease has been determined empirically, based on observations from large numbers of individuals.

In contrast, women at high risk have multiple cases of breast cancer in close relatives. The age of onset of disease tends to be one to two decades earlier than in the general population (frequently 45 or less). The affected relatives are closely related, with one or more affected first-degree relatives, and additional affected individuals in two or more succeeding generations. Some affected members may have more than one primary cancer, i.e. bilateral breast cancer or breast and ovarian cancer. Some individuals have a very early age of onset, i.e., before the age of 40, and some affected individuals are male. Other cancers are observed in these families, including those of the colon, prostate, and pancreas.[42] The findings are compatible with the idea that cancer susceptibility results from inheritance of a highly penetrant autosomal dominant gene. The cancer develops as the result of additional mutations in breast or ovarian tissue; however, the inherited mutation acts as a first hit, lowering the age at which cancer develops and also lessening the threshold for cancer development in each of the susceptible tissues.

Table 1. Breast Cancer Risk Estimates for Members of
Moderate-Risk Families

Affected Relative	Age of Affected Relative	Cumulative Risk (%) by Age 80
One first-degree	<50	13–21
	≥50	9–11
One second-degree	<50	10–14
	≥40	8–9
Two first-degree	Both <50	35–48
	Both ≥50	11–24
Two second-degree	Both <50	21–26
	Both ≥50	9–16

Hoskins, et al. 1995 JAMA 273:577
adapted from Claus et al. 1994 Cancer 73:643.

4.2. Risk Prediction Models for Individuals at Moderate Risk

For women at moderate risk for developing breast cancer, empirical risk estimates are provided either as relative risks or cumulative risks. Relative risk is the rate of disease in a group that has been exposed to a specific factor, compared to a second group that has not been exposed to that factor. This is a very useful measure for the relative magnitude of effect of a specific risk factor, and thus is more useful for describing the risk to a population rather than an individual. Cumulative risks provide an estimate for the likelihood of developing disease over a fixed span of time, such as for the next 20 years or for a fixed life span. This estimate is more useful in clinical practice.

Four models of risk prediction based on family history have been developed: Anderson,[45] Gail,[46] Claus,[47] and the Nurses Study.[48] Each of the models was based on a different study design and uses different factors for calculating risks. Hence, the estimates that are provided by each of these models differ somewhat. Although the risks provided by these models are not completely consistent, they tend to provide similar estimates. The Anderson, Gail, and Claus models tend to overestimate risks compared to the Nurses Health Study. For clinical counseling, it is useful to calculate risks derived from several models, and to offer these to patients as a range.

5. COUNSELING PROTOCOL

Genetic counseling is appropriate for any individual who perceives herself to be at increased risk for breast or ovarian cancer (Table 2). Generally such perception is based on family history, although some individuals with early-onset or multi-organ disease may be told by their physicians that they are at risk for other malignancies. Genetic counseling is a multi-step procedure for assessing and modifying risk.

The detailed protocol used in the Human Genetics Program at New York University Medical Center begins with a first patient contact that is usually by phone. The overall process is explained and procedures are put into place for obtaining accurate information that will be utilized for the counseling. At the first consultation session, the patient learns about the elements of the consultation, including the number of sessions

Table 2. Individuals Who Might Consider Testing

1. A woman under the age of 50 who has a diagnosis of invasive breast carcinoma, with or without a family history.
2. A woman with a family history of one or more affected first-degree relatives when at least one of the relatives was less than 50 at the time of diagnosis.
3. A woman/man with a family history of male breast cancer.
4. A woman with a personal or family history of more than one primary tumor, i.e. bilateral breast cancer, breast/ovarian cancer.
5. A woman with breast cancer who has a relative with ovarian cancer or an aggregation of other cancers such as those of the colon, prostate, or pancreas.

and their content, how the diagnosis will be validated, how the information will be provided (only in person), and the availability of other specialists, including oncologists and psychotherapists. A detailed family history is obtained, including information about all malignancies in the family. In addition, general medical and genetics histories are obtained to learn about other conditions for which the patient is at risk. Based on this information, a hypothetical diagnosis is provided and the possibilities for additional testing, counseling, and follow up are discussed.

If the family is a candidate for testing (i.e., high risk), then a full explanation is provided for the testing procedures. This includes information about the likelihood that a positive result will be found, the frequency and significance of false positives, the implications of a negative result, the type of information that the patient will receive (cumulative probability, etc.), the recommendations for monitoring and prevention following testing, and the benefits and drawbacks of testing. If the patient is part of a family group, then an opportunity is provided for each person to meet individually with the physician or counselor during this time. Note that blood is usually not drawn during this session; this provides the patient an opportunity to reflect on the information. If the family is not a candidate for testing, or chooses not to be tested, then risk assessment is still provided, the applicability of surveillance and preventive measures is discussed, and the opportunity to bank DNA is provided.

Following the first counseling session, the medical records are reviewed. The histological sections are reviewed to determine if there is any doubt about the diagnosis, and information about genetic testing and prevention is updated by literature search. The information for this family is then presented to a team of physicians and genetic counselors in a case conference. The team makes recommendations about testing, counseling, and surveillance. At the second genetic counseling session, the patient is presented with the conclusions of the case management conference and the details of genetic testing are reviewed. The patient has the opportunity to indicate his/her decision privately and if testing has been chosen, blood is drawn.

Once the results have been obtained, the patient is invited for a third genetic counseling session. The result is provided alone or in the presence of other individuals previously designated. The patient is provided with emotional support. The counselor or physician needs to be prepared not only for anger or depression among those who learn about an increased risk, but also for paradoxical responses. Patients who are told of positive results may express a sense of relief, because the uncertainty with which they have lived has now been resolved. Patients who are told of negative results may experience a sense of "survivor's guilt," especially if other family members are told of positive results. Acute depressive reactions have been rarely observed under such circumstances, although the physician or counselor should have made arrangements to obtain emergency psychiatric consultation, should this be required. The indications for surveillance by diagnostic imaging and screening tests are discussed. The role of estrogen replacement therapy for prevention of coronary artery disease and osteoporosis is discussed and balanced against possible increased risks for breast cancer.

6. TESTING

6.1. Testing Procedures

Ideally, for families at high risk for whom testing is appropriate, an affected individual should be tested first. If a mutation is identified in this affected person, then other family members wanting to know their carrier status may be tested. Any unaffected relative who does not have the family mutation knows that her chance of developing breast/ovarian cancer is no different from that of anyone else in the population.

Mutations in BRCA1 and BRCA2 can be detected with molecular techniques that utilize the polymerase chain reaction (PCR) to amplify portions of the genes for analysis (Fig. 1). For individuals of Ashkenazi heritage, direct mutation detection for the three common mutations in the two genes 185delAG, 5382insC, and 6174delT is an efficient approach. This is ordinarily done using allele specific oligonucleotide hybridization (ASO) or direct DNA sequencing of the appropriate amplified portion of the gene. The ASO procedure uses short oligonucleotide probes that are identical to the mutated sequence or to the normal sequence to determine the sequence of the amplified gene fragment that has been spotted onto a membrane for the analysis. Because of the large size of each of these genes, this direct mutation detection procedure represents a significant shortcut that is estimated to detect about 50% of mutations in Ashkenazi Jewish families.[15]

If a mutation is not detected using this mutation specific procedure, then broader screening of the genes must be undertaken. Single-stranded conformational polymorphism (SSCP) analysis together with targeted sequencing or high throuput sequencing may be used. SSCP is a screening test that compares differences in electrophoretic

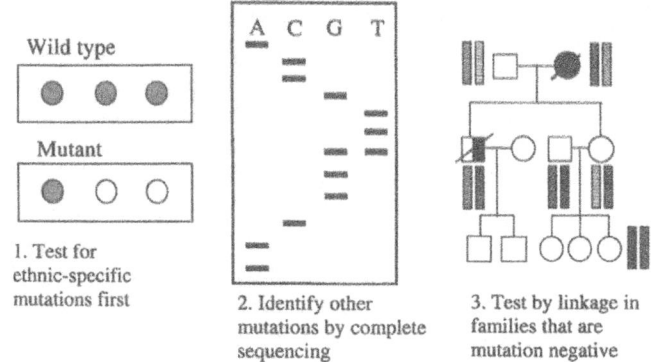

Figure 1. Strategies for mutation detection in breast cancer predisposing genes.

mobility of unknown sequences with normal sequences and must be followed by sequencing to determine the exact nucleotide change.

If an affected individual from a "high risk" family is negative for the initial mutation analysis, then it may be prudent to test another affected member, since the first individual may constitute a sporadic case within a hereditary breast family.

6.2. Mutations versus Polymorphisms

Patients should be prepared for the possibility of an ambiguous result even if a sequence change is detected. If a detected sequence change has been observed before and is known to be associated with disease, as in the case of the founder mutations, then the clinical significance is clear. However, many individuals with BRCA1 or BRCA2 mutations will have new mutations and others will have previously undetected polymorphisms that do not predispose to disease. Sequences that result in premature chain termination of the protein, alternative splicing of the mRNA, or in an amino acid change, are more likely to have clinical significance, particularly if associated with affected individuals in the family. This association may, however, be difficult to detect because of the incomplete penetrance of mutations in these genes.

Some clinically significant mutations may be particularly difficult to detect because they are DNA sequence changes that do not result in any change in the protein they encode, but nonetheless increase the potential for subsequent mutations. An example of this is the I1307K mutation (Fig. 2) in the APC gene which predisposes to colon cancer.[49] This mutation is also a founder mutation in the Ashkenazi Jewish population that occurs at high frequency (6%) and represents a new "three hit" mechanism for conferring cancer predisposition.

6.3. Undetected Mutations and Other Genes

If an affected individual from a "high risk" family is negative for the initial mutation analysis, then it may be prudent to test another affected member since the first individual may constitute a sporadic case within a hereditary breast family. Further evaluation may be indicated, and a limited linkage analysis could be carried out in the family to determine whether the cancer predisposition appears to be linked to either

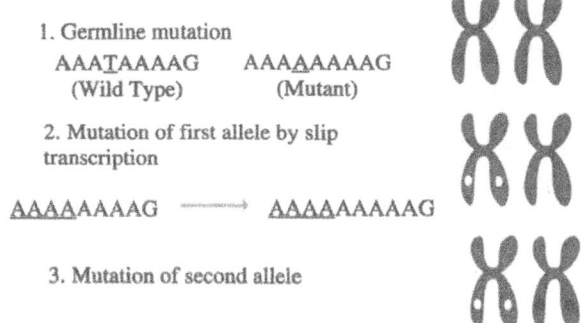

1. Germline mutation

AAATAAAAG   AAAAAAAAG
(Wild Type)   (Mutant)

2. Mutation of first allele by slip transcription

AAAAAAAAG ⟶ AAAAAAAAAG

3. Mutation of second allele

Figure 2. The I1307K mutation in the APC gene creates a predisposition to cancer by producing a hypermutable sequence rather than altering the encoded protein. Cancer develops when the inherited sequence change and the other allele each become mutated as separate additional events or "hits".

chromosome 17 or 13. If linkage is detected, it might suggest that theirs may constitute an undetected mutation in one of these genes or to another closely linked gene. There is evidence for another gene on chromosome 17. There have been many families identified in which there do not appear to be linkage to either of these genes, thus providing strong evidence for the existence of other breast cancer loci.[16] The estimate of risk for that individual should be based on an assessment of the probability that breast cancer is heritable in the individual/family together with an assessment of the sensitivity and specificity of the test.

7. RECOMMENDATIONS FOR INDIVIDUALS AT HIGH RISK

Although the implications of inheriting a mutation in either BRCA1 or BRCA2 are uncertain, it is still possible to provide some risk assessment to carriers. This should be individualized, taking into account the personal medical history of the patient, the family constellation of cancer, the ethnic origin and the specific mutation. The care provider should investigate the latest studies and extrapolate from them information that is most relevant. He/she should provide a range of risks derived from multiple studies with an explanation of the limitations of these results with respect to the given individual. Patients should be educated about surveillance and, although there have been no recommendations about prophylactic surgery for carriers, depending on their personal history, they may wish to consider it as a preventive measure.[50] These recommendations are applicable to patients identified as carriers or who remain at high risk, even in the absence of a detectable mutation. In addition, risk assessment or testing and recommendations for screening may be applicable to other family members and should be offered.

Affected women with BRCA1 mutations should be advised of their increased risk for a second primary tumor, either breast and/or ovarian, and referred for appropriate monitoring, as outlined in the next five sections of this chapter. Unaffected women who are carriers of the mutation or who remain at high risk in the absence of a detectable mutation should understand the range of risks to which they are subject. Men carrying a BRCA1 mutation should be monitored for colon and prostate cancer, although it has not been demonstrated that there is an early age of onset.

Affected and unaffected women carrying the BRCA2 mutation should be advised similarly, as above, with the caveat that the probability of ovarian cancer, while higher than for others in the general population, is lower than that of BRCA1 carriers. Men who are carriers should also be examined regularly by their internists for signs of breast cancer. The benefit of mammography in men at high risk is unknown. Males and females should be screened for signs of colon cancer and monitored for symptoms of pancreatic cancer (i.e., unexplained abdominal pain). Currently there are no recommended screening tests for pancreatic cancer. In addition, males should be monitored for signs of prostate cancer.

7.1. Breast

The major recommendations for increased surveillance for prevention of breast cancer are breast self examination and mammography.[51] Monthly breast self-examination should begin in early adult life and should be supplemented by semiannual or annual clinical examination beginning at age 25–35 years. Up to 10% of breast cancers can be detected by clinical examination alone.[52]

Mammography is useful for identifying early cancers that may not be palpable by physical examination. For women who are at moderate or high risk, annual mammography is recommended beginning at age 25 to 35 years.[50] Whenever possible, the mammograms should be performed at the same location with prior films available for comparison. Studies on the risks and benefits of mammography have been based on women with average risk; hence the risks and benefits of mammography before age 50 have not been established.[53] Although not proven, the estimated 20-fold increase in risk for developing breast cancer for BRCA1 and BRCA2 mutation carriers suggests that mammography screening may be of benefit. Mammography should be supplemented where indicated by sonography.

Two major concerns have been voiced with early use of mammography.[54,55] First, early and frequent exposure to radiation may, in fact, increase the risk of breast cancer. Second, mammography is less useful for identifying small masses in younger women, whose breasts are dense than those of older women. MRI and PET scanning could also be used for screening, but these tests tend to be more expensive and their sensitivity has not been evaluated. For carriers of mutations in these genes, the risk of other malignancies is also increased, and therefore, surveillance for carriers should include monitoring for ovarian, colon, and prostate cancer.

7.2. Ovarian

Two major screening methods are available for detection of early stage ovarian cancer in BRCA1 mutation carriers: vaginal ultrasound and measurement of the serum marker, CA-125. Vaginal ultrasound can detect masses as small as 2mm in diameter, that is, at a stage where they may not be palpated during physical examination.[56] Two analytical methods have been applied to improve the discrimination between malignant and benign lesions: 1) application of a morphology index based on ovarian volume, cyst wall thickness, and septal structure and 2) use of color flow Doppler, which can reliably distinguish the lower impedance to blood flow of ovarian neoplasms.[57,58]

CA-125 is a glycoprotein that is shed into the blood by malignant cells, most commonly of ovarian epithelial origin.[59] Baseline measurement with elevation on a subsequent measurement may be indicative of the development of an ovarian cancer.[60] Unfortunately, both false positive and false negative results occur with a measurable frequency, suggesting that CA125 is not a stand alone technique to screen for early stage ovarian cancer.

7.3. Prostate

The benefits of screening for prostate cancer have not been proven to reduce morbidity or mortality, and some organizations, including the U.S. Preventive Services Task Force, have declined to recommend screening.[61] In contrast, the American Cancer Society recommends annual digital rectal examination and measure of serum prostate-specific antigen (PSA) for men aged 50 and older.[62]

7.4. Colon

For risk of colon cancer, the major screening methods are fecal occult blood screening and colonoscopy, which can detect precancerous adenomas and early cancers.[63] Fecal occult blood screening should be performed every 12 months and colonoscopy should be performed every 3–5 years, beginning at age 50. If a polyp is detected during the colonscopy it can be removed; early polypectomy is protective against subsequent development of colon cancer.[64]

7.5. Surgery

Some individuals at increased genetic risk may choose to have prophylactic surgery for prevention of breast and ovarian cancer. The benefits are not proven; however, an NIH Consensus Conference recommended that women with two or more relatives with ovarian cancer be offered prophylactic oophorectomy following child bearing at age 35. This was based on the fact that the mean age of onset of ovarian cancer in such families is in the mid- to late 40s.[65] In addition, a meta analysis calculated, depending on the cumulative risk, that 30 year old women with BRCA1 or BRCA2 mutations may gain 2.9 to 5.3 years of life expectancy from prophylactic mastectomy and 0.3 to 1.7 years from prophylactic oophorectomy. Women could delay prophylactic oophorectomy until age 40 too without loss of benefit. With increasing age, these gains diminish and are negligible for 60 year old women.[66] Breast tissue is left behind following simple mastectomy and breast tissue may occur in ectopic sites; hence prophylactic surgery cannot convey absolute protection against subsequent development of breast cancer.[67] Some concern has been expressed that carcinoma of the coelomic epithelium has been observed in a few women at increased genetic risk following prophylactic oophorectomy.[68] Nonetheless, recent studies suggest that the lifetime risk of ovarian cancer is reduced for women who have prophylactic surgery.[69,70]

7.6. Hormone Replacement Therapy

Hormone replacement therapy (estrogen alone or estrogen-progestin combination) is used to treat menopausal symptoms and to prevent cardiac disease and osteoporosis. Because family history and estrogen exposure are the two major known risk factors for development of breast cancer, concerns have been expressed about providing estrogen replacement to women who are at increased risk. Estrogen use for less than 5 years is not associated with increased risk of developing breast cancer. Combination hormone replacement therapy has no incremental effect on the risk of developing breast cancer and lessens the risk of uterine cancer among women who have not had hysterectomies.[71] In addition, previous short-term use of estrogens has not been identified as a risk factor for breast cancer; hence, short-term replacement therapy for relief of the vasomotor symptoms is indicated for most post-menopausal women.[72]

When deciding about long-term use of hormone replacement therapy, the risk factors for coronary heart disease, hip fracture and breast cancer should be weighed. Most women at high risk for osteoporosis will benefit from hormone replacement therapy. Likewise, most women at high risk for coronary heart disease, including those with first degree relatives with breast cancer, will benefit.[73,74] However, the risks of estrogen replacement are unlikely to outweigh the benefits for most women who have two or more first degree relatives with breast or ovarian cancer or who themselves are BRCA1 or BRCA2 mutation carriers.[74]

8. OTHER CONSIDERATIONS

Many individuals who are at high risk for a genetic predisposition to breast cancer choose not to have testing. Some may cite a desire "not to know" whereas others express concerns about potential misuse by third parties, including insurers and employers.[75] Given the sensitive nature of this information, there are several steps that the health care provider can take. First, he or she can provide the patient with a guarantee of confidentiality which is only waived when the patient signs a request directing her information to a third party.

Second, the provider can advise patients that several forms of legal protection exist on both the Federal and state levels.[75] There are two major Federal laws that may be invoked: the Americans with Disabilities Act of 1990 and the Health Insurance and Portability and Accountability Act of 1996, which states that genetic information shall not be considered a preexisting condition, nor may insurers refuse to renew or continue coverage because of this information. In recent years, certain states have enacted protective legislation that limit the use of genetic testing by insurers and employers.[76]

Third, providers can anticipate adverse psychological outcomes of their patients. Prior to undertaking genetic testing, it is advisable to review how the patient may handle the results and to arrange for psychiatric support should an adverse psychological outcome occur.

The identification of genetic risks for development of breast and ovarian cancer is a potential public health benefit, as it leads to the identification of those at risk prior to the development of disease. Judiciously applied preventive strategies could have a major impact for those at highest risk. Given the novelty of this field, many kinks need to be worked out for developing sensitive tests, cost-effective testing strategies and protections from potential misuse of genetic information. Development in each of these areas is likely to occur during the next several years, and it may be necessary for health care providers to consult sources beyond this chapter.

REFERENCES

1. American Cancer Society: Cancer facts and figures:1995. Atlanta, GA, 1995
2. Wingo PA, Landis S, Ries LA: An adjustment to the 1997 estimate for new prostate cancer cases. Cancer 80:1810–1813, 1810
3. Ries L, Miller B, Hankey T, et al: Cancer statistics review 1973–91: tables and graphs. Bethesda, MD, 1994
4. Struewing JP, Abeliovich D, Peretz T, et al: The carrier frequency of the BRCA1 185delAG mutation is approximately 1 percent in Ashkenazi Jewish individuals Nature Genet 11:198–200, 1995
5. Newman B, Austin MA, Lee M, et al: Inheritance of human breast cancer: evidence for autosomal dominant transmission in high-risk families. Proceed Natl Acad of Sci USA 85:3044–3048, 1988
6. Egan K, Newcomb P, Longnecker M, et al: Jewish religion and risk of breast cancer. Lancet 347:1638–1639, 1996
7. Hall JM, Lee MK, Newman B, et al: Linkage of early-onset familial breast cancer to chromosome 17q21. Science 250:1684–1689, 1990

8. Miki Y, Swensen J, Shattuck-Eidens D, et al: A strong candidate for the breast and ovarian cancer susceptibility gene BRCA1. Science 266:66–71, 1994

9. Wooster R, Neuhausen SL, Mangion J, et al: Localization of a breast cancer susceptibility gene, BRCA2, to chromosome 13q12–13. Science 265:2088–2090, 1994

10. Wooster R, Bignell G, Lancaster J, et al: Identification of the breast cancer susceptibility gene BRCA2 Nature 378:789–792, 1995

11. Couch F, Farid L, DeShano M, et al: BRCA2 germline mutations in male breast cancer cases and breast cancer families. Nature Genet 13:123–125, 1996

12. Vehmanen P, Friedman LS, Eerola H, et al: A low proportion of BRCA2 mutations in Finnish breast cancer families. Am J Hum Genet 60:1050–1058, 1997

13. Krainer M, Silva-Arrieta S, FitzGerald MG, et al: Differential contributions of BRCA1 and BRCA2 to early-onset breast cancer. New Engl J Med 336:1416–1421, 1997

14. Struewing JP, Hartge P, Wacholder S, et al: The risk of cancer associated with specific mutations of BRCA1 and BRCA2 among Ashkenazi Jews. New Engl J Med 336:1401–1408, 1997

15. Tonin P, Weber B, Offit K, et al: Frequency of recurrent BRCA1 and BRCA2 mutations in Ashkenazi Jewish breast cancer families. Nature Med 2:1179–1183, 1996

16. Schubert EL, Lee MK, Mefford HC, et al: BRCA2 in American families with four or more cases of breast or ovarian cancer: recurrent and novel mutations, variable expression, penetrance, and the possibility of families whose cancer is not attributable to BRCA1 or BRCA2. Am J of Hum Genet 60:1031–1040, 1997

17. Thorlacius S, Sigurdsson S, Bjarnadottir H, et al: Study of a single BRCA2 mutation with high carrier frequency in a small population. Am J of Hu Genet 60:1079–1084, 1997

18. Narod SA, Ford D, Devilee P, et al: An evaluation of genetic heterogeneity in 145 breast-ovarian cancer families. Breast Cancer Linkage Consortium. Am J of Hum Genet 56:254–264, 1995

19. Couch F, DeShano M, Blackwood M, et al: BRCA1 mutations in women attending clinics that evaluate the risk of breast cancer. New Engl J Med 336, 1996

20. Li FP, Fraumeni JF, Jr: Soft-tissue sarcomas, breast cancer, and other neoplasms. A familial syndrome? Annals of Internal Med 71:747–52, 1969

21. Swift M, Morrell D, Massey RB, et al: Incidence of cancer in 161 families affected by ataxia-telangiectasia. New Engl J Med 325:1831–6, 1831

22. Easton D: Cancer risks in A-T heterozygotes. Int J Radiat Biol 66:S177–S182, 1994

23. Bishop DT, Hopper J: AT-tributable risks? Nature Genet 15, 1997

24. Wooster R, Mangion J, Eeles R, et al: A germline mutation in the androgen receptor gene in two brothers with breast cancer and Reifenstein syndrome. Nature Genet 2:132–134, 1992

25. Phelan CM, Rebbeck TR, Weber BL, et al: Ovarian cancer risk in BRCA1 carriers is modified by the HRAS1 variable number of tandem repeat (VNTR) locus. Nature Genet 12:309–311, 1996

26. Couch F, Weber B, and the Breast Cancer Information Core: Mutations and polymorphisms in the familial early-onset breast cancer (BRCA1) gene. Hum Mut 8:8–18, 1996

27. Stratton MR: Recent advances in understanding of genetic susceptibility to breast cancer. Hum Mol Genet 1515–1519, 1996

28. Shattuck-Eidens D, McClure M, Simard J, et al: A collaborative study of 80 mutations in the BRCA1 breast and ovarian cancer susceptibility genes. Implications for presymptomatic testing and screening. JAMA 273:535–541, 1995

29. Gayther SA, Mangion J, Russell P, et al: Variation of risks of breast and ovarian cancer associated with different germline mutations of the BRCA2 gene. Nature Genet 15:103–105, 1997

30. Hakansson S, Johansson O, Johansson U, et al: Moderate frequency of BRCA1 and BRCA2 germline mutations in Scandinavian breast cancer families. Am J Hum Genet 60:1068–1078, 1997

31. Peelen T, van VM, Petrij-Bosch A, et al: A high proportion of novel mutations in BRCA1 with strong founder effects among Dutch and Belgian hereditary breast and ovarian cancer families [see comments]. American Journal of Human Genet 60:1041–1049, 1997

32. Serova O, Montagna M, Torchard D, et al: A high incidence of BRCA1 mutations in 20 breast-ovarian cancer families. Am J of Hum Genet 58:42–51, 1996

33. Gao Q, Neuhausen S, Cummings S, et al: Recurrent germline BRCA1 mutatuions in extended African American families with early onset breast cancer. Am J Hum Genet 60:428–433, 1997

34. Easton DF, Ford D, Bishop DT: Breast and ovarian cancer incidence in BRCA1-mutation carriers. American Journal of Human Genet 56:265–271, 1995

35. FitzGerald MG, MacDonald DJ, Krainer M, et al: Germ-line BRCA1 mutations in Jewish and non-Jewish women with early-onset breast cancer. New Engl J of Med 334:143–149, 1996

36. Langston A, Malone K, Thompson J, et al: BRCA1 mutations in a population-based sample of young women with breast cancer. New Engl J Med 334:137–142, 1996
37. Oddoux C, Struewing JP, Clayton CM, et al: The carrier frequency of the BRCA2 6174delT mutation among Ashkenazi Jewish individuals is approximately 1%. Nature Genet 14:188–190, 1996
38. Roa B, Boyd A, Volcik K, et al: Ashkenazi Jewish population frequencies for common mutations in BRCA1 and BRCA2. Nature Genet 14:185–187, 1996
39. Neuhausen S, Gilewski T, Norton L, et al: Recurrent BRCA2 6174delT mutations in Ashkenazi Jewish women affected with breast cancer. Nature Genet 13:126–128, 1996
40. Friedman LS, Szabo CI, Ostermeyer EA, et al: Novel inherited mutations and variable expressivity of BRCA1 alleles, including the founder mutation 185delAG in Ashkenazi Jewish families. Am J of Hum Genet 57:1284–1297, 1995
41. Gayther S, Harrington P, Russell P, et al: Frequently occuring germline mutations of the BRCA1 gene in ovarian cancer families from Russia. Am J Hum Genet 60:1239–1242, 1997
42. Ford D, Easton DF, Bishop DT, et al: Risks of cancer in BRCA1-mutation carriers. Breast Cancer Linkage Consortium. Lancet 343:692–695, 1994
43. Tonin P, Ghadirian P, Phelan C, et al: A large multisite cancer family is linked to BRCA2. J of Med Genet 32:982–984, 1995
44. Hoskins KF, Stopfer JE, Calzone KA, et al: Assessment and counseling for women with a family history of breast cancer. A guide for clinicians. JAMA 273:577–585, 1995
45. Anderson D, Badzioch M: Risk of familial breast cancer. Cancer 56:383–387, 1985
46. Gail MH, Brinton LA, Byar DP, et al: Projecting individualized probabilities of developing breast cancer for white females who are being examined annually. J Natl Cancer Inst 81:1879–1886, 1879
47. Claus EB, Risch N, Thompson WD: Autosomal dominant inheritance of early-onset breast cancer. Implications for risk prediction. Cancer 73:643–51, 1994
48. Colditz GA, Willett WC, Hunter DJ, et al: Family history, age, and risk of breast cancer. Prospective data from the Nurses' Health Study [published erratum appears in JAMA 1993 Oct 6;270(13):1548]. JAMA 270:338–343, 1993
49. Laken SJ, Petersen GM, Gruber SB, et al: Familial colorectal cancer in Ashkenazim due to a hyper-mutable tract in APC. Nature Genet 17:79–83, 1997
50. Burke W, Daly M, Garber J, et al: Recommendations for follow-up care of individuals with an inherited predisposition to cancer II. BRCA1 and BRCA2. JAMA 277:997–1003, 1997
51. Anonymous: Reports of the working group to review the National Cancer Institute—American Cancer Society breast cancer detection project. J Natl Cancer Inst 62:639–709, 1979
52. Greenwald P, Nasca P, Lawrence C, et al: Estimated effect of breast self examination and routine physician examinations on breast cancer mortality. New Engl J Med 299:271–273, 1978
53. Kerlikowske K, Grady D, Rubin S, et al: Efficacy of screening mammography: a meta-analysis. JAMA 273:149–154, 1995
54. Fletcher S, Black W, Harris R, et al: Report of the international workshop on screening for breast cancer. J Natl Cancer Inst 85:1644–1656, 1995
55. Mettler F, Upton A, Kelsey C, et al: Benefits versus risks from mammography. Cancer 77:903–909, 1996
56. van Nagell J, Higgins R, Donaldson E, et al: Transvaginal sonography as a screening method for ovarian cancer. Cancer 65:573–577, 1990
57. Daly M: The epidemiology of ovarian cancer. Hematol Oncol Clin N Amer 6:729–738, 1992
58. Kurjak A, Zalud I, Alfirevic Z: Examination of adnexal masses with transvaginal color ultrasound. J Ultrasound Med 10:295–297, 1991
59. Jacobs I, Bast R, Jr: The CA-125 tumor-associated antigen. Hum Reprod 4:1–12, 1989
60. Skates S, Feng-Ji X, Yin-Hua Y, et al: Toward an optimal algorithm for ovarian cancer screening with longitudinal tumor markers. Cancer 76:2004–2010, 1995
61. US Preventive Services Task Force: Guide to Clinical Preventive Services. Baltimore, 1996
62. Mettlin C, Jones G, Averette H, et al: Defining and updating the American Cancer Society Guidelines for cancer-related check-up. Cancer J Clin 43, 1993
63. Levin B, Murphy G: Revision in American Cancer Society recommendations for the early detection of colorectal cancer. Cancer J clin 42:296–299, 1992
64. Selby J, Freedman G, Queensberry C, Jr., et al: A case-control study of screening sigmoidoscopy and mortality from coorectal cancer. New Engl J Med 326:653–657, 1992
65. Cancer NCPoO: Ovarian cancer screening, treatment, and follow-up. JAMA 273:491–497, 1995
66. Schrag D, Kuntz K, Garber J, et al: Decision analysis—Effects of prophylactic mastectomy and

oophrectomy on ife expectancy among women with BRCA1 and BRCA2 mutations. New Engl J Med 336:1465–1471, 1997

67. Billimoria M, Morrow M: The woman at increased risk for breast cancer: evaluation and management strategies. Cancer J Clin 45:263–278, 1995
68. Tobachman J, Tucker M, Kase R: Intraabdominal carcinomatosis after prophylatic oophrectomy in ovarian cancer prone families. Lancet 2:795–797, 1982
69. Piver M, Jishi M, Tsukada Y, et al: Primary peritoneal carcinoma after prophylactic oophrectomy in women with a family history of ovarian cancer. Cancer 71, 1993
70. Struewing JP, Watson P, Easton DF, et al: Prophylactic oophorectomy in inherited breast/ovarian cancer families. Journal of the National Cancer Institute. Monographs 17:33–35, 1995
71. Colditz G, Hankinson S, Hunter D, et al: The use of estrogens and progestins and the risk of breast cancer in postmenopausal women. New Engl J Med 332:1589–1593, 1995
72. Cancer CGoHFiB: Breast cancer and hormonal contraceptives. Lancet 347, 1996
73. Gradym D, Rubin S, Petitti D, et al: Hormone therapy to prevent disease and prolong life in post-menopausal women. Ann Int Med 117, 1992
74. Col N, Eckman M, Karas R, et al: Patient-specific decisions about hormone replacement therapy in postmenopausal women. JAMA 277, 1997
75. Ostrer H, Allen W, Crandall L, et al: Insurance and genetic testing: Where are we now? Am J Hum Genet 52, 1993
76. Rothenberg K, Fuller B, Rothstein M, et al: Genetic information and the workplace: legislative approaches and policy changes. Science 275, 1997

6

TESTING MINORS FOR INHERITED CANCER RISK

Mary Z. Pelias

Professor of Genetics
Louisiana State University Medical Center

INTRODUCTION

Recent advances in the technology of molecular genetics have extended the powers of individuals and health care professionals to control the ravages of genetic disease. These powers now include a spectrum of genetic tests that can predict future disease or disease susceptibility. Accurate prediction of future disease was first realized when detection of the gene for Huntington disease became a medical reality.[1] This first step was subsequently expanded to include tests for some cancers, including familial ademomatous polyposis[2] and Von Hippel-Lindau syndrome.[3] Particularly dramatic in determining disease susceptibility has been the development of tests for genes that cause breast and ovarian cancer—tests that determine an increased probability, though not a certainty, of developing these dreaded diseases.[4] These and other molecular genetic tests are now used for determining the genetic status of current patients as well as for pre-conception and prenatal testing for the purpose of avoiding the birth of children destined to suffer serious genetic diseases.

The issue of genetic testing in children erupted in 1990 when researchers in neurogenetics asserted that no minors should ever be tested for the gene that causes Huntington disease.[5] The justifications for this assertion included the fact that Huntington disease is an adult-onset, neurodegenerative disease for which no treatment or cure is yet available. Further justification was an assertion that children who learned of their own inevitable debilitation and lingering, degrading death would suffer serious psychosocial consequences. The authors asserted an obligation to protect the future auton-

Address communications to: Dr. Mary Z. Pelias, Department of Biometry and Genetics, Louisiana State University Medical Center, 1901 Perdido Street, New Orleans, Louisiana 70112-1393, Phone: (504) 568-6151, Fax: (504) 568-8500, E-mail: mpelia@lsumc.edu

Cancer Genetics for the Clinician, edited by Shaw.
Kluwer Academic / Plenum Publishers, New York, 1999.

omy of children and further contended that parents should be treated as third parties with respect to decisions about testing their own children for the Huntington gene. Somewhat later another group of geneticists suggested a similar moratorium on the testing of minors for the gene, or genes, that cause breast and ovarian cancer.[6] These proposals generated heated debate among genetics professionals about the relative rights and duties of parents and health care professionals in providing genetic services, including genetic testing of families and especially children.

The individual issues that have been dissected and examined over the past 8 years have sorted out into 4 broad areas of concern. The first, and perhaps the most important, is concern for children and their welfare, both present and future. The second is consideration of the authority of parents in relation to making decisions for their own minor children and in relation to their position in the physician-patient relationship. The third is an examination of the role of genetics professionals in the arena of genetic counseling and genetic testing. Finally, the fourth includes several observations about continuing and emerging variables in the practice of medical genetics. This paper examines these four areas of concern with a view to synthesizing policy that will protect all parties who interact in medical genetics and genetic counseling.

CONCERN FOR CHILDREN

The question of genetic testing in children and adolescents generates intense concern largely because of their position of dependency as persons who are not yet competent to act as their own decision makers. Their incapacity heightens the awareness of adults in their efforts to provide care and protection for these developing but immature persons. In the narrower confines of medical genetics and genetic counseling, genetics professionals are appropriately mindful of the welfare of children, both as a matter of individual health and as a matter of their interpersonal relationships. The genetics community was quick to acknowledge the implications of genetic testing for children and adolescents.[7] Professional geneticists have agreed that the primary justification for testing minors is the opportunity to provide an immediate medical benefit for the child whose genotype confers an imminent risk of disease. Such benefits include, for example, medical monitoring for the appearance of polyps when a child is determined to be at risk for early onset colorectal cancer.[8] Conversely, children who are determined not to be at risk for this disease also enjoy a benefit when they are released from uncomfortable monitoring procedures.

In addition to emphasizing the primary objective of realizing immediate medical benefits, genetics professionals have carefully examined other consequences of genetic testing in minors, most notably the impact of genetic information on the psychosocial development of children and adolescents. These less tangible sequelae have been the subject of concern since the early days of genetic counseling. They may include the alteration of a child's self image, changes in the child's perceptions of prospects for the future, and shifts in the child's relationships with parents, siblings, and persons outside of the family. Geneticists are careful and correct to note that insensitive or inappropriate use of genetic information could well damage both the child as an individual and the child's interactions in the social milieu.[9]

Although minors are generally presumed to be incompetent for purposes of making major decisions about medical care and life directions, the law has acknowledged limited decisional capacity under "mature minor rules" that permit minors to seek medical treatment, on their own initiative, for sexually transmitted diseases and pregnancy.[10] An increasingly significant factor in genetic testing and genetic counseling is the acknowledgement of the child as an individual participant in the testing process. Indeed in some situations the inclusion of the child in a decision to proceed with testing is an altogether logical step. Depending on the minor's apparent level of maturity, geneticists who seek to engage the child in the decision making process may seek the child's *assent*, or an adolescent's *consent*, to proceed with testing. How these situations unfold will depend on the complex set of circumstances that exist within the family and that surround the family in the counseling scenario.

Most discussions of the negative psychosocial consequences of genetic testing in children rest on the presumption that parents will invariably disclose to their children information about the tests themselves and about the meaning of test results. This presumption is extended to the assertion that testing children will foreclose "their freedom to make these choices for themselves once they reach adulthood."[11] Such conclusions are, however, not necessarily valid. Parents may, for example, view such candor as inadvisable, and they may elect not to disclose test results until some future time, if at all. In such situations the parents may use the genetic information of their children to make their own personal plans, or their own personal provisions for the future of their children, without necessarily revealing to the children their genetic status or prognosis.

Finally, in urging caution about the many and often unpredictable consequences of genetic testing in children, some genetics professionals emphasize exclusively the goal of providing a "timely medical benefit" as the "primary justification" for pursuing testing. However, while this language implies that "secondary" justifications may exist, little or no attention is afforded to these undefined factors.[12] More thorough examination could, however, define less rigorous but nevertheless valid justifications for testing minors, including, but not limited to, providing funds for a child's later inevitable health care needs, or seeking more favorable social and health care environments for the management of an illness that may or will appear at a later time.

RESPECT FOR PARENTS

The family is the basic social unit of human society, and it has been remarkably stable over the centuries. Traditionally the family unit has been headed by the father, whose role has been that of protector and provider, but who also, as head-of-household, has exercised the power of life and death over his spouse and children as well as the power to sell them as property. The mother has traditionally fulfilled the role of managing the home and tending the children. Children have traditionally been subservient to the parents and have contributed their labor to the welfare of the family. Until only recently women enjoyed very few rights, and children next to none.[13] Gradually, however, during the 20th century, women have gained recognition of their status as co-equals, and both women and children have become persons and individuals in the eyes of society and the law.

In the shifting balance of personhood and authority within the family, society has consistently supported first the fathers, and now the parents, as the individuals who are entitled to make decisions on behalf of their own families. The depth of this support is found in decisions of the United States Supreme Court that address questions of parental authority to guide the education and medical care of minor offspring. In questions of educational choices, the Court has affirmed a "liberty" interest of the individual to include "the right of the individual to contract, to engage in any of the common occupations of life, to acquire useful knowledge, to marry, establish a home and bring up children."[14] A second decision affirmed the "liberty of parents and guardians to direct the upbringing and education of children under their control."[15] A third decision affirmed the authority of Amish parents to remove their children from state schools at the end of eighth grade so that the children could finish their education and training within the Amish community.[16] These early cases establish firm support for parental authority within the family—support that withstands the attempt of state legislation to undermine the parental prerogative.

While decisions by the Supreme Court supporting parental authority in educational questions are distantly removed from the dilemmas of genetic testing in children, a more recent holding applies directly to decisions about health care for children. In the early 1980's, on several occasions, parents of severely impaired newborns elected to forego medical or surgical treatment for their infants for one anomaly because such treatment would bring no improvement in the infant's overall diminished quality of life. After a series of lawsuits and appeals, the Supreme Court again affirmed the parental prerogative: the right to make the difficult decisions about severely compromised infants ultimately rests with their parents. In noting that "[s]tate law vests decisional responsibility in the parents, in the first instance," the Court supported parents as the persons charged with making difficult—often immensely difficult—decisions for their own minor children.[17]

Attention to constitutional support for parental authority, from education to health care, does not, however, imply unbridled parental authority. Nor does it support a constitutional right to demand genetic tests for children, as some geneticists have mistakenly concluded.[11] Indeed, the Supreme Court limited what parents may demand from the medical profession when it held that "the parents cannot always have absolute and unreviewable discretion to decide whether to have a child institutionalized. They . . . retain plenary authority to seek such care for their children, *subject to a physician's independent medical judgment*"[18] (emphasis added). Although committing a child to a mental institution may be far more serious than requesting a genetic test, the two cases about making health care decisions for minors should be read in concert and interpreted to extend broad deference to parental authority. Such authority can indeed be limited by the professional *medical* judgment of the health care professional, but parents should appropriately retain the authority to make non-medical decisions that are not directly derived from professional medical judgment.

With respect to the concept of parental prerogative, or parental autonomy, our legal and social institutions allow parents great latitude in making decisions for their own minor children, limited only by statutory provisions that protect children from unlawful abuse and neglect. This latitude acknowledges the automomy of parents as individuals and in their role as caregivers for their own children, and it rests on the presumption that parents act in the best interests of the child. A policy that presumes to rest on the *future* autonomy of the child denies the *real and present* interests that parents have in making autonomous decisions for themselves and on behalf of their families.

Health care professionals who propose a moratorium on genetic tests for minor children argue from four tenuous assumptions that collectively abrogate the authority that society vests in parents. The first is the assertion that the professional is more qualified than parents to make at least some hard decisions, even non-medical decisions, about testing minors. The second assumption is that parents may not, or should not, or perhaps even *cannot*, make appropriate decisions about testing their own children. The third assumption is that the *only* reason for testing a child is to provide an immediate medical benefit of the child. The fourth assumption is that information about the child's genotype will inevitably be used by the parent to the detriment of the child. After 8 years of debate these assumptions remain good fuel for argument, even as they seek to negate the role of parents as the primary guardians of and caregivers for their own children.

ROLE OF HEALTH CARE PROFESSIONALS

A physician-patient relationship is created when a patient seeks medical care and the physician agrees to provide it. The relationship is based on the concept of implied contract, with both parties advancing expectations and accepting duties when the relationship is joined.[19] The physician accepts the duty of providing appropriate care for the patient and expects cooperation and remuneration from the patient. The patient accepts the duty of assisting in medical management and expects the physician to provide suitable care. Over and above this reciprocity, however, is the *fiduciary* nature of the interactions between physician and patient and the imbalance that characterizes a fiduciary relationship. This imbalance is associated with the superior training and expertise of the professional and the patient's relative lack of medical knowledge: the patient must place some *faith* in the physician, who is obligated, because of his superior position, to act for the benefit of the patient.[20] In the context of medical genetics, the fiduciary relationship rests on the genetics professional, who has a thorough knowledge of the field and the ability to convey relevant information to those who seek it.

In the specialized and highly charged atmosphere of genetic counseling, the persons who appear in genetics clinic usually include one or both parents, often with one or more of their children, sometimes accompanied by one or more grandparents and possibly other relatives or friends as well. The challenge for the genetics professional is providing information that will clarify the uncertainties that underlie the family's appearance in clinic. As the fiduciary in the professional-patient relationship, the genetics professional has the duty to communicate information that the family seeks to those members of the family who can reasonably understand the information and respond to it. In most counseling situations these persons are the parents, although the counselor knows that the information can have an impact on other members of the family as well. Indeed, "[i]n genetics, the patient is really the family rather than the individual," so that the "traditional view about doctor-patient relationships may have to change."[21] The "patient" becomes a group of persons, with varying ages, competency, autonomy rights, and decisional authority.

With the family as the patient, the genetics professional must meet the challenge of providing appropriate care for not one, but several persons. Although some of the care provided in the genetics clinic is medical treatment, much of the care offered by the genetics professional is provided in the form of information about the genetic problem that brought the family to the genetics clinic. Such information is conveyed to the parents, usually according to the tradition of the "non-directive" counseling *process* that allows the family to consider and decide, based on complete information, about how to cope with the genetic problem that has appeared in their family. An early definition of genetic counseling emphasized that the goal of counseling is to help patients "choose the course of action which seems appropriate to them in view of their risk and their family goals and [to] act in accordance with that decision."[22]

The *content* of counseling includes a spectrum of information about medical diagnosis and prognosis, recurrence risks, psychological factors, and community services and support groups. In addition to providing information, the diligent geneticist takes care to inquire about other circumstances in the family, including educational background, employment and financial factors, religious affiliation, and other social details that may indicate the direction that the family may follow in coping with their specific genetic legacy. With an appreciation of the medical as well as social circumstances of the family, the geneticist may then be prepared to reinforce both the articulated and the implied decisions of parents who are charged with the awesome duty of providing for their family. Once the geneticist has provided a complete package of information about the genetic problem, about the possible psychosocial sequelae of testing children, and has helped the family find its own orientation in dealing with its own genetic legacy, the geneticist has done all that can be done and *should* be done. The ultimate decision about proceeding with testing should rest with the persons who will live with that decision for the rest of their lives.[23]

As genetic knowledge and the availability of genetic tests continue to expand at an increasingly rapid rate, the task of the health care professional becomes increasingly onerous. At the very least, the health care professional must know whether a particular health problem is hereditary and detectable by genetic testing. If parents are requesting genetic tests for their children, the genetic evaluation and counseling protocol should include detailed information, *before* testing, about both the positive and negative ramifications of generating genetic information.[24] Parents should be aware that genetic information may have a decidedly negative impact on children. Parents should also understand that some children want to know about their situation and that some children experience a great sense of relief when uncertainly is removed, one way or the other. Parents should also know that some children may not want to know, and may never want to know, about their genetic endowment. Finally, however, geneticists should respect the decisions of parents, who may or may not reveal test results to their children, depending on what the parents decide is best for *their* children and *their* family.

In addition to directing both the process and content of genetic counseling and genetic testing, the health care professional should also be at least aware of legal consequences that may ensue after the birth of children with predictable inherited disorders. Since the right to privacy was expanded to include the right of a woman to decide to terminate a pregnancy, and since the new genetic technologies permit prenatal diagnosis of numerous hereditary disorders, the options for ensuring the birth of healthy children have increased dramatically. As parents have become increasing informed about these options, they have become quick to assert their right to have healthy children, within the limits of the new technologies. Litigation in medical malpractice for failure to inform patients about these options has resulted in numerous judgments in favor of parents who have successfully asserted injury resulting from the birth of children with predictable impairments.[25] This line of reasoning could reasonably be expanded to acknowledge claims by parents and their children who may have benefited from early genetic testing but were denied access to tests. Legal injury from loss of potential benefits may first focus on medical issues but may also include psychological or social injuries as well: all that is needed for successful prosecution is a legally cognizable claim, a skillful lawyer, and a sympathetic judge or jury. For genetics professionals to deny categorically this possibility is a disservice to fellow professionals as well as to the patients and families who seek genetic testing as a means to managing their own lives and future.[11]

CONTINUING VARIABLES IN MEDICAL GENETICS

The practice of medical genetics and genetic counseling has evolved over 5 decades to accommodate the explosion of knowledge about human genes. Even as the compendium of information has expanded, however, several fundamental variables in practical clinical genetics have remained unchanged. These variables include biological and medical factors, social factors, and the ethical and legal dilemmas of genetics practice.

Biological and medical variables in clinical genetics include mode of inheritance and the probability of developing a serious disease based on what is known about age-of-onset, penetrance, and variation in expression of any gene. Biological questions may also include queries about gene frequencies, about interactions between genes and the environment, and about predicting genetic susceptibility to disease as well as genetic certainty. Further, patients and families may also have a critical interest in medical factors, such as the possibility and effectiveness of any treatment that is available for their disorder. These approaches to coping with genetic disease include evaluating dietary management and medical or surgical treatments as well as consideration about a patient's quality of life after any of these solutions is implemented.

Testing newborns and children for carrier status for recessive diseases is problematic because of the specter of stigmatizing the child or creating the mistaken impression that the youngster is in some way ill or should be avoided by peers. Testing young persons for untreatable, adult-onset dominant diseases presents problems similar to testing for recessive carrier status, but with the additional difficulty of determining the child's apparently inevitable fate, possibly many years in the future. On the other hand, testing young people for treatable, early-onset dominant diseases is approached with caution and optimism—caution about negative effects on family relationships, and optimism about successful treatment modalities. Finally, testing persons of any age for treatable recessive diseases generally meets with approval because of the great benefits that may accrue to the individual, and possibly to society as well. Thus, the variables of how the gene causes disease, and when, and the possibility of therapy continue to factor into every scenario in genetic counseling.

In addition to ever-present biological and medical factors as influences in the practice of genetics, so too are *social factors*, particularly the age and circumstances of the person, or family, who requests genetic testing. Genes that cause diseases in minors may be part of state-mandated newborn screening programs, or, in the case childhood cancers such as retinoblastoma or Li-Fraumini syndrome, may be the focus of early testing in families that have positive histories these diseases. Some families, on the other hand, may be managed by parents who are reluctant to have their children tested, even in the face of disease that could clearly harm or even cause the death of the child. In other families, the children may seek information about what they perceive to be the family health problem, and responses may vary significantly from one sibling to the next. Some youngsters seem to cope well with knowledge of a deleterious genotype, and they may even experience a new sense of "belonging" when they learn that they share the deleterious gene with other members of the family. Conversely, some children may experience emotions of "survivor guilt" when they learn that they are likely to out-live their siblings who have a deleterious gene.[7] Indeed, the range of emotional responses to learning about personal genotypes may be as broad as the whole range of human emotions. The genetics practitioner must always be mindful that each family presents a unique constellation of circumstances and should therefore be treated and managed within its own conceptual context, with special attention to the health and security of the minor children. Achieving an appropriate balance in the interests of children, parents, and the family as a whole demands skill and sensitivity from the professional in the fiduciary relationship.

Finally, the continuing variables in the practice of genetics include *ethical and legal issues*. From the view of the professional, the issues of beneficience and doing no harm are of continuing concern, as is the issue of avoiding allegations of medical negligence. From the view of patients and families, the issues focus on autonomy, competence, comprehension, and respect for persons, both adults and minors. Requests for genetic testing in children will generally be initiated by parents, who are endowed by society with the authority to request information and to act on that information, presumably in the best interests of their family. The genetics professional should, however, expect to encounter occasional parental requests that are wholly contradictory to his or her personal and professional code of conduct. In such circumstances the genetics professional is under no obligation to comply with requests that are unequivocally inappropriate, although a professional duty may extend to referring the patient or family to another professional. A policy of deference to parental requests does not imply blind compliance with any and all requests for testing minors.

CONCLUSIONS

The continuing debate about genetic testing in children has permitted the development of several principles that should govern the practice of medical genetics and genetic counseling as it relates to genetic testing in children and adolescents. What is incumbant on the genetics professional is at least the pursuit of *reasonable* courses of action that acknowledge the heavy burden that parents must bear in making decisions for their children and for themselves. Careful, thorough genetic counseling is the first and most important activity of the genetics professional, with a view to deferring to parental autonomy in all but the most egregious circumstances.

Over the past several years much attention and thought have focused on the difficult questions raised by the prospects of genetic testing in children. Professionals who favor one policy or another have heatedly debated the issues and listened to vastly disparate arguments, always with a view to protecting the interests of children in questions of exploring their genotypes. Indeed, the most striking feature of these debates is the persistent common denominator of concern for the welfare of children. The most striking disparity has been the ongoing disagreement about the relative roles of parents and genetics professionals in making decisions about testing minors. The fact that these controversies continue to thrive serves to underscore the many variables that enter into decisions about pursuing genetic testing. Since our expanding knowledge of the human genome continually introduces new variables into the practice of medical genetics and genetic counseling, the interrelationships of children, parents, and genetics professionals become increasingly complex, and this complexity may direct our attention to the simple fact that each family represents a unique set of circumstances and values, and, as such, a unique set of solutions to a particular genetic problem.

As genetics professionals continue to grapple with questions about testing children, some truisms are emerging. First, health care professionals are never required to do something that is morally and personally repugnant. Thus, a refusal to authorize genetic testing of children in the face of clearly inappropriate parental motivations is justifiable, although such a refusal may well carry a duty to refer the patient or family to another professional. Second, the genetics professional should work from the traditional premise of providing thoughtful, thorough genetic counseling so that parents are equipped to make fully informed decisions about the immediate issue of testing children and about the future directions of their family life. Beyond such counseling, however, the professional should defer to the parents as the decision makers for their own minor children. Third, with respect to principles of constitutional law, the Constitution of the United States clearly supports the parental prerogative, although nowhere in constitutional history do we find a "constitutional right" for parents to demand a genetic test for their children. Such a claim is a misinterpretation of those constitutional principles which do support the parental prerogative in making educational decisions and most health care decisions for their own children. Finally, the recent history of medical malpractice litigation in the United States indicates that caution and circumspection may serve the genetics professional well. To deny the possibility of litigation when parents are denied opportunities to do what they are convinced is good for their families is to invite the wrath of the courts in response to allegations of medical malpractice.

Our expanding knowledge of technology in molecular genetics heightens our awareness of the psychosocial impact that genetic information can have on individuals and families. Since our knowledge of both the technical and the interpersonal factors in the world of human genetics is likely to remain incomplete and is likely to shift in emphasis as we learn more about our genetic legacies, we must be careful to retain a firm grasp on the values and interrelationships that we encounter and serve in the practice of medical genetics and genetic counseling.

REFERENCES

1. Brandt J, Quaid KA, Folstein SE, Garber P, Maestri NME, Abbott MH, Slavney PR, et al: Presymptomatic diagnosis of delayed-onset disease with linked DNA markers: the experience in Huntington's disease. JAMA 261:3108–3114, 1989
2. Nishisho I, Nakamura Y, Miyoshi Y, Miki Y, Ando H, Horii A, et al: Mutations of chromosome 5q21 genes in FAP and colorectal cancer patients. Science 253:665–669, 1991
3. Latif F, Tory K, Gnarra J, Yao M, Duh F, Orcutt ML, et al: Identification of the von Hippel-Lindau disease tumor suppressor gene. Science 260:1317–1320, 1993
4. King MC, Rowell S, Love SM: Inherited breast and ovarian cancer: What are the risks? What are the choices? JAMA 269:1975–1980, 1993
5. Block M, Hayden MR: Opinion; Predictive testing for Huntington disease in childhood: challenges and implications. Am J Hum Genet 46:1–4, 1990
6. Biesecker BB, Boehnke M, Calzone K, Markel MS, Garber JE, Collins FS, Weber BL: Genetic counseling for families with inherited susceptibility to breast and ovarian cancer. JAMA 269:1970–1974, 1993
7. ASHG/ACMG Report. Points to consider: Ethical, legal, and psychosocial implications of genetic testing in children and adolescents. Am J Hum Genet 57:1233–1241, 1995
8. Peterson GP, Francomano C, Kinzler K, Nakamura Y: Presymptomatic direct detection of adenomatous polyposis coli (APC) gene mutations in familial polyposis coli. Hum Genet 91:307–311, 1993

9. Wertz DC, Fanos JH, Reilly PR: Genetic testing for children and adolescents: Who decides? JAMA 272:875–881, 1994

10. Holder AR: Disclosure and consent problems in pediatrics. Law, Med, Health Care 16(3–4):219–228, 1988

11. Clayton EW: Removing the shadow of the law from the debate about genetic testing of children. Am J Med Genet 57:630–634, 1995

12. Holtzman NA, Watson MS, eds: Promoting Safe and Effective Genetic Testing in the United States: Final Report of the Task force on Genetic Testing. Bethesda, MD: The National Institutes of Health, 1997

13. McLaughlin MM: Survivors and surrogates: Children and parents from the ninth to the thirteenth centuries, in deMause L (ed): The History of Childhood. New York, Harper & Row, p 140, 1970

14. *Meyer v. Nebraska*, 262 US 390, 399, 1929

15. *Pierce v. Society of Sisters*, 268 US 510, 535, 1925

16. *Wisconsin v. Yoder*. 406 US 205, 1972

17. *Bowen v. American Hosp Ass'n*. 476 US 610, 627, 1986

18. *Parham v. J.R.* 422 US 584, 1978

19. *Hankerson v. Thomas*, 148 A.2d 583, D.C. 1959

20. Gifis SG: Dictionary of Legal Terms. New York, Barron's Educational Series, Inc., p 180, 1983

21. Wertz DC, Fletcher JC: Ethics and genetics: An international survey. Hastings Ctr Rprt Supp 19(4):20–24, 1989

22. American Society of Human Genetics Ad Hoc Committee on Genetic Counseling. Genetic counseling. Am J Hum Genet 27:240–241, 1975

23. Pelias MZ, Blanton SH: Genetic testing in children and adolescents: Parental authority, the rights of children, and the duties of geneticists. Univ of Chicago Law School Roundtable 3(2):525–543, 1996

24. Chapman MA: Canadian experience with predictive testing for Huntington disease: Lessons for genetic testing centers and policy makers. Am J Med Genet 42:491–498, 1992

25. Pelias MZ: Medicolegal aspects of prenatal diagnosis, in Milunsky A (ed): Genetic Disorders and the Fetus: Diagnosis, Prevention, and Treatment. Baltimore, MD, Johns Hopkins, 4th ed, 972–998, 1998

7

THE LABORATORY ANALYSIS OF CANCER SUSCEPTIBILITY GENES

Comprehensive Sequencing of BRCA1 and BRCA2

Brian E. Ward

Vice President of Operations
Myriad Genetics Laboratories
Salt Lake City, Utah

Laboratory analysis for genetic susceptibility to cancer is a rapidly evolving discipline. This chapter will provide a brief overview to the types of clinical laboratory tests that are currently being performed for characterization of mutational status in cancer susceptibility genes. The latter portion will focus on comprehensive sequencing of the breast and ovarian cancer susceptibility genes BRCA1 and BRCA2 as a representative model of predispositional testing for inherited cancer and to demonstrate the complexity of current diagnostic tests.

It has been known for several decades that certain cancers cluster in families. Investigation into these families has led to identification of over 25 common autosomal dominant familial cancer syndromes (Table 1). Additionally six common autosomal recessive familial cancer syndromes are known plus a smaller number of familial clustered cancer syndromes with uncertain modes of inheritance. Identification of familial cancer syndromes and characterization of their mode of inheritance has resulted in the appreciation that a proportion of cancer can be directly attributed to genetic causes. This realization coupled with the dynamic progress in molecular genetics has resulted in the identification of specific genes associated with some of these cancer syndromes. It is now possible to perform laboratory analysis to diagnose germ line mutations that may predispose an individual to development of a specific cancer.

In this age of rapidly developing technology and discoveries it should be realized that scientific advances in research are often not rapidly transferable to the clinical laboratory. After a gene is discovered there are numerous challenges and obstacles that must be overcome prior to the introduction of a clinical test. Assays must not only be clinically accurate, but the results of the test should have the potential to be clini-

Cancer Genetics for the Clinician, edited by Shaw.
Kluwer Academic / Plenum Publishers, New York, 1999.

Table 1. Common Familial Cancer Syndromes

Autosomal Dominant	Autosomal Recessive	Uncertain Inheritance
Adenomatous Polyposis	Ataxia-telangiectasia	Carcinoid, familial
Basal Cell nevus syndrome	Bloom syndrome	Hodgkin's disease, familial
Breast/Ovarian Cancer	Fanconi's anemia	Pancreatic cancer, familial
BRCA1 & BRCA2		
Carney syndrome	Rothmund-Thomson	Testicular carcinoma
Chordoma, familial	Werner's syndrome	
Colon cancer syndrome	Xeroderma pigmentosum	
Cowden syndrome		
Esophageal cancer with tylosis		
Gastric cancer, familial		
Li-Fraumeni syndrome		
Melanoma, familial		
Multiple endocrine neoplasia type 1 & 2		
Neurofibromatosis type 1 & 2		
Osteochondromatosis		
Paraganglioma familial		
Peutz-Jeghers syndrome		
Prostate cancer		
Renal cancer, familial		
Retinoblastoma		
Tuberous sclerosis		
Von Hippel-Lindau disease		
Wilms' tumor		

(From N.M. Lindor and M.H. Green. The concise handbook of family cancer syndromes. J Nat'l Ca Inst 1998,90:1039–1071.)

cally useful. Assay selection has a direct bearing on accuracy and therefore on clinical utility. The method of analysis of predispositional testing for a specific syndrome or gene is dependent on a host of factors including assay sensitivity, specificity, positive predictive value of the test, known genotype/phenotype correlation, the existence of mutational hot spots within the gene, speed of analysis, and cost of performing the analysis.

Currently, the vast majority of diagnostic molecular genetic predispositional cancer tests are considered to be "Investigational". As such, results of clinical genetic testing should only be given to a patient if the analysis was conducted in a laboratory that meets the standards for the Clinical Laboratory Improvement Act or was conducted as part of an approved research protocol. Laboratories providing such diagnostic services have the responsibility to validate both the technology utilized and the laboratory's sensitivity and specificity of the particular diagnostic assay.

It is an ongoing challenge for clinical laboratory scientists to match the appropriate clinically applicable methodology to the gene being studied and the type of diagnostic analysis required. A small number of cancer syndromes are diagnosable by cytogenetic analysis. These include syndromes such as Fanconi's anemia, Bloom Syndrome and Ataxia Telangataisia.

There are also a growing number of familial cancer syndromes that are known to be associated with the presence of deleterious mutations in specific genes. The diagnosis of the presence of deleterious mutations in these genes can be accomplished by a number of different protocols. Several methods currently exist for the detection of mutations. These methodologies include allele specific oligonucleotide hybridization (ASO), heteroduplex analysis, protein truncation assays, denaturing gradient gel electrophoresis (DGGE), single-strand conformation (SSCP) analysis and DNA sequencing (Table 2). Different laboratory methods examine differing proportions of the gene in question.

Mutation detection by ASO examines very small regions of the gene and detects specific known sequence changes. In the field of predisposition cancer testing, ASO's

Table 2. Methods of Mutation Detection

Testing Method	Description	Advantages	Disadvantages
DNA sequencing	Direct determination of nucleotide sequence of DNA	Most sensitive method of mutation detection	May not find mutations in promoter regions or introns
			May miss large deletions or insertions
Single-strand conformation analysis (SSCP)	Mutation detection based on the different mobilities of denatured PCR products.	Rapid, simple, and widely available for many genes	Subsequent DNA sequencing needed to characterize mutation
			Sensitivity drops with longer DNA sequences
Denaturing gradient gel electrophoresis (DGGE)	Mutation detection of partially denatured double stranded DNA are electrophoresced in denaturing gradient gels.	Sensitive. Better resolution than SCCP	Not efficient for analyzing large DNA fragments. Labor-intensive to set up
Protein truncation assays (also called in vitro synthesized protein assay)	A method of mutation detection that translates mRNA into a radiolabeled protein after PCR amplification of cDNA	Identifies mutations that truncate proteins and are apt to be harmful	Cannot detect nontruncating mutations which can be harmful
			Subsequent sequencing needed to characterize mutation Misses mutations that are near either end of the gene
Heteroduplex analysis	Denatured PCR products are allowed to cool creating unique secondary structure which can be detected by gel electrophoresis.	Sensitive (>90%) Rapid, simple, and widely available for most genes	Subsequent DNA sequencing needed to characterize mutation
Allele-specific-oligonucleotide (ASO) hybridization	A method of specific mutation detection that employs a short single-stranded DNA segment that binds to a normal or mutant sequence	Panels of ASO probes useful in detecting common mutations	Each ASO probe detects only one specific sequence
		Sensitive method for detecting known mutations	Most useful for small sequence changes

cDNA = Complementary DNA mRNA = Messenger RNA: PCR = Polymerase chain reaction.

are currently most commonly used to detect the presence of very specific mutations such as the two deleterious mutations in BRCA1 (187delAG and 5382insC) and the one deleterious mutation in BRCA2 (6174delT) that are associated with a increased risk for breast and ovarian cancer in the Ashkenazi Jewish population.

Assays based on base pair mismatches within the DNA molecule have the potential to examine a significant proportion of the gene. These technologies, i.e. SSCP and CSGE, are based on the knowledge that DNA sequence changes can alter the three-dimensional shape and/or physical size of specific sections of DNA within a gene following amplification, denaturation and reassociation. The altered DNA fragments migrate through a charged gel at different rates than non-mutated DNA fragments. Such technologies are evolving into initial screening assays, which are designed to indicate the potential presence of deleterious mutations in large genes. SSCP and DGGE have been used as screening tests for the presence of deleterious mutations in hereditary nonpolyposis colon cancer, TP53, BRCA1, and BRCA2.

Protein truncation assays indirectly examine a major portion of a specific gene via examination of protein products from a specific gene. RNA is isolated and used as a template to create complimentary DNA (cDNA) for specific portions of the gene. The cDNA is transcribed into mRNA that is translated in vitro to generate protein fragments that are then electrophoretically separated. The presence of normal protein segments and of abnormal, truncated protein products indicate the potential presence of a deleterious mutation. Due to the large size of the currently identified predispositional genes and associated technical problems, protein truncation typically is not capable of examination of the entire gene. Routinely protein truncation tests examine 1/2 to 3/4 of the gene in question. Protein truncation assays have been successfully utilized for screening MLH1 and MSH2 for the presence of abnormal truncated proteins indicating deleterious mutations.

Finally, comprehensive DNA sequencing directly determines the nucleotide sequence within the DNA molecule and can accurately diagnose genetic mutations within the entire coding region of a gene. Sequencing is the most sensitive method of mutation detection and is consistently utilized to characterize the exact DNA changes that are provisionally identified by other technologies. Additionally, sequencing can be used in a targeted manner for sequence analysis of mutational "hot spots" within a specific gene. Such partial sequencing strategies have been successfully used to diagnose deleterious mutations within a region of the RET proto-oncogene. Comprehensive DNA sequencing is considered the most rigorous of laboratory testing protocols for gene analysis and is therefore considered to be the "gold standard" of diagnostic analysis. It is also the most challenging type of test to manage from an Informatics standpoint. The application of sequencing technologies for diagnosis of deleterious mutations in large genes is a recent advance in molecular genetics and is best illustrated by comprehensive sequencing of BRCA1 and BRCA2.

As previously described, there are genetic syndromes which predispose an individual to developing tumors at an early age or rare tumors. One of the current primary goals of cancer research in these syndromes is to identify the specific gene or genes responsible for the genetic predisposition. The first breast and ovarian cancer susceptibility gene was discovered in 1994. This gene, BRCA1, is located on the long arm of chromosome 17 (Fig. 1). The BRCA1 gene spans nearly 100 kilobases of DNA. The coding region of this gene extends over 24 exons, contains over 5580 base pairs, which encodes a protein of 1863 amino acids. The second predispositional breast and ovarian cancer gene, BRCA2, was isolated the following year. BRCA2 (Fig. 1) is located on the

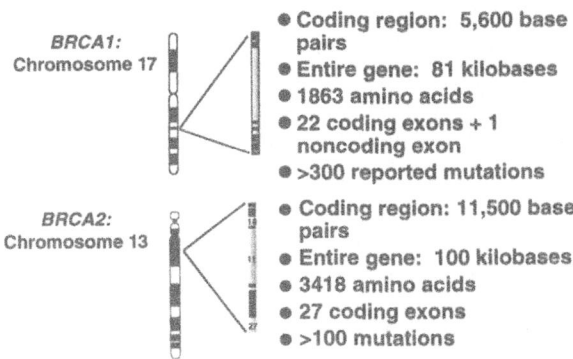

BRCA1:
Chromosome 17

- Coding region: 5,600 base pairs
- Entire gene: 81 kilobases
- 1863 amino acids
- 22 coding exons + 1 noncoding exon
- >300 reported mutations

BRCA2:
Chromosome 13

- Coding region: 11,500 base pairs
- Entire gene: 100 kilobases
- 3418 amino acids
- 27 coding exons
- >100 mutations

Figure 1. Characteristics of breast/ovarian cancer predispositional genes.

long arm of chromosome 13 and contains 27 exons spanning 80 kilobases of DNA. The coding sequence of BRCA2 is over 10,200 base pairs, encoding a protein of 3418 amino acids.

Deleterious mutations in either the BRCA1 or BRCA2 gene are correlated with an increased genetic predisposition to breast and ovarian cancer. The discovery of the genetic sequence for these two cancer predispositional genes was subsequently followed by the development of clinical assays, which would diagnose the presence of deleterious mutations in high-risk patients. The most accurate and thorough laboratory analysis for the presence of deleterious mutations in these genes relies on DNA sequencing. Comprehensive DNA sequence analysis of large genes, such as BRCA1 and BRCA2, is an emerging technology within the clinical laboratory and has been made possible through the development of new sequencing strategies. These new strategies include extensive use of laboratory automation, miniaturization of the reaction process, robotic manipulation of specimens, development of new sequence analysis algorithms, and the creation of a computerized tracking system which positively tracks specimens through a process requiring over 1000 reactions per patient. The incorporation of these new strategies into the clinical laboratory setting now allows comprehensive sequence analysis of BRCA1 and BRCA2 as a robust clinical laboratory analysis.

DNA sequence analysis is designed to detect changes (mutations) within the DNA molecule. Generally mutations can be characterized as deleterious, uncertain variants, or of no clinical significance. Deleterious DNA mutations lead to the creation of non-functional or truncated protein products. Deleterious mutations include nonsense mutations, frameshift mutations caused by insertions or deletions, splice site mutations that lead to abnormal RNA products, and regulatory mutations. Mutations that are of no clinical significance include: silent mutations, where a DNA base change does not change the amino acid sequence; polymorphisms, where a common mutation leads to an amino acid change that has been shown not to alter the functionality of the protein; and mutations at the splice site junctions that do not alter the RNA products generated by the gene. Uncertain variants describe a class of mutations where a change in the DNA sequence results in an amino acid substitution where the effect on the functionality of the protein is unknown at this time.

An increased predisposition to breast and ovarian cancer is a result of the presence of normal and abnormal proteins, produced as a consequence of the presence of mutated DNA. The presence of abnormal functioning proteins has the potential to result in a cascade of events leading to aberrant replication patterns within those cells and eventually uncontrolled cellular proliferation.

Hereditary breast/ovarian cancer has a different phenotype than typical post-menopausal breast cancer. Within families where breast and ovarian cancer cluster, the presence of hereditary components to breast and ovarian cancer is indicated by a vertical transmission from generation to generation of the breast or ovarian cancer. Hereditary cancer is also characterized by earlier diagnosis, increased severity, and the presence of both breast and ovarian cancer in the same family. Additionally, male breast cancer, bilateral breast cancer and an increased incidence of secondary tumors are hallmarks of hereditary breast cancer.

Of the 180,000 new cases of breast cancer every year, approximately 7% can be considered to be hereditary. In addition, 10% of the 25,000 cases of ovarian cancer diagnosed annually are hereditary. It is currently estimated that 90–95% of hereditary breast cancer is genetic and is associated with deleterious mutations in BRCA1 or BRCA2. There are families that demonstrate a strong hereditary component and are not shown to have mutations within BRCA1 or BRCA2. It is presumed that the cancer predisposition in these families is the result of another one of the cancer syndromes or due to a deleterious mutation in a " private" familial gene which is not ubiquitous in nature but limited to a single family.

The risk of developing breast or ovarian cancer in the presence of a deleterious mutation is significant. The risk in the general population that a woman will be diagnosed with breast cancer before age 50 is approximately 1 in 50. However, if a woman carries a deleterious mutation in BRCA1 or BRCA2 her risk rises to 1 in 2. In a parallel manner, the general population risk of a woman being diagnosed with ovarian cancer before 50 years of age is approximately 1 in 100 but mutation carriers have up to a 1 in 3 risk of being diagnosed with ovarian cancer prior to age 50.

Clinical laboratory tests for BRCA1 and BRCA2 are designed to diagnose deleterious mutations in individuals at increased risk for breast and ovarian cancer so that they may begin to employ intervention strategies and to improve survival.

The gold standard of DNA based testing is comprehensive sequence analysis. Although sequence analysis may be more costly than other types of screening methodologies, it is required to achieve appropriate levels of specificity and sensitivity for detection of deleterious mutations in breast and ovarian cancer genes. Sequence analysis of BRCA1 and BRCA2 is currently recommended because these genes have some rather unique characteristics. First, deleterious mutations have been demonstrated throughout the entire gene for both BRCA1 and BRCA2 (Fig. 2). Almost every exon contains deleterious mutations. There are no "hot" spots of mutations with the limited exceptions of three mutations with increased prevalence in the Ashkenazi Jewish population, one deletion within the Icelandic population and two common deletions within the Dutch population. Secondly, over 550 mutations have been identified in BRCA1 and over 330 in BRCA2. In addition, all types of mutations have been described in BRCA1 and BRCA2 including truncating mutations, frame shift, missence, insertions, deletions, and splice site mutations. Finally, comprehensive sequence analysis routinely discovers new, previously undescribed deleterious mutations. To date, over 40% of the deleterious mutations identified in BRCA1 and BRCA2 have been uncovered by sequencing during clinical analysis. These attributes preclude the use of screening methodologies such as protein truncation and single base pair mismatch for mutation detection in BRCA1 or BRCA2. These attributes concordantly support the approach

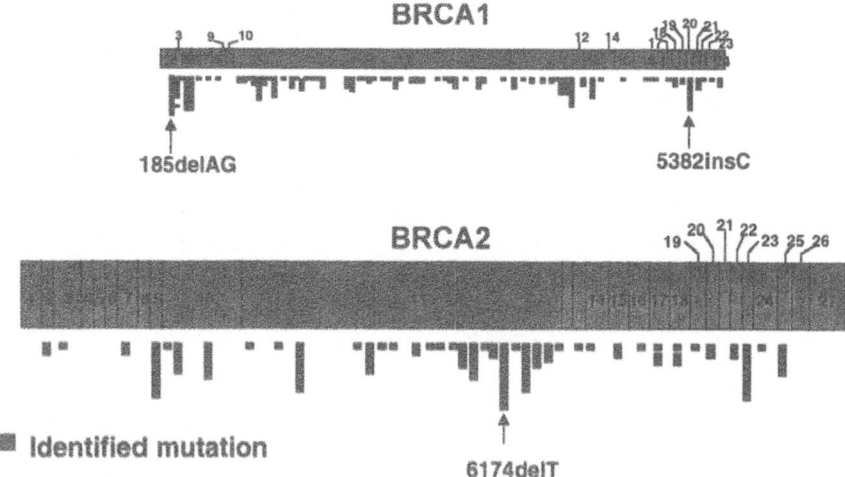

Figure 2. Mutations are found throughout the BRCA1 and BRCA2 genes.

that comprehensive sequencing is most appropriate for clinical diagnosis of deleterious mutations until such time as the molecular biology of these genes is understood at a deeper level.

Comprehensive sequence analysis of BRCA1 and BRCA2 employs methodology that examines each DNA base of the open reading frame for both genes plus a significant amount of the sequence surrounding the exon/intron borders within these genes. This requires analysis of more than 17,500 bases in both the forward and the reverse direction for a total of more than 35,000 base pairs. Generation of this amount of sequence data is a considerable challenge. Approximately, 1000 unique reactions are required per analysis and more than 300 different reagents are required. Such complex analysis is only possible in a highly automated laboratory environment.

Diagnostic platforms that are capable of performing the magnitude of sequence analysis required for BRCA1 and BRCA2 have only recently been developed. The diagnostic platform that allows accurate, timely completion of comprehensive sequencing relies on positive specimen tracking throughout the laboratory process using bar coded specimens and interactive data base specimen tracking through all reaction steps. Specimen manipulation and creation of reaction mixtures occurs robotically to minimize human interaction and eliminate human error. Data analysis is accomplished via a proprietary interactive computerized program. The flow of a patient's specimen through the laboratory process for comprehensive sequencing for predispositional testing for breast and ovarian cancer is schematically presented in Fig. 3. The diagnostic platform was developed in a laboratory specifically designed for clinical, diagnostic sequencing. Design parameters of this specialized laboratory include creation of positive pressure clean rooms where all pre-PCR procedures are performed. Such precautions minimize the potential of cross contamination of amplified products between specimens.

Typically, whole blood or extracted DNA specimens arrive in the laboratory with a bar code label attached. This bar code corresponds to an identical label on the test requisition form. The bar code is scanned into the database and associated with a laboratory processing number. Thereafter, sample handling is automated and is tracked by bar code transfers. Such rigorous control allows for precise monitoring of the sample

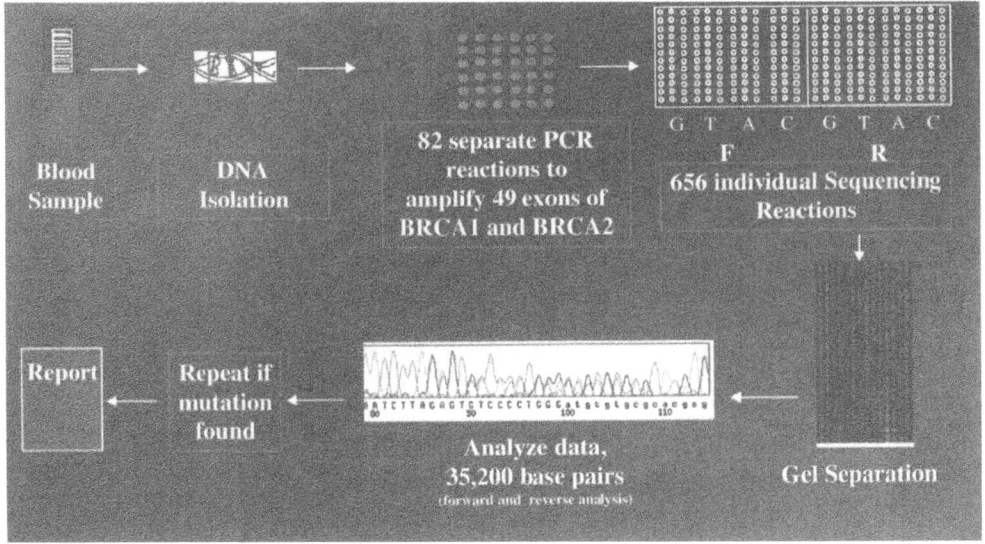

Figure 3. BRCA1 and BRCA2 sequence analysis.

as it progresses through the complex DNA sequencing process. This process also creates numerous quality control measurements, which allows continuous monitoring and improvement of the diagnostic process.

Mononuclear blood cells are isolated from the whole blood specimen and serve as the source for obtaining genomic DNA. Following DNA isolation, 82 separate amplification reactions plus appropriate controls are initiated. These reactions allow for amplification of the entire coding regions of the 49 exons of BRCA1and BRCA2. Each of the amplified PCR products is then subjected to dye primer thermocycle sequencing, which requires 656 sequencing reactions per patient. The products from these sequencing reactions are resolved on conventional slab gels with fluorescent detection via high-throughput sequencers. Each patient analysis results in the generation of approximately 200 gel lanes of DNA sequencing data. The fluorescent sequence signals are transformed into a waveform signal as displayed. It is these waveforms that are presented to data analysists who identify and confirm the presence of deleterious mutations.

One of the most critical parts of the testing process is the data analysis. Routine analysis of 35,000 base pairs of data in a clinical environment would be nearly impossible without extensive computer assistance. Initially the database queries the sequencing machine's computers to identify and capture the sequence data. A proprietary data review application analyzes the sequence for polymorphisims and potential mutations. These sequence variations are presented to technologists specifically trained to interpret such data. A normal sequence will appear as a clean, single peaked waveform at each base position. Potential mutations appear as double waveforms at specific base positions. A DNA mutation is a disruption in the DNA base pattern. We each have two copies of each gene, one maternally derived and one paternally derived. When both copies of the gene posses the normal sequence, there is agreement between the waveforms generated by the sequence data. However, if a potential mutation is present, there is disagreement between maternal and paternal gene copies

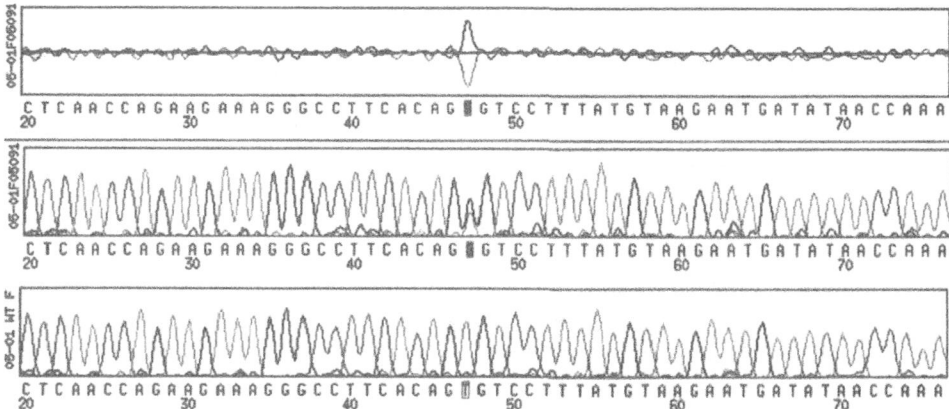

Figure 4. Computer-assisted analysis of sequence information.

which results in a disruption in the wave form beginning at point of the mutation. Once an analyst has verified a sequence variation, it is noted in the database. Two independent analysts review all data in a blinded manner. A unique computer algorithm, developed at Myriad Genetics, "subtracts" the sequence of the patient from a composite wild type generated from analysis of over 1000 chromosomes. As depicted in Fig. 4 when the patient's sequence (the middle waveform) is equivalent to the expected normal sequence (the lower waveform) the subtraction algorithm presents a flat line. However, when the sequence differs, a unique waveform is generated (top waveform). If the sequence variation is interpreted to be a deleterious mutation, a repeat analysis is initiated. The patient's DNA is re-sequenced and re-analyzed. Following confirmation of the mutation, the Laboratory Director reviews the data and a final report is generated.

All Investigational tests require careful quality control and quality assurance monitoring. Laboratory automation and computerization allow for extensive monitoring. Internal quality control begins with reagent preparation. All newly formulated reagents are controlled against reagents in use. Reaction conditions are reported to the database by reagent tracking software that also monitors equipment performance. Quality control of the sequence reactions is monitored through the use of numerous unique sequence algorithms such as signal-to-noise ratio, expected patient base pair alignment to normal sequence score, signal intensities, and number of potential heterozygous locations per patient sequence. Quality assurance programs include peer review and inspections by outside agencies, processing of samples with known deleterious mutations in a blinded fashion and performance of validation studies. Such intense monitoring has resulted in the creation of a diagnostic platform with an analytical sensitivity and specificity of greater than 99%.

Following the analytical validation of the specificity and sensitivity of this computerized, highly automated platform and prior to the clinical introduction of comprehensive sequencing for predispositional genetic risk assessment for breast and ovarian cancer, two research trials were performed. The first trial included BRCA1 sequencing in over 800 individuals. The second trial included 14 collaborating institutions from across the United States and comprised 238 women diagnosed with breast cancer before the age of 50 or a diagnosis of ovarian cancer with at least one relative with either breast or ovarian cancer. These patients submitted three generation family histories. Comprehensive sequencing of BRCA1 and BRCA2 was performed on all women. The data was analyzed in such a manner as to allow the creation of modeled probabilities for characterization of the risk of carrying a deleterious mutation in BRCA1 or BRCA2 given a specific family history. Table 3 presents these modeled probabilities. These modeled probabilities suggest that there is a high likelihood (greater that 25%) of a deleterious mutation being present in a patient diagnosed with breast cancer before the age of 50 if the patient has one or more relatives who was also diagnosed with breast cancer before the age of 50. The probability of the presence of a deleterious mutation segregating within the family increases with increasing numbers of affected individuals, the presence of bilateral breast cancer, and particularly in the presence of ovarian cancer in the family. As shown in Table 3, the probability that a particular affected patient carries a deleterious mutation increases to 89% in families with strong history of bilateral breast cancer plus ovarian cancer. This study concluded that the risks of a deleterious mutation for BRCA1 or BRCA2 segregating in a family where two or more individuals diagnosed with breast cancer prior to age 50 were higher than originally predicted and all such families are potential candidates for predispositional genetic testing.

The clinical experience currently totals greater than 1000 patients submitted to the laboratory for comprehensive BRCA1 and BRCA2 sequence analysis. This experience has affirmed the philosophy that comprehensive sequence analysis for BRCA1 and BRCA2 is most efficacious at the current time. Clinical analysis has diagnosed over 80 distinct deleterious mutations spread throughout the entire lengths of BRCA1 and BRCA2. Over 40% of these mutations had not been previously described prior to clinical analysis. These mutations include nonsense mutations, deletions, insertions, and splice site deleterious mutations.

Additionally, the proportion of patients with deleterious mutations diagnosed in the clinical setting has validated the risk calculations proposed by the modeled probabilities. Although complete ascertainment of family history is not possible in a clinical reference laboratory setting, it was anticipated that approximately 25% of patients who were referred with a diagnosis of breast cancer prior to age 50 and who indicated any family history of breast cancer would have a deleterious mutation. Analysis of the clin-

Table 3. Probabilities of a Deleterious Mutation in BRCA1 or BRCA2 In a Women With Breast Cancer under 50 Years of Age

Relatives with BrCa < 50?	Relatives with OvCa?	Proband: Bilateral BrCa or OvCa?	Proband: BrCa < 40?	Modeled Probability
+	−	−	−	25%
+	−	−	+	40%
+	−	+	−	51%
+	−	+	+	75%
+	+	−	−	35%
+	+	−	+	59%
+	+	+	−	71%
+	+	+	+	89%

Frank et al. J Clin Onc 1998: 16, 2417.

ical database demonstrates that 25.4% of such patients had a deleterious mutation. The close correlation between the actual mutation rate and the proposed modeled probabilities validates the use of such modeled probabilities in a clinical setting.

It is the ultimate goal of molecular diagnosis for a predisposition to specific types of cancer to effect changes in patient management. For those patients at increased risk for breast and/or ovarian cancer based on a genetic predisposition due to a deleterious mutation in BRCA1 or BRCA2, that goal is within reach. The discoveries of these genes were the first step. These discoveries were followed by applied research, which allowed a deeper understanding of the molecular biology of these genes and the proposed role of deleterious mutations in the cancer process. Eventually a clinical assay was developed that relied on the creation of a diagnostic platform which utilizes automation, positive patient tracking, and computer assisted sequence analysis to accurately diagnose deleterious mutations in BRCA1 and BRCA2. The final step in achieving this goal is the application of the knowledge obtained in the clinical laboratory toward reducing the risk of ovarian and breast cancer. As basic and applied research progresses, effective interventions will continue to be discovered and improved.

REFERENCES

Aitkin M, Anderson D, Francis B, Hinde J: Statistical modelling in *glim*. Walton Street, Oxford, England OX2 6DP: Oxford University Press, 1989

Beaudet AL, Tsui LC: A suggested nomenclature for designating mutations. Hum Mut 2:245–248, 1993

Berchuck A, Cirisano F, Lancaster JM, et al: Role of BRCA1 mutation screening in the management of familial ovarian cancer. American Journal of Obstetrics & Gynecology 175:738–746, 1996

Breast cancer facts, and figures 1996. Atlanta: American Cancer Society, 1995:3

Breast Cancer Information Core. http://www.nhgri.nih.gov/ Intramural_research/Lab_transfer/BIC, 1997

Burke W, Daly M, Garber J, et al: Recommendations for follow-up care of individuals with an inherited predisposition to cancer. II. BRCA1, and BRCA2. Cancer Genetics Studies Consortium. JAMA 277: 977–1003, 1997

Chapman MS, Verma IM: Transcriptional activation by *BRCA1*. Nature 382:678–679, 1996

Claus EB, Schildkraut JM, Thompson WD, et al: The genetic attributable risk of breast and ovarian cancer. Cancer 77:2318–2324, 1996

Cotton RGH: Mutation Detections, Oxford Univ. Press 1997

Couch FJ, DeShano ML, Blackwood MA, et al: BRCA1 mutations in women attending clinics that evaluate the risk of breast cancer [see comments]. New England Journal of Medicine 336:1409–1415, 1997

Cummings S, Olopade O: Predisposition Testing for Inherited Breast Cancer: Oncology, Vol.12, Number 8, Aug. 1998

Easton DF, Bishop DT, Ford D, et al: Genetic linkage analysis in familial breast, and ovarian cancer: results from 214 families. Am J Hum Genet 52:678–701, 1993

Easton DF, Ford D, Bishop DT, et al: Breast, and ovarian cancer incidence in BRCA1-mutation carriers. Am J Hum Genet 56:265–271, 1995

Easton DF, Steele L, Fields P, et al: Cancer risks in two large breast cancer families linked to BRCA2 on chromosome 13q12–13. Am J Hum Genet 61:120–128, 1997

Ford D, Easton DF, Bishop DT, et al: Risks of cancer in *BRCA1*-mutation carriers. Lancet 343:692–695, 1994

Friedman LS, Ostermeyer EA, Szabo CI, et al: Confirmation of *BRCA1* by analysis of germline mutations linked to breast, and ovarian cancer in ten families. Nature Genetics 8:399–404, 1994

Gayther SA, Warren W, Mazoyer S, et al: Germline mutations of the *BRCA1* gene in breast and ovarian cancer families provide evidence for a genotype-phenotype correlation. Nature Genetics 11:428–433, 1995

Krainer M, Silva-Arrieta S, FitzGerald MG, et al: Differential contributions of BRCA1 and BRCA2 to early-onset breast cancer. New England Journal of Medicine 336:1416–1421, 1997

Lindor NM, Greene MH, Mayo Familial Cancer Program: The Concise Handbook of Family Cancer Syndromes. Journal of the National Cancer Institute, Vol.90, NO.14, 1998

Mazoyer S, Dunning AM, Serova O, et al: A polymorphic stop codon in *BRCA2*. Nature Genetics 14:253–254, 1996

McCancer KL, Jorde LB: Evaluating the Genetic Risk of Breast Cancer: The Nurse Practitioner, Aug. 1998

Miki Y, Swensen J, Shattuck-Eidens D, et al: A strong candidate for the breast and ovarian cancer susceptibility gene *BRCA1*. Science 266:66–71, 1994

Milner J, Ponder B, Hughes-Davies L, et al: Transcriptional activation functions in BRCA2. Nature
386:772–773, 1997

Narod SA, Ford D, Devilee P, et al: An evaluation of genetic heterogeneity in 145 breast-ovarian cancer
families. Breast Cancer Linkage Consortium. Am J Hum Genet 56:254–264, 1995

NIH Consensus Development Panel on Ovarian Cancer: Ovarian Cancer. Screening, treatment, and follow-
up. JAMA 273:491–497, 1995

Phelan CM, Lancaster JM, Tonin P, et al: Mutation analysis of the BRCA2 gene in 49 site-specific breast
cancer families. Nature Genetics 13:120–122, 1996

Robson ME, Offit K: New *BRCA2* mutation in an Ashkenazi Jewish family with breast and ovarian cancer.
Lancet 350:117–118, 1997

Scholl T, Pyne MT: High Throughput Automatic DNA Sequence Analysis of the Breast/Ovarian Cancer
Susceptibility Genes BRCA1 and BRCA2, Personal Communication

Serova OM, Mazoyer S, Puget N, et al: Mutations in BRCA1 and BRCA2 in breast cancer families: are there
more breast cancer-susceptibility genes? Am J Hum Genet 60:486–495, 1997

Shattuck-Eidens D, Oliphant A, McClure M, et al: *BRCA1* sequence analysis in women at high risk for susceptibility mutations: risk factor analysis and implications for genetic testing. JAMA 278:1242–1250, 1997

Shen MR, Frank TF, Gumpper K, Deffenbaugh A, Ward BE: Novel mutations in BRCA1 and BRCA2 genes
detected by automated high throughput sequencing. Am J Hum Genet 63

Statement of the American Society of Clinical Oncology: genetic testing for cancer susceptibility. J Clin Oncol
14:1730–1736, 1996

Stoppa-Lyonnet D, Laurent-Puig P, Essioux L, et al: BRCA1 sequence variations in 160 individuals referred
to a breast/ovarian family cancer clinic. Institut Curie Breast Cancer Group. Am J Hum Genet 60:
1021–1030, 1997

Struewing JP, Hartge P, Wacholder S, et al: The risk of cancer associated with specific mutations of BRCA1,
and BRCA2 among Ashkenazi Jews. New England Journal of Medicine 336:1401–1408, 1997

Tavtigian SV, Simard J, Rommens J, et al: The complete *BRCA2* gene and mutations in chromosome 13q-
linked kindreds. Nature Genetics 12:333–337, 1996

Tessaro I, Borstelmann N, Regan K, et al: Genetic testing for susceptibility to breast cancer: findings from
women's focus groups. Journal of Womens Health 6:317–327, 1997

Tonin P, Weber B, Offit K, et al: Frequency of recurrent *BRCA1* and *BRCA2* mutations in Ashkenazi Jewish
breast cancer families. Nature Med 2:1179–1183, 1996

Vasen HFA, Mecklin J-P, Meera Khan P, et al: The international collaborative group on hereditary nonpolyposis colorectal cancer (ICG-HNPCC). Dis Colon Rectum 34:424–425, 1991

Ward BE, Manley S, McClure M, et al: Clinical diagnostic laboratory experience with BRCA1 and BRCA2
utilizing DNA sequencing technology. Am J Hum Genet: 61

Wijnen J, Meera Khan P, Vasen H, et al: Hereditary non-polyposis colorectal cancer families not complying
with the Amsterdam criteria show extremely low frequency of mismatch-repair-gene mutations. Am J
Hum Genet 61:329–335, 1997

Wooster R, Bignell G, Lancaster J, et al: Identification of the breast cancer susceptibility gene BRCA2. Nature
378:789–792, 1995

Wu LC, Wang ZW, Tsan JT, et al: Identification of a RING protein that can interact in vivo with the BRCA1
gene product. Nature Genetics 14:430–440, 1996

Yancik R: Ovarian cancer. Age contrasts in incidence, histology, disease stage at diagnosis, and mortality.
Cancer 71:517–523, 1993

8

PROPHYLACTIC SURGERY AND INHERITED CANCER PREDISPOSITION

Kevin S. Hughes, Moshe Z. Papa, Timothy Whitney, and
Robert McLellan

*The Risk Assessment Clinic
 The Lahey Clinic, Peabody, Massachusetts, USA
+The Chaim Sheba Medical Center
 Sackler School of Medicine
 Tel Aviv University
 Tel Hashomer, Israel

The purpose of this chapter will be to discuss the role of prophylactic oophorectomy and prophylactic mastectomy in the management of patients with hereditary breast and ovarian cancer syndrome. The approach described here can serve as a template in reviewing the efficacy of prophylactic surgery for other hereditary cancer syndromes.

The cloning of the BRCA1 and BRCA2 genes has opened the door to the identification of women at high risk for developing breast or ovarian cancer. It is problematic that our understanding of how to manage these patients has not kept pace with our ability to identify them.

In order to determine appropriate management strategies, it is important to know the penetrance of the gene mutation, and the expected age at which that cancer will develop. In general, women with a BRCA1 mutation are thought to have a 19.1% risk of developing breast cancer by the age of 40, an 85% risk of developing breast cancer by the age of 70, and between a 26% and 85% risk of developing ovarian cancer by the age of 70.[1,2,3,4] Women with a BRCA2 mutation are thought to have a similar risk of developing breast cancer to BRCA1, though perhaps beginning at a later age,[2,5] and a 10 to 16% risk of developing ovarian cancer by the age of 70.[2,6]

In determining the efficacy and advisability of prophylactic surgery, we must compare it to the efficacy of the alternatives, screening and chemoprevention. The efficacy of screening will vary with the type of cancer, and would be expected to be

Address all correspondence to: Kevin S. Hughes, M.D., The Risk Assessment Clinic, 1 Essex Center Drive, The Lahey Clinic, Peabody, Massachusetts, USA

Cancer Genetics for the Clinician, edited by Shaw.
Kluwer Academic / Plenum Publishers, New York, 1999.

quite different for breast cancer and ovarian cancer. Breast cancer screening is justified in the general population probably after the age of 40, and certainly after the age of 50. Intensive screening in the BRCA1 and BRCA2 mutation carriers is likely to be indicated and effective if begun at an early age,[5] but with our current technology, a finite number of women will develop advanced cancer and die despite intensive screening. Chemoprevention of breast cancer is in its infancy, and while the Breast Cancer Prevention Trial has suggested that tamoxifen can decrease the risk of breast cancer, it is not yet known if it will be effective in BRCA1 and BRCA2 mutation carriers. Prophylactic mastectomy seems to be effective in preventing cancer, but its protective effect is not absolute.

Ovarian cancer screening is not effective for the general population.[7] Ovarian cancer screening in the BRCA1 and BRCA2 mutation carriers seems appropriate, but the efficacy of this screening in detecting cancer early is unknown.[5] It would be predicted that a large proportion of those intensively screened will progress to an incurable stage before detection. Chemoprevention by the use of oral contraceptives does appear to be effective for the general population, but its efficacy in the BRCA1 and BRCA2 mutation carrier is not known.[8] Similar to breast cancer, prophylactic oophorectomy seems to be effective in preventing ovarian cancer, but its protective effect is not absolute.[9,10]

This would suggest that under the current circumstances for the BRCA1 and BRCA2 mutation carriers, intensive screening for breast cancer, with or without chemoprevention, may be close in efficacy to prophylactic mastectomy in preventing cancer death, but that prophylactic oophorectomy is likely to be much more effective than screening in preventing ovarian cancer death.

Due to these intrinsic differences, we will begin by discussing cancer of the breast and cancer of the ovary separately, and then conclude by synthesizing a coordinated approach to these two problems.

1. MANAGEMENT OF BREAST CANCER RISK

Relative to her breast cancer risk, the woman found to harbor a mutation in the BRCA1 and BRCA2 gene can be managed by intensive observation (with or without chemoprevention), or by prophylactic mastectomy, with or without reconstruction (Fig. 1). Chemoprevention, while a seemingly ideal approach, is not currently well understood. In choosing a management strategy, the strengths and weaknesses of each approach must be considered.

Relative to her breast cancer risk, the woman found to harbor a mutation in the BRCA1 and BRCA2 gene can be managed by intensive observation (with or without chemoprevention), or by prophylactic mastectomy, with or without reconstruction.

The discussion can be framed in the context of a set of questions that need to be answered, which include: Is effective chemoprevention available? What is the efficacy of screening? With screening, how often will cancer be identified at an early, curable stage? What is the efficacy of prophylactic mastectomy? How often will women who have had this procedure develop cancer and how many of those will die? What type of mastectomy should be done? When should this surgery be done? Should the patient undergo reconstruction, and if so, what type? What will the psychosocial effect of this procedure be on the patient and her family?

We will attempt to define the state of the art as it relates to these questions. Many

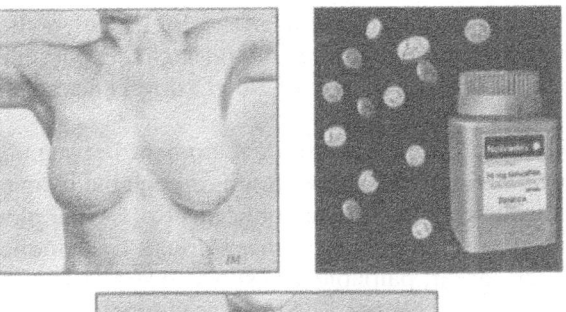
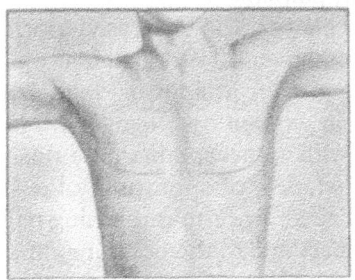
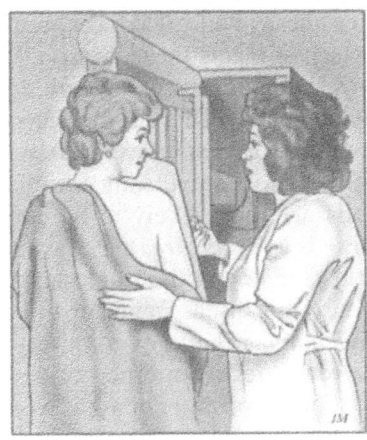

Figure 1. Options for mutation carrier.

of the questions are not able to be answered at our current level of knowledge, and continued research is essential.

1.1. Chemoprevention

Chemoprevention is defined as the utilization of a drug or a chemical to prevent the development of cancer. While this may be the ideal approach in the future, no proven agent is currently available. The Breast Cancer Prevention Trial has suggested that tamoxifen is effective in preventing breast cancer. However, it is unclear if it will be effective in the population carrying a BRCA1 or BRCA2 mutation or at what age tamoxifen should be begun, how long it should be continued, or what the long term effects will be. It will be many years before extended use of this or any agent has been tested in a young population.

1.2. Screening

It is tempting to recommend intensive screening rather than prophylactic mastectomy to the woman who carries a BRCA1 or a BRCA2 mutation, as this would appear to be a much less distressing and mutilating approach. However, it is important to remember that intensive screening does not work by preventing cancer (primary prevention), but rather works by detecting cancer at an earlier, more treatable stage (secondary prevention). Efficacy is dependent on the ability of intensive screening to detect cancer early enough that surgery, chemotherapy, and/or radiation is able to cure the cancer. If cure rates were not stage dependent, then early detection would not be necessary.

The efficacy of screening in the woman who carries a BRCA1 and BRCA2 mutation has not been tested. While there is currently no data specific to BRCA1 and BRCA2 carriers, we can make some broad predictions relative to this group.

Effective surveillance is dependent on an adequate incidence of cancer, a silent early phase, adequate treatment, and adequate technology.[11] Breast cancer screening after the age of 50 is accepted universally as a means of decreasing cancer death because it meets these criteria.[12]

Women over 50 have an *adequate incidence* of cancer development between age 50 and death.[13] There is a *silent, early phase* of breast cancer that is detectable by mammography. Breast cancers often go through a ductal carcinoma in-situ (DCIS) phase that is almost universally curable, but even small invasive cancers found by mammography are more likely to be cured than larger, palpable invasive cancers (BCDDP). There is *adequate treatment* available for breast cancer. The decreased mortality found with screening in the randomized trials of women over 50 is dependent on our ability to cure this disease, and for the cure rate to be greater at a lower stage. Finally, there is *adequate technology* to detect breast cancer in women over age 50. Mammography is a very effective method of detecting cancer with an acceptable false positive rate.

In the postmenopausal woman, there is a window of opportunity, the silent, early phase, when the mammogram will identify the cancer prior to it reaching palpable size. This time can range from 1 to 3 years. This is in part due to the doubling time of tumors in this age group. Assume that a single cell begins the process of development of a tumor. Using volume calculations, 20 doublings will need to take place to reach a 1 mm diameter, and 10 more doublings will need to take place to go from a 1 mm diameter to a 1 cm diameter.[14,15]

The threshold size for cancer detection by mammography is about 1–2 mm (about 20 doublings), and the threshold size for cancer detection by palpation is about 1 cm (about 30 doublings). Spratt has estimated a doubling time of 103 to 191 days for node negative invasive cancers in women over age 50. Using an estimate of 125 days, and using volume calculations, the time from inception to mammographic detection would be about 2500 days (6.8 years), and from mammographic detection to clinical detection by palpation would be an additional 1250 days (3.4 years) (Fig. 2). This produces a window of opportunity of over 3 years during which cancers will be detectable by mammography, but will not be detectable by palpation. In general, the longer this window is, the more effective screening mammography will be. In addition, most women go through a phase of DCIS before developing invasive cancer, which adds to the window of opportunity.

In post-menopausal women, the growth rate of cancers is slower, depicted in figure 2 by a doubling time of 125 days, and the window of mammographic detection is relatively long. In pre-menopausal women, the growth rate of cancers is faster, and the window of mammographic detection is shortened.

We should not be complacent relative to breast cancer screening over the age of 50. We need to improve the treatment of breast cancer to increase the cure rate to 100% and we need to improve the technology to decrease both the false negative and the false positive rate. This proviso not withstanding, we do have good reason to recommend screening in this group.

1.3. Efficacy of Surveillance in Hereditary Breast Cancer Patients

As many as 19% of female BRCA1 and BRCA2 mutation carriers will develop breast cancer by the age of 40, and as many as 50% will develop breast cancer by the age of 50.[1,2,3,4] Two factors will have a negative effect upon the length of the mammographic detection window in this population. First, the rate of growth of breast cancer

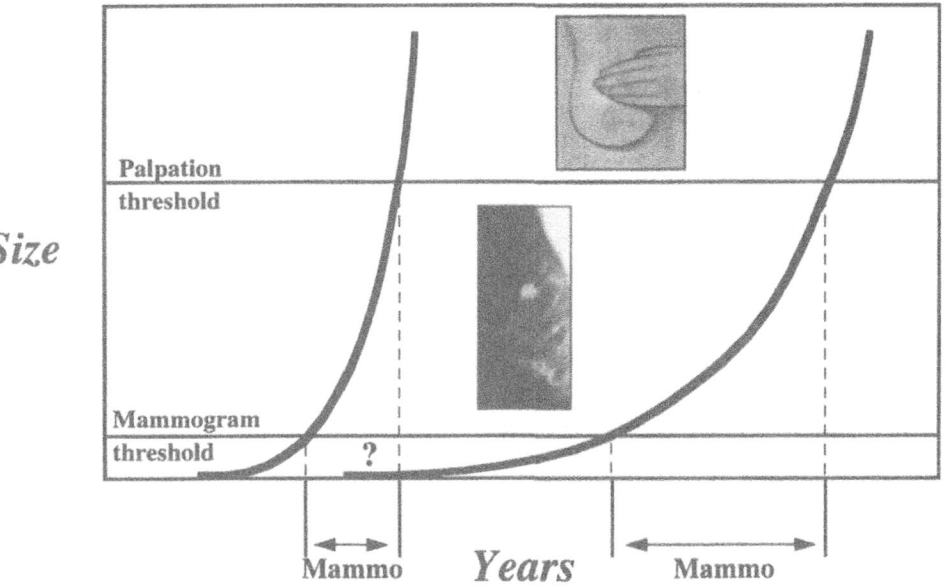

Figure 2. Doubling time of 50 days vs 125 days.

is faster in younger women, and second, the breast parenchyma is denser in younger women, making mammographic detection more difficult.

Spratt has estimated a doubling time of 50 to 64 days for node negative invasive cancers in women in their 30's. Using 50 days, and assuming the same mammographic and palpation thresholds discussed earlier, the time from inception to mammographic detection would be about 1000 days (2.7 years), and from mammographic detection to clinical detection by palpation would be an additional 500 days (1.35 years) (Fig. 2). This produces a window of a little over one year during which cancers will be detectable by mammography, but will not be detectable by palpation.

The problem, however, is that young women tend to have denser breast tissue, and therefore the ability to see cancers on mammograms is diminished and the ability to feel cancers in compromised (Fig. 3). In fact, Dr. Barbara Smith has found in over 100 women under age 40 treated for breast cancer at the Massachusetts General Hospital, that 30% had negative mammograms. This means that the mammographic and palpation threshold are most likely larger in the younger population, and up to one-third may not be detectable by mammography.[16]

In pre-menopausal women, the density of breast tissue increases the mammographic threshold, and can also shorten the window of mammographic detection.

We lack data regarding BRCA1 and BRCA2 mutation carriers. They may, or may not, have denser breast tissue on mammography than the non-carrier, but it would seem reasonable to assume that their breast tissue density is commensurate with their age.

In regards to growth rate, it is likely that BRCA1 mutation carriers will have rapidly growing cancers. Foulkes, et al.[17] found that Ashkenazi Jewish women who carry one of the two established mutations (185 delAG and 5382insC) were more likely to have grade 3 tumors (11/12 were grade 3) in carriers vs. 29/100 in non-carriers), were more likely to be node positive (45.5% in carriers vs. 31.1% in non-carriers) and were larger in diameter (mean size 2.48 cm in carriers vs. 1.71 cm in non-carriers). Other

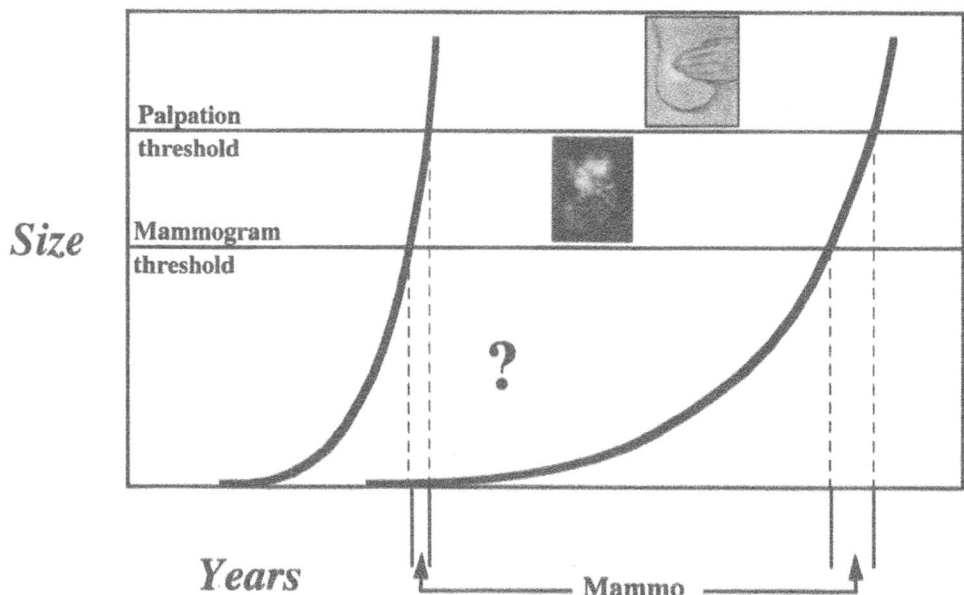

Figure 3. Dense breast tissue.

studies have found cancers in carriers to be more likely estrogen receptor negative,[18,19] and P53 positive.[20] Therefore, BRCA1 mutation carriers will likely have faster growing cancers that will pass through the mammographic window rapidly. BRCA2 breast cancers also seem to be of higher grade than sporadic cancers, and will also likely grow faster and be less easily identified when small.[21]

Therefore, we would expect that BRCA1 and BRCA2 mutation carriers will have rapidly growing tumors that will be difficult to identify by mammography or palpation, especially while they are under the age of 40. Therefore, despite intensive screening with our current technology, we can expect to find these cancers later and larger. It is reasonable to assume that a finite number will have metastasized by the time they are detected.

Regardless of growth rate, screening will not be effective if there is poor compliance with screening recommendations. Dr. Lermann has found that among women found to carry a BRCA1 or BRCA2 mutation, less than half followed the recommendations for mammography when evaluated 6 months after testing.[22] In the absence of compliance, screening will be ineffective.

1.4. Possible Outcomes of Screening

The possible outcomes of screening are depicted in Fig. 4. If all women carrying mutations in BRCA1 and BRCA2 receive a recommendation for intensive screening, the current technology will allow the majority of those who comply to be detected at a stage when they are still curable. In the postmenopausal patient, about 80 to 90% of the patients screened can be cured (BCDDP). In this pre-menopausal group, with dense breast tissue, fast growing cancers and possibly poor compliance, the number detected when curable will most likely be much lower. The size of the arrows are roughly proportional to the number of women predicted to go along each path. The size of the

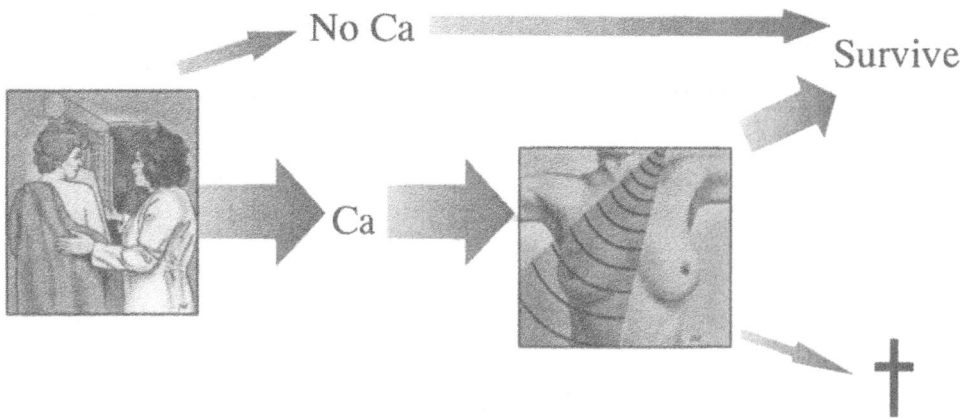

Figure 4. Possible outcomes of screening the breast.

arrows will change as we increase our understanding of the natural history and treatment of those patients. The number of women who develop breast cancer will be decreased when adequate chemoprevention becomes available. The number of those who develop breast cancer and are cured will increase with better screening technology (finding earlier stage cancer) and improved treatment (more cancers cured stage for stage).

If all women carrying mutations in BRCA1 and BRCA2 are screened, the level of the current technology will allow the majority of them to be detected at a stage when they are still curable. In the postmenopausal patient, about 80 to 90% of the patients screened can be cured. In this pre-menopausal group, with dense breast tissue and fast growing cancers, the number detected when curable will most likely be less than 80%. This must be taken into account when recommending screening to this group. The size of the arrows is a gross approximation of the number expected to move down each pathway. The exact size of the arrows will be determined by future research.

2. PROPHYLACTIC SURGERY FOR BREAST CANCER RISK

Prophylactic mastectomy is the only currently available method that appears to decrease life-time breast cancer risk to a significant degree. Efficacy is dependent on the ability to remove the majority of breast tissue, and on the supposition that residual cancer risk is proportional to the amount of residual breast tissue. While prophylactic mastectomy is a disfiguring approach that the medical profession would prefer to avoid, it must be compared objectively to screening in terms of the ultimate result.

There is a perception that the literature has called into question the efficacy of prophylactic mastectomy. While at first glance, the literature (Table 1),[23–36] would seem to suggest that prophylactic mastectomy is not completely effective, in actuality, the efficacy of prophylactic mastectomy has not been adequately studied. While several series and case reports appear in the literature, the combined data does not provide a compelling argument for or against this procedure. The factors that might lead to an underestimate of efficacy in these reports include the type of mastectomy performed, technical thoroughness of the mastectomy, incomplete follow-up of patients, and lack of a denominator.

Table 1. Series and Case Reports of Prophylactic Mastectomy in the Literature

Author	Cases	Denominator	Mastectomy	Time to Cancer	Mean Follow-up	Cancer Developed	Reference
Case reports							
Holleb	2	?	Total	10y, 12y		Flap,Flap	23
Ziegler	1	?	Total	18y		Flap	24
Goodnight	1***	?	Subcutaneous	3y		Flap	25
Bowers	2	?	Subcutaneous	3y, 10y	N/A	Flap,Flap	26
Mendez-Fernandez	1	?	Subcutaneous	8y	N/A	Nipple	27
Elder	1	?	Subcutaneous	6y	N/A	Flap	28
Jameson	1	?	Subcutaneous	42y	N/A	Under Nipple	29
Series							
Humphrey	3	16	Subcutaneous	N/A	N/A	Flap	30
Pennisi	6	1232**	Subcutaneous	N/A	N/A	Unknown	31
Woods	5	1500	Subcutaneous	N/A	22y	Unknown	32
Slade	1	83****	Subcutaneous	10y	N/A	Under Nipple	33
Fredericks	1	39*****	Subcutaneous	5y	N/A	Flap	34
Amaaki	1	9*	Subcutaneous	N/A	N/A	N/A	35
Hartmann	7	950	89% Subcutaneous	17Y	N/A	N/A	36

Patients were excluded as not truly prophylactic if they had contralateral or ipsilateral cancer at the time of the initial procedure.
* 8' excluded as had cancer at initial procedure.
** 268 excluded as had cancer at initial procedure.
*** 3 excluded as had cancer at initial procedure.
**** 5' excluded as had cancer at initial procedure.
***** 1 excluded as had cancer at initial procedure.

To understand the importance of the type of mastectomy performed on efficacy of prophylactic mastectomy, it is essential that the technical differences and resulting residual tissue be discussed. Removal of all breast tissue is probably not possible, but the extent of residual tissue is dependent on the procedure performed, and the meticulousness of the technique.

The most extensive mastectomy is the radical mastectomy, which removes the nipple-areolar complex and surrounding skin, "all" breast tissue, the pectoralis major and minor muscles, and the axillary lymph nodes. Even with a radical mastectomy, some breast tissue remains, and new primary breast cancers can develop.[37] The radical mastectomy is a deforming operation that makes reconstruction difficult, and has no role in prophylactic surgery.

The modified radical mastectomy removes the nipple-areolar complex and surrounding skin, "all" breast tissue, and the axillary lymph nodes, but does not include removal of the pectoralis major and minor muscles. (In the past, the pectoralis muscle was removed by some surgeons.) The modified radical mastectomy is really not necessary for prophylactic surgery, and formal dissection of the lymph nodes adds morbidity, without increasing the efficacy of the procedure. Some surgeons believe that removing the nodes is necessary to totally remove the breast tissue contained in the tale of Spence, but more likely than not, this area is removed with a good, technical total mastectomy.

The total or simple mastectomy removes the nipple-areolar complex and surrounding skin, and "all" breast tissue, but does not include removal of the axillary lymph nodes, or the pectoralis major and minor muscles. This is the operation most commonly performed for prophylactic surgery today.

The subcutaneous mastectomy is performed through an incision made in the inframammary crease. Dissection is than performed separating the skin and nipple from the breast tissue. It is technically difficult to produce thin flaps, and to remove the breast tissue found in the tale of Spence, therefore leaving behind breast tissue in this area, but, by definition, the nipple and its underlying breast tissue are left behind on purpose.

In subcutaneous mastectomy, a large amount of breast tissue is left beneath the nipple. In subcutaneous and total mastectomy, breast tissue can be left adherent to the skin flaps, and on the pectoralis fascia. The amount of residual tissue on the skin flaps is technique dependent. The thinner the flap is made (the less subcutaneous fat is left on the flap), the less breast tissue will be left, but as the flap loses some of its blood supply, the less viable the flap will be. A thicker flap (more subcutaneous fat left on the flap) will have a better blood supply, and be less subject to ischemia or necrosis, but will have more residual breast tissue. In addition, leaving behind the pectoralis fascia makes the surgery easier and decreases blood loss, but breast tissue is left behind on and in the fascia. While it is tempting to do lesser surgery in these patients who do not have cancer, meticulous technique will limit the amount of residual tissue, and hopefully therefore decrease the future risk.

If the assumption is made that the efficacy of prophylactic mastectomy is inversely proportional to the amount of breast tissue left behind, than it is obvious that a total mastectomy with thin skin flaps and removal of the pectoralis fascia provides the maximum acceptable operation for prophylaxis while minimizing residual tissue.

In terms of the type of mastectomy performed, most series report on subcutaneous mastectomy. Where site of recurrence is recorded for subcutaneous mastectomy, 3 of the 11 patients developed cancer in the residual tissue below the nipple, and the other 8 developed cancer under the flap.[23–30,33] The large amount of tissue left beneath the nipple accounts for the recurrence in that area, while recurrence beneath the flap is explained by residual breast tissue left on the flap. While all 3 cases of breast cancer after total mastectomy occurred under the flap,[23,24] it is technically more difficult to remove the axillary tale of Spence and harder to make thin flaps during a subcutaneous mastectomy performed through an inframammary crease incision. Therefore, while we are unable to cull this conclusion from the literature, it is reasonable to assume that subcutaneous mastectomies will also lead to a greater incidence of cancer under the flap than a total mastectomy.

The length of follow-up and the ages of the patients are critical factors in determining the number of breast cancers expected in patients undergoing prophylactic mastectomies, and to thus quantitate the efficacy of the procedure. The number of cancers that would have developed in this population is dependent on the age of the patient (older women are expected to develop more cancers in a given year then younger women) and on the length of time each patient is followed. Only Hartman's series[36] takes this into account, and finds a 91% reduction in breast cancer risk, despite the fact that 90% of the mastectomies were subcutaneous. The other series do not provide individual information on age, risk, and follow-up, and in one series, 30% of the patients were lost to follow-up.[31] The case reports[23–29] are unable to provide a denominator, so the per cent failing cannot be ascertained.

Factors that might lead to an overestimate of the efficacy of prophylactic mastectomy include inadequate risk assessment, and marginal indications for surgery (by today's standards). Today we consider women with LCIS, or a very strong family history suggestive of BRCA1 or BRCA2 mutations to be at high risk of breast cancer. Women with atypical hyperplasia are felt to be at moderate risk. In the literature reports, the indication for prophylactic mastectomy was often something that we would feel had little or no impact on risk, such as persistent breast nodules, ductal hyperplasia, papillomatosis, significant macrocystic disease, severe dysplasia on mammogram, or multiple biopsies.[31] While some prophylactic mastectomies were done for positive family history, the definition of a strong family history was marginal by today's standards. Woods defined a positive family history as "a maternal history of breast cancer in one or more primary relatives.[32] In Hartman's series,[36] of the 950 bilateral prophylactic mastectomy patients, 35% did not have a family history, 34% had a family history that was not considered significant by today's standards, and 31% had a strong family history as suggested by multiple relatives, young age at diagnosis, or the presence of ovarian cancer. Judging by this series, less than half of the women undergoing prophylactic mastectomy would have a had a significant family history by today's standards, and, in the absence of genetic testing, less than half of them would have been mutation carriers.

2.1. Types of Mastectomy

Subcutaneous mastectomy is almost uniformly followed by submuscular insertion of implants, and requires about 3 to 5 hours of operative time. In general, the cosmetic result is excellent, but sensation in the nipple is usually diminished or absent. Assuming efficacy is proportional to the amount of breast tissue removed, this procedure is likely to be inadequate. The mammogram in Fig. 5 gives an idea of how much residual breast tissue remains after this procedure.

This mammogram demonstrates the amount of breast tissue left behind the nipple following a subcutaneous mastectomy.

The initial morbidity of the procedure is low, and is proportional to the amount of breast tissue removed. The most serious complication is slough or loss of the nipple areolar complex. This occurs if the nipple areolar complex is devascularized by removal of the breast tissue below the nipple, and can be prevented by leaving larger amounts of residual breast tissue. This means that the more breast tissue removed, the more effective the procedure will be in preventing breast cancer, but the greater the risk of loss of the nipple areolar complex. Conversely, leaving more residual breast tissue will minimize the risk of loss of the nipple areolar complex, but will increase the risk of breast cancer in the future.

Long term morbidity is dependent on the method of reconstruction. The use of submuscular implants, which have a limited life expectancy, will necessitate replacement every 5 to 15 years.[38,39] As patients undergoing this procedure are in their 30's, they can expect to have 4 to 8 future operations on each side for exchange of implants over a lifetime. While much has been made regarding the risk of silicone implants, recent studies do not corroborate the initial concerns. Despite this, the tendency currently is to use saline filled prostheses, which while having less theoretical risk, do not have the same consistency or natural feel as silicone, and thus give a less pleasing cosmetic result in this situation. Saline implants are adequate for breast augmentation because they are placed beneath normal skin, breast tissue, and muscle, which together hide the texture of the implant. After subcutaneous mastectomy, the implant is only covered by muscle and skin, and its consistency is obvious to the touch.

Due to the large amount of residual breast tissue, these patients require routine mammography and frequent physical examinations at the schedule appropriate to their risk category. The efficacy of screening to detect cancers early will be compromised by

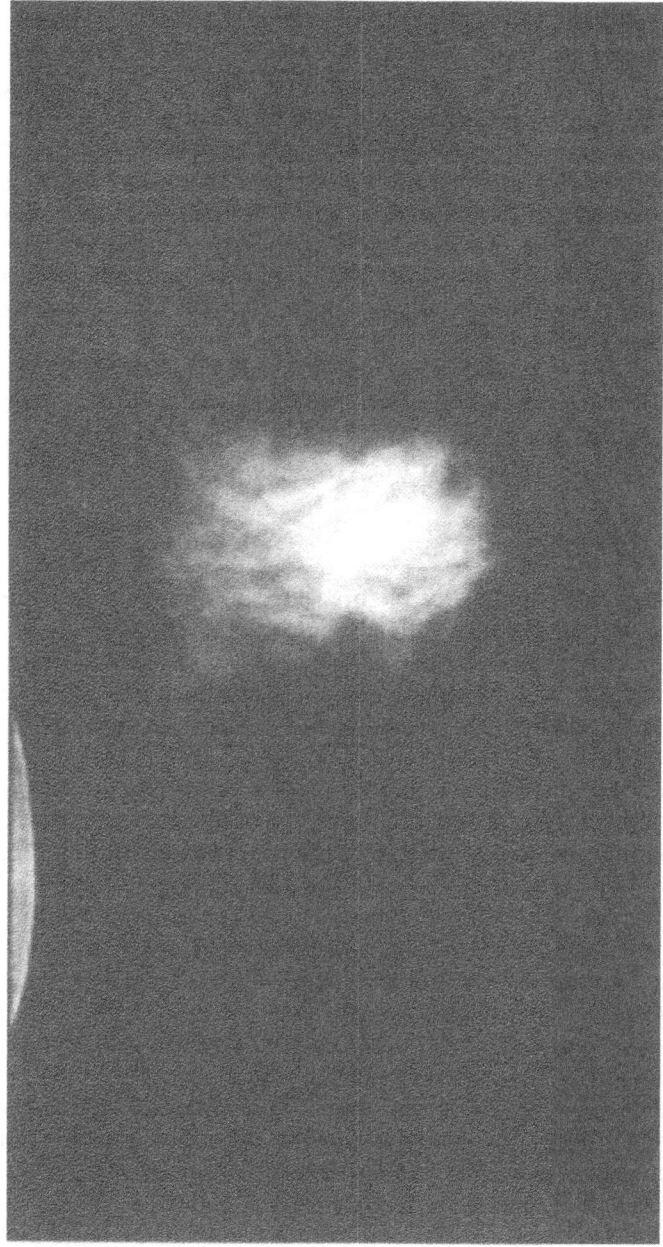

Figure 5. This mammogram demonstrates the amount of breast tissue left behind the nipple following a sub-cutaneous mastectomy.

the presence of an implant. In doing mammography, special distraction views must be undertaken to assure adequate visualization of all breast tissue. In women who undergo augmentation, some breast tissue is not seen on mammography. The per cent of breast tissue missed on mammography in women who have undergone subcutaneous mastectomy will most likely be less, but it is unclear how much less. The area below the nipple will be well visualized, but residual tissue high in the flaps and axillae will be obscured by the implant. Physical examination may be aided, as the implant below the muscle pushes the breast tissue forward where it may be more accessible, but on the other hand, the soft implant gives a poor basis on which to examine, and a breast mass could be obscured as it is pressed into the soft background.

The false positive rate (positive findings suggestive of cancer) for physical examination and mammography will most likely be increased due to the scarring and calcification caused by the initial surgery. This will likely generate additional biopsies in this high-risk population. While in the average woman a breast biopsy can be done under local anesthesia with sedation, it will be necessary to use general anesthesia in this population with an implant, as the needle used to inject local anesthetic could potentially damage the implant.

In summary, due to the large amount of residual breast tissue, the risk of cancer after subcutaneous mastectomy appears too high to endorse this procedure. Women who have already had this done need intensive monitoring with mammography and physical examination, not dissimilar to any woman in her risk category.

2.2. Total Mastectomy

Total mastectomy (removal of the breast tissue and the nipple areolar complex), when performed without reconstruction, requires about 2 to 4 hours of operative time. In general, the cosmetic result is poor, as there is no breast form present and an external prosthesis must be used. Assuming efficacy is proportional to the amount of breast tissue removed, this procedure is likely to be very effective, as 90 to 95% of the breast tissue is removed.

The initial morbidity of the procedure is low, but is dependent on the amount of breast tissue removed. The most troubling complication is slough of the skin flap. This occurs if the skin flap is made too thin causing devascularization. This tends to be a self-limiting problem and can be prevented by leaving larger amounts of subcutaneous fat with the flap. This means that the more breast tissue removed, the more effective the procedure will be in preventing breast cancer, but the greater the risk of skin loss. Conversely, leaving more residual breast tissue will minimize the risk of skin loss, but will increase the risk of breast cancer in the future.

In follow-up, mammography is not necessary. Physical examinations by a clinician and self-examination by the patient is all that is necessary.

In the event of cancer developing, the efficacy of screening to detect cancers early will be quite good. Physical examination may be aided, as the breast tissue lies directly against the pectoral muscle, with minimal intervening skin or fat. The chest wall provides a firm surface that makes palpation easy.

The false positive rate for physical examination will be quite low if most breast tissue has been removed. A suboptimal procedure will leave behind residual breast tissue that may cause incorrect diagnosis of masses in the future, and lead to unnecessary biopsies.

3. TYPES OF RECONSTRUCTION

3.1. Breast Reconstruction after Total Mastectomy

Current practices in breast reconstruction are designed to restore the breast mound after mastectomy in one of two ways: the use of an implant or the use of auto-

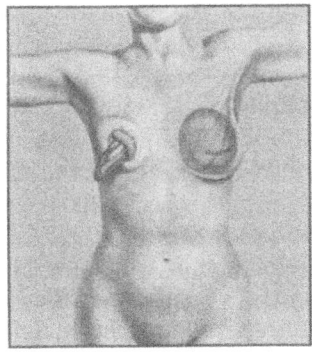
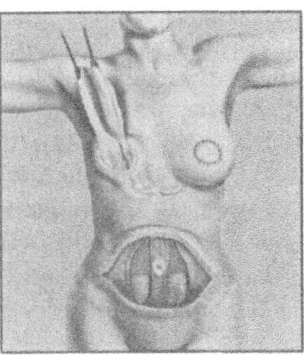
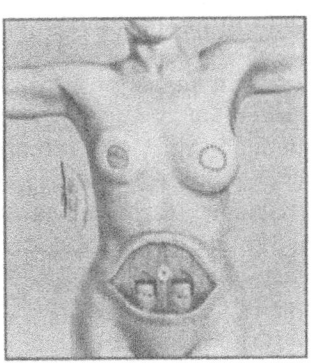

| Mastectomy and Implants | Mastectomy and Rotation TRAM | Mastectomy and Free TRAM |

Figure 6. The most commonly used reconstruction methods after total mastectomy include: submuscular implant, pedicle TRAM flap, and free TRAM flap.

genous tissue. Once a patient has chosen to undergo reconstruction, the patient and her surgeon must decide 1) timing of reconstruction (immediate vs. delayed), 2) type (expander/implant, their own tissue or some combination) and 3) donor site, if autogenous tissue is selected. Each reconstructive method carries a unique set of risks and benefits, and must be selected with the patient's age, general health and operative risks in mind (Figs. 6 and 7).

The most commonly used reconstruction methods after total mastectomy include: submuscular implant, pedicle TRAM flap, and free TRAM flap.

Cosmetic results after total mastectomy and reconstruction. All underwent delayed nipple reconstruction. The arrows shown in the rotation (pedicle) TRAM depict a grossly visible area of fat necrosis.

3.2. Total Mastectomy with Immediate Implants

At the completion of total mastectomy, as part of the same operation, reconstruction can be accomplished by the immediate placement of implants. In general, this procedure is reserved for patients with smaller breasts without significant ptosis, as it

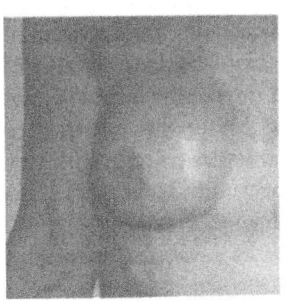
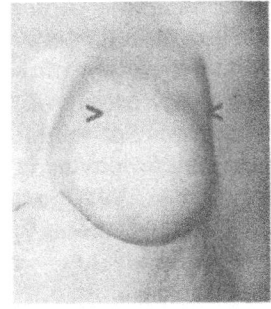
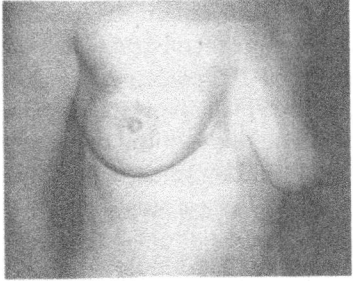

| Mastectomy and Implants | Mastectomy and Rotation TRAM | Mastectomy and Free TRAM |

Figure 7. Cosmetic results after total mastectomy and reconstruction. All underwent delayed nipple reconstruction. The arrows shown in the rotation (pedicle) TRAM depict a grossly visible area of fat necrosis.

is difficult to avoid post-operative skin slough if the native breast skin flaps are closed with tension over a large implant. In the past, implants were placed immediately into the subcutaneous position, leading to a high complication rate of 25–50%, including exposure, infection, and capsular contracture.[40,41] This technique has largely been abandoned, and the preferred approach today is to place the implant into a submuscular pocket behind the pectoralis muscle, utilizing rectus fascia and serratus muscles to completely cover the infero-lateral positions of the implant.[42,43]

Immediate placement of the permanent prosthesis requires accepting a smaller breast size, as the nipple-areolar complex and some adjoining skin will have been removed, decreasing the size of the breast mound. This is seldom acceptable in the case of unilateral reconstruction, where the remaining breast cannot be adequately matched and the reconstructed breast is markedly smaller than the unaffected side. In the case of bilateral mastectomy and reconstruction, this approach is acceptable if the patient is amenable to a reduction in breast size. Immediate submuscular implants can provide reasonable results if bilateral reconstruction is required. In general, this reconstructive method adds only 1–2 hours to operative time when performed immediately after mastectomy. Nipple-areolar reconstruction or tattooing will require a second operation several months later.

3.3. Total Mastectomy with Staged Expander-Implant Reconstruction

The use of balloon tissue expanders allows the recreation of the pre-operative breast size. It requires serial outpatient expansion followed by a second procedure to remove the expander and place the permanent prostheses. Expanders are placed into the submuscular space following mastectomy, and the native skin flaps are closed. Using a buried inflation port, saline is instilled percutaneously to stretch the skin and muscular pocket. In general, the expander is filled beyond the volume required to restore the pre-operative cup size, to create enough residual skin to recreate the inframammary fold. Although the initial morbidity of the procedure is low, complications including infection of the expander, hematoma, skin necrosis, and exposure of the prosthesis can occur, which would require the expander to be removed completely and another reconstructive approach considered.[40]

Long term morbidity is similar to patients who undergo immediate final prosthesis placement or cosmetic augmentation and is primarily related to the implant. These include wrinkling, scarring, and capsular contracture which can lead to a hard mound, a poor aesthetic appearance, or implant rupture. The implants are likely to require replacement of every 5–15 years.[38,39] In a young patient in her 30's with bilateral implant reconstruction, normal life expectancy of the prosthesis may result in the need for 4–8 replacement procedures for each breast over a lifetime. The need for serial implant replacement must be discussed as one of the factors influencing the choice of reconstructive method prior to undertaking prophylactic mastectomy. Due to the FDA moratorium on silicone gel implants begun in 1991, the majority of current implants in use in the US are single lumen, saline filled prostheses.[39] Although considered to be of minimal risk, patients must be made aware that they will still be exposed to the polymerized silicone shell of the saline filled implant.

Long term follow-up after implant reconstruction is straightforward, and rare areas of residual breast tissue within the skin flaps or pectoralis fascia can be easily palpated over the submuscular implant by self exam or by the surgeon. Mammography of the reconstructed breast is not necessary, but palpable masses may require biopsy, which should be performed under general anesthesia, to avoid needle puncture of the implant. In general, implant reconstruction lacks the extent of ptosis seen in the mature breast. The asymmetry seen in unilateral reconstruction may worsen over time as capsular contracture around the implant reduces the ptosis recreated at the original surgery. This is less of an issue with bilateral reconstruction, but one implant may develop more contracture than the other and result in asymmetry.

3.4. Autogenous Tissue Reconstruction

Advances in surgical technique and a dissatisfaction with the complications and results of implant reconstruction have led to increasing popularity of autogenous tissue methods of reconstruction, particularly among younger patients. Controversy over the use of silicone gel implants has added to the public anxiety over implant use, although current scientific data has failed to establish a causal link between silicone implants and connective tissue diseases.[44] Tissue reconstruction can be performed immediately or after a delay, and has several advantages over implant reconstruction. Of particular importance, autogenous tissue provides the ability to create a more mature, ptotic breast mound, combined with the ability to restore lost skin to the mastectomy wound and eliminate the implant associated problems of capsular contracture and rupture. Long term symmetry after unilateral or bilateral reconstruction is more common with tissue reconstruction than with implants.

All methods of tissue reconstruction add significantly to the duration of surgery, adding 4–8 hours onto the anesthetic time following mastectomy, a risk which must be weighed against the patient's physiologic status. This is seldom a major deterrent in young women undergoing prophylactic mastectomy.

If a patient chooses their own tissue for reconstruction, a variety of reconstructive methods including rotation or pedicle flaps and microsurgical transplantation are available, harvesting tissue from an arsenal of donor sites including abdomen, back, buttock, and thigh.[45]

3.5. Pedicle Transverse Rectus Abdominis Myocutaneous (TRAM) Flap Reconstruction

Pedicle TRAM flap breast reconstruction is currently the most popular method of autogenous tissue reconstruction, introduced by Hartrampf, Scheflan, and Black in 1982.[46] The flap uses the skin and subcutaneous fat of the lower abdomen to replace the breast mound, rotated to the breast defect based on the vascular pedicle of the superior epigastric artery contained within the rectus abdominis muscle.[47] (Fig. 8). The breast mound is reconstructed after total mastectomy within the native breast skin envelope, replacing resected skin as needed. While the procedure sounds extensive, the harvesting of the donor fat and skin is the same procedure used in a cosmetic abdominoplasty ("tummy tuck"). The procedure, therefore, also improves abdominal contour and firmness, a benefit universally popular among patients.[44] In this procedure, the rectus abdominis muscle is transected at or near the pubis, capturing the peri-umbilical perforators to the skin coming through the rectus muscle. The abdominal fascia is either closed primarily, or buttressed with synthetic mesh to reduce abdominal wall laxity or herniation.[48] Although uncommon in unilateral reconstruction, harvest of both rectus muscles for bilateral breast reconstruction increases the impact

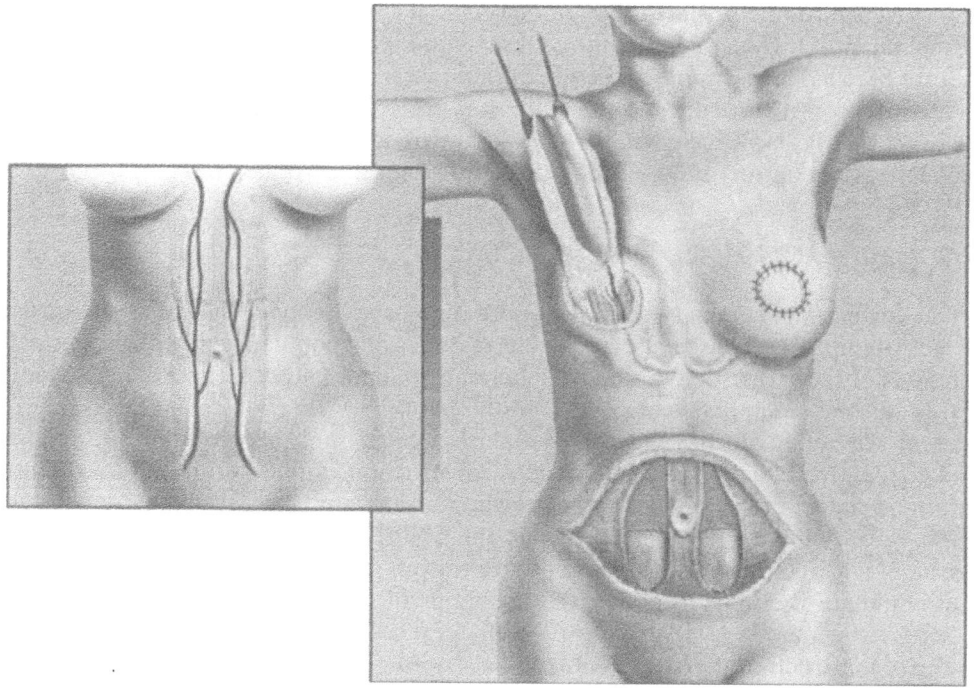

Figure 8. Pedicle TRAM flap breast reconstruction uses the skin and subcutaneous fat of the lower abdomen to replace the breast mound. The skin and fat are rotated to the breast defect based on the vascular pedicle of the superior epigastric artery contained within the rectus abdominis muscle. The inferior epigastric artery is transected and ligated.

on abdominal wall strength and function, which may compromise exercise or lifting capacity.[49]

Pedicle TRAM flap breast reconstruction uses the skin and subcutaneous fat of the lower abdomen to replace the breast mound. The skin and fat are rotated to the breast defect based on the vascular pedicle of the superior epigastric artery contained within the rectus abdominis muscle. The inferior epigastric artery is transected and ligated.

In the TRAM procedure for bilateral reconstruction, restoration of the breast mound is limited by the availability of abdominal pannus or fat, which must be split in the midline to provide symmetry. Therefore, the final breast size may be smaller than the preoperative size. Compared to implant reconstructions, the extent of surgery prolongs both hospitalization (4–7 days) and perioperative recovery (4–6 weeks). Flap associated complications, particularly partial flap loss and fat necrosis can affect up to 30% of TRAM patients.[50,51] This often leads to additional procedures to remove fat necrosis or scar tissue, both for cosmetic result and to rule out the possibility that these areas represent cancer. Long term follow-up requires serial exams. Mammography of the TRAM flap is not necessary, and may even be confusing, as fat necrosis causes scar and calcifications which may be mistaken for tumor and lead to unnecessary biopsies. As more experience is gained, mammography of the reconstructed breast may help to reduce anxiety if typical features of fat necrosis are seen.[52] The presence of the flap does not permit easy examination of the pectoral fascia, which should be removed with the mastectomy specimen. This procedure has been proven to be oncologically safe in the treatment of breast cancer and does not obscure recurrence of disease.[53,54]

3.6. Microsurgical TRAM Flap Reconstruction

In pedicle TRAM reconstruction as described above, the volume of the breast which can be reconstructed is limited by several factors, including the blood supply, the patient's body habitus, and the presence of previous abdominal surgical scars. The blood supply is of particular significance, as the procedure depends on the adequacy of the secondary circulation to the rectus muscle through the superior epigastric artery. The primary blood supply coming from the deep inferior epigastric artery to the abdominal skin and fat is transected. Reconstructive surgeons have attempted to improve flap circulation by either 1) "super-charging" the TRAM flap by augmenting the superior epigastric blood flow with microsurgical anastomoses of the inferior epigastric system to axillary vessels,[55] or by complete microsurgical transplantation of the abdominal tissue based on the deep inferior (dominant) epigastric pedicle, the so called "free" TRAM.[56] Microsurgical free TRAM flap reconstruction has several advantages over conventional pedicle techniques, despite the increased duration and complexity of the procedure. The extent of abdominal surgery is less, the need for full muscle harvest and tunneling is abrogated, the amount of muscle harvested can be greatly reduced, and restoration of the primary blood supply through the deep inferior epigastric artery has resulted in a reduction in fat necrosis.[57,58] Although not without risks,[57] the frequency of flap loss, partial skin loss, fat necrosis and abdominal herniation can be reduced to 1–5%, well below that seen in conventional pedicle TRAM flaps.[51,58,59]

Microsurgical breast reconstruction adds additional surgical time to the mastectomy (6–12 hours), and carries with it the risk of vessel thrombosis leading to complete loss of the reconstruction. Despite this, flap loss is uncommon,[50,58] and cosmetic results are excellent. The free mobility of the flap allows superior shaping and the inframammary fold remains intact as tunneling is unnecessary. Follow-up requires a similar approach to pedicle TRAM, with serial physical examination. Due to the marked decrease in fat necrosis, the rate of false positive findings on physical examination, and the rate of secondary biopsies would be markedly decreased.

3.7. Other Reconstruction Approaches

In patients without adequate tissue for TRAM or free TRAM reconstruction, or in whom previous abdominal surgery precludes use of the abdominal tissue, other free flap donor sites can be used to provide breast mound reconstruction, including superior and inferior buttock, lateral thigh, and iliac crest.[45]

3.8. Latissimus Flap Reconstruction

In selected patients, the latissimus flap can be used for breast reconstruction, with or without the addition of an implant. This method harvests the latissimus muscle and the overlying soft tissue from the back based on the thoracodorsal artery and vein, which is transposed anteriorly to recreate the breast mound. If adequate soft tissue is available to build a smaller breast, the flap can be shaped to complete the reconstruction. Otherwise an implant is placed behind the muscle flap to restore adequate volume.[39] Bilateral reconstruction is more difficult, requiring repositioning of the patient intraoperatively from one side to the other to permit exposure of the back, axilla, and breast. Unilateral reconstruction can be quite effective, allowing patients who do not wish serial expansion and subsequent second stage implant placement to complete their reconstruction in one stage. Unfortunately, although quite reliable, this method of reconstruction combines the risks of a flap (longer surgery, donor site harvest, hematoma) with those related to implants, such as capsular contracture and implant rupture.

Long term follow-up is similar to TRAM reconstruction, primarily through serial physical examination. With implant use, the implant remains deep to the muscle layer, permitting detection of developing tumors over the implant by palpation.

3.9. Possible Outcomes of Prophylactic Mastectomy

The efficacy of prophylactic mastectomy in the woman who carries a BRCA1 or BRCA2 mutation has not been tested. Women with mutations need to be followed intensively, and the rate of cancer development, the morbidity of treatment, and the rate of death must be monitored. While instances of new primary breast cancer after prophylactic mastectomy do exist, overall the rate of breast cancer does seem to be decreased by this procedure. While it is not possible to remove all breast tissue, the question remains whether removal of 90 to 95% of the breast tissue removes 90 to 95% of the risk, and whether the results in low risk patients can be extrapolated to BRCA1 and BRCA2 mutation carriers.

The possible outcomes of prophylactic mastectomy are depicted in Fig. 9. If all women carrying mutations in BRCA1 and BRCA2 undergo prophylactic mastectomy, theoretically a large number will not develop breast cancer and therefore not die of breast cancer. However, some undetermined number will develop breast cancer in the flap, will be treated by excision plus radiation, and will either be cured or die. The size of the arrows are roughly proportional to the number of women predicted to go along each path. The size of the arrows will change as we increase our understanding of the natural history and treatment of those patients.

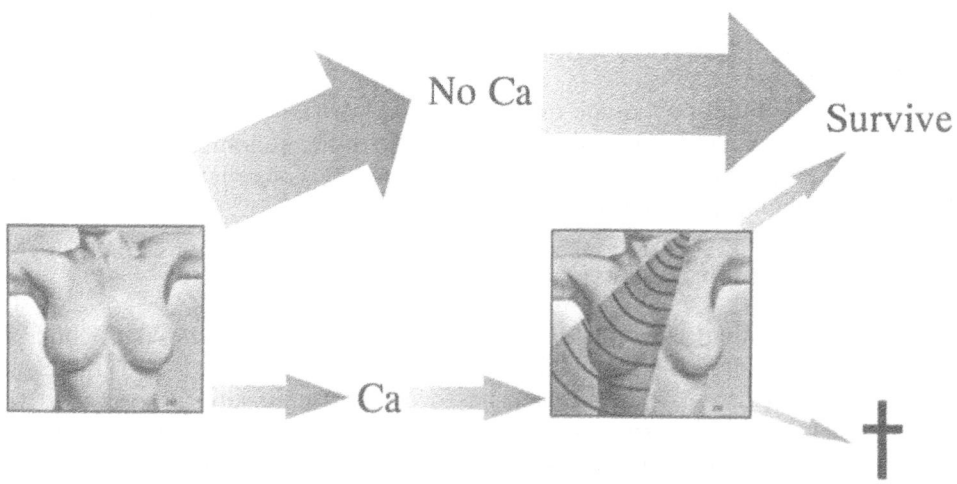

Figure 9. Possible outcomes of prophylactic mastectomy.

Table 2. Types of Reconstruction

Total Mastectomy and Implants		Total Mastectomy and Rotation Tram		Total Mastectomy and Free Tram	
Operation	4 to 6 hours	**Operation**	6 to 8 hours	**Operation**	3 to 5 hours
Cosmetic result	Good	**Cosmetic result**	Very good	**Cosmetic result**	Excellent
Efficacy	Removes 90–95% of tissue	**Efficacy**	Removes 90–95% of tissue	**Efficacy**	Removes 90–95% of tissue
Follow-up	Physical Exam	**Follow-up**	Physical exam	**Follow-up**	Physical exam
False negative	Low	**False negative**	High	**False negative**	Moderate
False positive	Low	**False positive**	Highest	**False positive**	Moderate
Morbidity		**Morbidity**		**Morbidity**	
Short term	Moderate	**Short term**	High	**Short term**	Very high
Long term	High	**Long term**	Moderate	**Long term**	Small

If all women carrying mutations in BRCA1 and BRCA2 undergo prophylactic mastectomy, theoretically a large number will not develop breast cancer and therefore not die of breast cancer. However, some undetermined number will develop breast cancer in the flap, will be treated by excision plus radiation, and will either be cured or die. The size of the arrows is a gross approximation of the number expected to move down each pathway. The exact size of the arrows will be determined by future research.

Women carrying mutations in BRCA1 and BRCA2 who undergo prophylactic mastectomy should undergo reconstruction at the same time. The attributes of the major types of reconstruction are summarized in Table 2. While this will theoretically mask the occurrence of new breast cancers arising in residual breast tissue, this risk is most likely small, and the psychosocial benefits of reconstruction are great. In terms of reconstruction, our preference is for autogenous tissue, ideally the free TRAM procedure.

4. MANAGEMENT OF OVARIAN CANCER RISK

Relative to her ovarian cancer risk, the woman found to harbor a mutation in the BRCA 1 and BRCA2 gene can be managed by intensive observation using transvaginal sonography and CA125 (with chemoprevention), plus oral contraceptives while premenopausal or by prophylactic oophorectomy (Fig. 10).

The discussion can be framed in the context of a set of questions that include: Is effective chemoprevention available? What is the efficacy of screening and how often will cancer be identified at an early, curable stage? How should the prophylactic oophorectomy be done? Should a hysterectomy be done at the same time? What is the efficacy of prophylactic oophorectomy, and how often will women who have had this procedure develop cancer and how many of those will die? When should this surgery be done? Should the patient receive hormone replacement therapy? What will the psychosocial effect of this procedure be on the patient and her family? What will the physiologic effect be on the patient?

We will attempt to define the state of the art as it relates to these questions. In

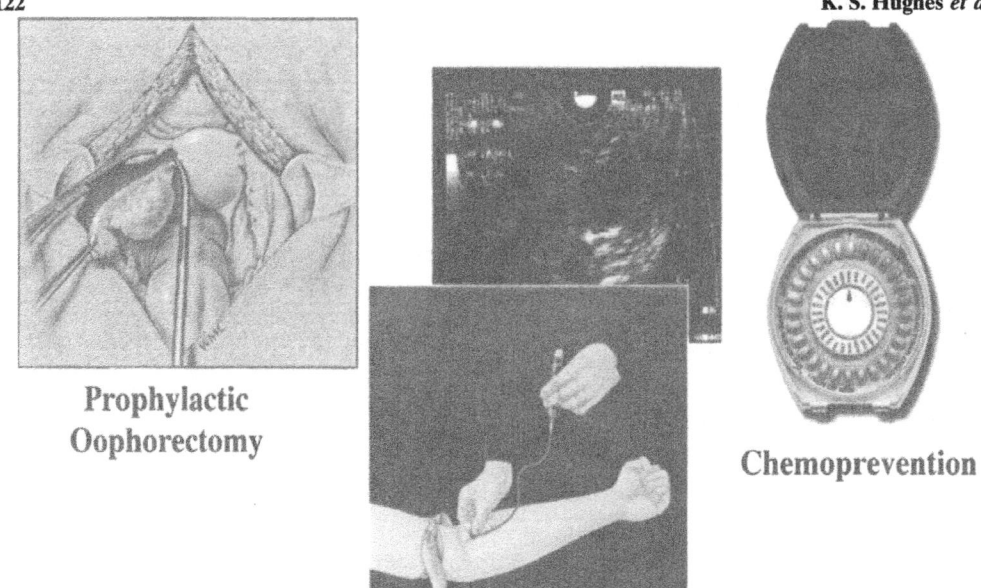

Prophylactic
Oophorectomy

Chemoprevention

Screening

Figure 10. Options for BRCA1, BRCA2 carrier.

general, our current level of knowledge allows only rudimentary answers and data gathering is essential.

4.1. Chemoprevention

The use of oral contraceptives has been associated with a decreased risk of ovarian cancer in the woman at average risk and women with positive family histories.[60] Incessant ovulation with subsequent monthly trauma to the epithelial cover of the ovary is associated with an increased risk of developing epithelial ovarian cancer. Oral contraceptives, as well as multiple full-term pregnancies, are believed to decrease this risk by the establishment of prolonged periods of anovulation. In the patient at high risk of hereditary breast and ovarian cancer, the efficacy of oral contraceptives in ovarian cancer prevention is unknown, but it is likely they will be at least partially effective. It therefore seems reasonable to consider oral contraceptives in women who are likely to harbor BRCA1 or BRCA2 mutations.

One concern, however, is that oral contraceptives may increase breast cancer risk in this population. Oral contraceptives have not been shown to increase the risk of breast cancer in the average risk woman to any significant extent,[61] but their effect on risk in the patient who harbors a BRCA1 or BRCA2 mutation is unknown. In the absence of data, it is reasonable to assume that, in this population, that oral contraceptives will decrease ovarian cancer risk while having no major impact on breast cancer risk. Over the next several years, this issue will be clarified, as more data accrues regarding women identified as BRCA1 & 2 carriers.

How long these women should take oral contraceptives is unknown. It appears the longer they are used, the greater the decrease in ovarian cancer risk. In a meta-analysis of 20 studies, the risk of ovarian cancer was reduced by 10–12% after one year of oral contraceptive use, while a 50% reduction in risk was observed after 5 years of use. This reduction in risk appeared to persist at least 10 years after discontinuation of oral contraceptives.[62] At what age one should begin oral contraceptives is also unclear, but presumably, the earlier, the better. When should one stop oral contraceptives? In the absence of data, continuing to menopause seems reasonable, if no contraindications exist. Relative contraindications to prolonged use of oral contraceptives include hypertension, cigarette smoking, obesity, and thromboembolic disease.

It may be reasonable to recommend that any woman, who has, or is likely to have, a BRCA1 or BRCA2 mutation (and whose ovaries have not been removed), should take oral contraceptives for a prolonged period of time while she is premenopausal, beginning as early as possible.

4.2. Efficacy of Surveillance in Hereditary Ovarian Cancer

Efficacy of ovarian screening to prevent cancer death is dependent on the ability of the technology to identify cancer early. It is well established that CA125 is elevated in about 50% of Stage I ovarian cancer.[63] Therefore, screening with CA125 alone will result in at least half of the patients advancing to higher stage disease prior to detection. Data on Transvaginal sonography is incomplete, but the sensitivity for detecting Stage I disease is most likely less than 80–90%.[64]

The use of transvaginal sonography plus CA125 every 6 months and rapid surgery based on an abnormality in either should theoretically decrease the death rate from ovarian cancer somewhat, but this has yet to be proven. Even assuming high sensitivity and excellent compliance, it must be recalled that even Stage I ovarian cancer has a 5 year survival of only 70–90%. Therefore, a significant number of women will die despite intensive screening. The magnitude of death must be established over the next few years.

Between 16% and 60% of BRCA1 mutation carriers will develop ovarian cancer.[1,6] The age of onset is skewed markedly toward the younger age population, with risk beginning to increase in the 30's. Approximately 16% of BRCA2 mutation carriers will develop ovarian cancer.[6] The age of onset appears to be older than the BRCA1 mutation carriers, but remains younger than the general population. Risk appears to begin to increase in the 40's. If we are to impact on the mortality of this disease in women who carry BRCA1 and BRCA2 mutations, intervention must begin early.

Ovarian cancer differs from breast cancer in many ways that make screening less likely to be effective. The lifetime risk of 1.7% is not high enough to justify population screening, a silent, treatable preclinical phase may not exist, treatment, in general, is inadequate, and adequate screening technology does not exist. Therefore, the American College of Obstetrics and Gynecology considers general population screening for ovarian cancer not justifiable.

On the other hand, the markedly increased frequency of ovarian cancer in the BRCA 1 and BRCA2 mutation carriers makes screening more appealing. The technology, however, remains inadequate.

CA125 is a glycoprotein present on the surface of most non mucin-producing ovarian cancer cells, as well as in many normal tissues. For serum CA125 to be effective, the cells must have this antigen, and they must shed this antigen into the bloodstream in sufficient amounts to be detectable. The chance of this happening with early ovarian cancer is about 50%. In studies of ovarian cancer, CA125 is elevated in 80% of all cancers, and 50% of stage I disease.[63] To add to the confusion, CA125 is relatively non-specific, and is often elevated in a number of benign and physiologic conditions, including, for example, menses, endometriosis, diverticulitis, liver disease, and pregnancy. Serial CA125 is more accurate, and noting trends in CA125 can decrease the false positive rate.

Similarly, transvaginal sonography has severe limitations for ovarian cancer screening. For transvaginal sonography to be effective, the ovarian cancer must have grown to a size that causes an anatomic change in the ovary that is above the threshold of transvaginal sonography. The false negative rate of transvaginal sonography in early ovarian cancer is not well studied. Most likely the sensitivity of this technique for detecting stage I ovarian cancer will be between 50 and 90%. To add to the confusion, transvaginal sonography is relatively non-specific, and is abnormal for any condition that produces an anatomic change in the ovary. Transvaginal sonography showed a persistent abnormality in 1.4% of the postmenopausal women screened, and of these patients, 93% were found not to have ovarian cancer (a false positive rate of 93%).[65]

The combination of CA125 and transvaginal sonography will increase the sensitivity, but also increase the false positive rate if every abnormality found on either test is evaluated independently. That is, more cancers will be found early, and more false positives will lead to more oophorectomies, if every CA125 elevation is acted upon whether or not the transvaginal sonography is abnormal, and if every transvaginal sonography abnormality is acted upon whether or not the CA125 is elevated.

On the other hand, the combination of CA125 and Transvaginal sonography will decrease the false positive rate and decrease the sensitivity if every abnormality found on either test must be corroborated by the second test, unless markedly and obviously abnormal. That is, cancers will not be found early if a CA125 elevation is only acted upon if the transvaginal sonography is abnormal (less than 90% sensitivity for Stage I), and if a transvaginal sonography abnormality is only acted upon if the CA 125 is elevated (50% sensitivity for Stage I). A markedly positive abnormality in either test could still generate evaluation independently. This will generate fewer false positives, but cancers detectable by only one of the 2 methods will be detected later.

Regardless, screening will not be effective if there is poor compliance with screening recommendations. Dr. Lermann has found that among women found to carry a BRCA1 or BRCA2 mutation, less than 10% followed the recommendations for CA-125 and transvaginal sonography when evaluated 6 months after testing.[22]

4.3. Possible Outcomes of Screening for Ovarian Cancer

A certain number of women carrying mutations in BRCA1 and BRCA2 will develop ovarian cancer. This number will be dependent on the penetrance of the BRCA1 and BRCA2 mutations, and might potentially be modified by the use of oral contraceptives. At the current level of screening technology and the current method of ovarian cancer treatment, many will be detected at a stage when they are not curable. The women who develop ovarian cancer will be treated with surgery alone or with surgical debulking plus chemotherapy. The majority of these will most likely die of their disease, unless screening is extremely effective at identifying cancer at an early and curable stage.

The vagaries and uncertainties are depicted in Fig. 11 by arrows of varying sizes. The exact size of each arrow will be determined by future research.

If all women carrying mutations in BRCA1 and BRCA2 are screened, the current level of screening technology and the current method of ovarian cancer treatment

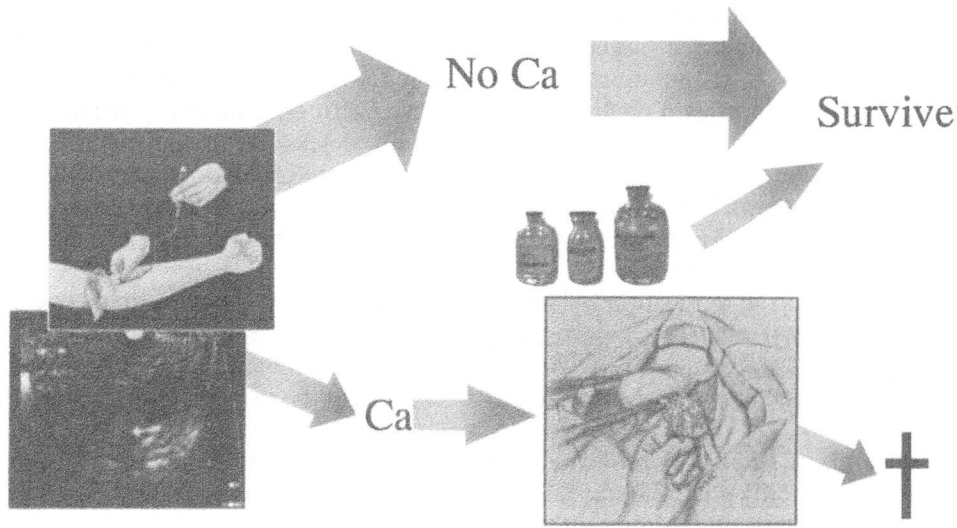

Figure 11. Possible outcomes of screening the ovary.

will mean that the majority of them will be detected at a stage when they are not curable. The size of the arrows is a gross approximation of the number expected to move down each pathway. The exact size of the arrows will be determined by future research.

4.4. Efficacy of Prophylactic Oophorectomy in Hereditary Ovarian Cancer

Prophylactic bilateral oophorectomy is most likely effective in preventing ovarian cancer. However, as with prophylactic mastectomy, it appears that it does not completely prevent cancer. Numerous cases of primary peritoneal carcinomatosis with histologic and clinical features similar to ovarian cancer, have been reported after prophylactic oophorectomy.[66,67] It is theorized that the coelomic epithelium which lines the peritoneal cavity is of the same origin as the ovarian epithelium, and is at similar risk of developing cancer. While the lifetime risk of developing this complication has been estimated to be 3–5%, it must be considered in the context of at least 16%–65% lifetime risk of ovarian cancer in BRCA1 mutation carriers with a cancer family syndrome.

Struewing has pooled data on high-risk families from the National Cancer Institute and Creighton University. When compared to the average risk population, those who had not undergone oophorectomy had 20.3 times the risk of ovarian cancer compared to the general population, while those who had undergone prophylactic oophorectomy only had 8.4 times the risk. This translates to a relative risk (RR) for those undergoing prophylactic oophorectomy of 0.44 with a range from 0.1 to 1.3. That is, the risk of ovarian cancer is decreased by about somewhere between 0 and 90%. This seems like a rather modest decrease in risk, and must be reevaluated as further data accumulates.

Prophylactic oophorectomy may be appropriately considered in women with hereditary breast-ovarian cancer syndrome and possibly in families with Lynch II-type syndromes (colorectal, endometrial, or ovarian cancers). Current evidence suggests the indications for prophylactic surgery are particularly strong in women who are carriers of BRCA1 or BRCA2 mutations. Consideration for prophylactic surgery may also include women with second or first-degree relatives with documented ovarian cancer or combinations of breast or ovarian cancer when at least one occurred premenopausally. Although women with only one first degree relative with documented ovarian cancer are, in general, not considered candidates for prophylactic surgery, mitigating circumstances such as limited access to family history must be considered in individualizing these recommendations.

Women who undergo prophylactic oophorectomy may also consider concomitant hysterectomy either by laparoscopy or open technique (either abdominal or vaginal). Such an approach offers the benefit of eliminating another at risk organ in patients with Lynch II-type syndromes as well as simplifying hormone replacement therapy.[68]

In terms of surgical approach, options include bilateral salpingo-oophorectomy vs total hysterectomy plus bilateral salpingo-oophorectomy. The surgical procedure can be done laparoscopically vs open.

If only bilateral salpingo-oophorectomy is opted for, the procedure should be done laparoscopically, whenever possible. The advantage of the laparoscopic approach is that it can be done on an out-patient basis, with relatively low morbidity. The rate of complications is quite low. Adhesions from prior abdominal surgery, or previous episodes of pelvic inflammatory disease or endometriosis may make this approach untenable. To avoid morbidity, careful patient selection, and a willingness to convert to an open procedure if difficulties arise, is essential.

If hysterectomy is opted for, open surgery may be more appropriate. A totally laparoscopic approach to hysterectomy is not usually possible and vaginal hysterectomy plus oophorectomy is unlikely to be an option in this young population. While oophorectomy can sometimes be accomplished during a vaginal hysterectomy, this is usually in older women who have had multiple vaginal deliveries. These older women tend to have a lax pelvic floor, and some degree of prolapse of the uterus. In a young patient population, most of whom have had few children (as is the current social trend), there will be little prolapse, and a relatively intact pelvic floor. In this young population, a laparoscopically assisted vaginal hysterectomy might be an option, but most likely an open procedure will be necessary.

4.5. Special Technical Considerations Due to the Risk of Breast Cancer

In undertaking the surgery, it is important to consider that the patient is also at high risk of developing breast cancer, and therefore may need breast reconstruction in the future, either for treatment or prophylaxis. Most patients in the general population choose breast conservation when breast cancer develops, but in this high risk group the number who opt for mastectomy, or even bilateral mastectomy (treatment on the affected side and prophylaxis on the contralateral side) will probably be higher. Of those who choose conservation, between 5 to 10% will recur in the breast and need mastectomy at a later date.

Therefore, it is imperative that the option of reconstruction not be lost. A free TRAM flap depends on intact inferior epigastric vessels, and both the free and rotation TRAMs depend on the perforating vessels that come through the rectus fascia. Damage to these vessels must be avoided. In doing laparoscopic surgery, the incisions should be placed so as to avoid injury to the inferior epigastric vessels. In open surgery, a lower midline incision is best. A Pfannenstiel incision (the transverse incision that is made below the panty line) is acceptable as long as the subcutaneous fat is not dissected free from the fascia, (which would transect the perforating vessels that come through the rectus fascia), and that the rectus muscles are not transected. In either incision, retraction on the rectus muscles should be delicate, and in closing the incision, sutures should not go so far from the edge of the incision as to damage the epigastric vessels.

4.6. Use of Hormone Replacement Therapy

To be effective, prophylactic oophorectomy will need to be done at an early age. The longer one delays the procedure, the fewer patients will benefit, as some will already have developed the disease. Data continues to accumulate, but it may be reasonable to assume at this time that prophylactic oophorectomy in the patient with a BRCA2 mutation may be put off until the 40's but for the patient with a BRCA1 mutation, this should be done in the 30's.

These young women will suddenly go through a severe surgical menopause, and the negative impact on quality and length of life for this population will be tremendous if left untreated. Women could expect to rapidly lose bone mass, and be at risk for fractures and kyphosis. The rate and severity of heart disease and stroke will increase markedly. In addition, these young women can expect hot flashes, vaginal dryness, urinary tract infection, dyspareunia, frequency of urination, decreased skin tone, and other problems.

To counteract these effects without the use of estrogen would include a pharmacopoeia that could include calcium, multivitamins, vaginal lubricants, skin creams, bellergal, raloxifine.

While the use of hormone replacement therapy could easily prevent these problems, there is concern that hormone replacement therapy could increase the risk of breast cancer in this high-risk population. While in the post-menopausal patient, hormone replacement therapy is felt to either have no effect on breast cancer risk, and at most, marginally increase the risk (RR 1.4),[69] it is not clear what the effect on risk will be in this population. The blood levels of estrogen in premenopausal women are significantly higher than the blood levels of estrogen produced by hormone replacement therapy. Therefore, if estrogen were an important factor in producing breast cancer in these women, hormone replacement therapy would produce an ameliorated effect. Without oophorectomy, depending on the penetrance of the mutations, up to 87% of patients will develop breast cancer by the age of 70. Oophorectomy might decrease that number slightly. Struewing initially reported a suggested decrease in breast cancer risk with oophorectomy, but this has not been confirmed. If oophorectomy does decrease breast cancer rate, hormone replacement therapy might modestly abrogate that benefit, so that the breast cancer rate is less than that seen without oophorectomy, but more than that seen with oophorectomy.

Even considering the inadequacy of breast screening discussed earlier for this population, most patients who do develop breast cancer are cured. Therefore, while the actual increase in breast cancer with hormone replacement therapy will be small at most, the increase in cancer death will be minimal to non-existent, and the health benefits will be tremendous. Therefore, we are inclined to recommend that a woman who undergoes oophorectomy in the premenopausal age group should use hormone replacement therapy, and currently we suggest that she should continue to use it through age 50. Use beyond age 50 will require further study.

4.7. Possible Outcomes of Prophylactic Oophorectomy

If all women carrying mutations in BRCA1 and BRCA2 undergo prophylactic oophorectomy, the majority will not develop ovarian cancer. Somewhere between 35 to 84% would not have developed ovarian cancer anyway due to the limited penetrance of the BRCA1 and BRCA2 mutations. Of the remaining patients, the number who are prevented from developing ovarian cancer will be dependent on the efficacy of this procedure. The women who develop ovarian cancer despite the procedure will be treated with surgical debulking plus chemotherapy (all would have Stage III disease), and the majority will die of their disease.

The vagaries and uncertainties are depicted in Fig. 12 by arrows of varying sizes. The exact size of each arrow will be determined in the future.

If all women carrying mutations in BRCA1 and BRCA2 undergo prophylactic oophorectomy, theoretically a large number will not develop ovarian cancer and therefore not die of ovarian cancer. However, some undetermined number will develop peritoneal carcinomatosis, will be treated by debulking plus chemotherapy, and will either be cured or die. The size of the arrows is a gross approximation of the number expected to move down each pathway. The exact size of the arrows will be determined by future research.

4.8. Incidental Oophorectomy

The function of the ovary in childbearing years is to act as a source of eggs, and to provide an appropriate level of female hormones. After childbearing is complete, the ovary continues to provide an appropriate level of female hormones for a short time and then ceases to function. The ovary is a unique organ in that it is virtually

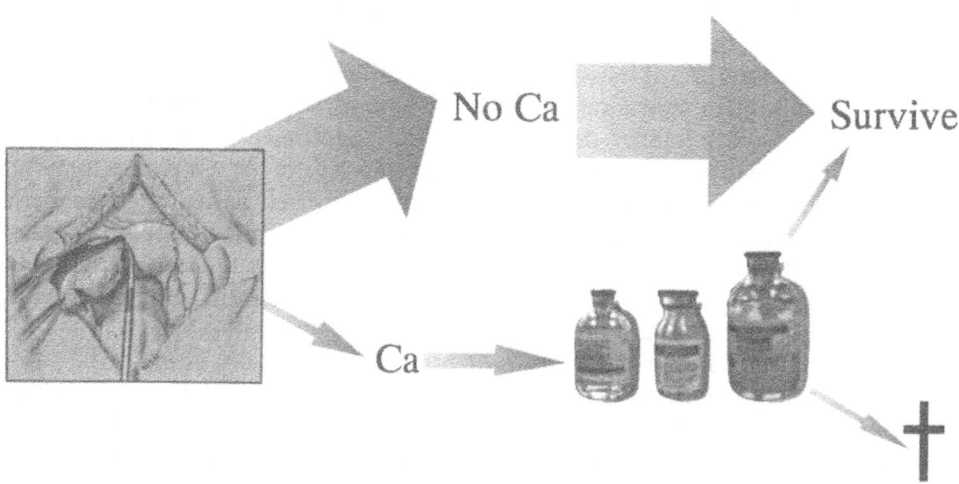

Figure 12. Possible outcomes of prophylactic oophorectomy.

without function after the age of 50, being unable to produce eggs or hormones. In general, function of hormone production is easily replaced pharmacologically once childbearing is complete. In addition, unlike the breast, absence of the ovaries has no effect on appearance or sexuality (if the hormonal function is replaced).

In the patient at moderate or undetermined risk (BRCA1 or BRCA2 mutation suspected), it may not be reasonable to suggest an invasive procedure to remove the ovaries, even if childbearing is complete. However, undertaking oophorectomy during another surgical procedure would be perfectly reasonable if it did not add undue morbidity. Therefore, in our patients who are at any increased risk of ovarian cancer, we recommend that they strongly consider incidental oophorectomy if they are undergoing hysterectomy, cholecystectomy, or any abdominal procedure. It is important to educate surgeons regarding this, as the surgeon and the patient must both be comfortable in proceeding in this manner.

5. GENETIC TESTING

Prophylactic surgery is not to be considered lightly. The morbidity and psychosocial consequences are not trivial, and this surgery should not be performed without a thorough understanding of the indications and consequences. While the utility of genetic testing is controversial, we feel that there should be no controversy in the woman who is contemplating prophylactic surgery. Prior to a prophylactic mastectomy or prophylactic oophorectomy, patients should be strongly encouraged to undergo genetic testing. Incidental oophorectomy can certainly be considered in the absence of genetic testing.

In the average risk woman, prophylactic mastectomy, or an invasive procedure with the sole purpose of removing the ovaries for cancer prevention is not indicated. Therefore, when it is possible to quantitate risk, and to determine whether a patient truly falls into a high-risk group, we are obligated to try to obtain this information.

In utilizing genetic testing to determine the need for prophylactic surgery, we need to examine the Jewish woman and the non-Jewish woman separately. If a non-Jewish woman wishes prophylactic surgery, we need to test an affected relative first. If the affected relative is found to carry a deleterious mutation, then we have identified the family specific mutation. The unaffected woman is then tested for that mutation. If she does not carry that mutation, then she is at the population risk and should not undergo prophylactic surgery. If she does carry the mutation, then prophylactic surgery is a reasonable approach, within the context of the information presented in this chapter.

If the affected relative does not carry a mutation, then either the family is not a hereditary cancer family, or the test as performed produced a false negative result. False negative tests can occur for several reasons, including testing the wrong gene (the family may carry a mutation in a gene other than BRCA1 or BRCA2), testing the wrong patient (the patient tested may be a sporadic case), or doing the wrong test (the mutation may have been missed by the test performed). Close scrutiny of the pedigree can help to elucidate the likelihood of each scenario.

In terms of testing the wrong gene, while the majority of breast ovarian cancer families are due to mutations in BRCA1 and 2, some are caused by mutations in p53, PTEN, or other genes. The absence of a BRCA1 or 2 mutation does not rule out a mutation in one of these other genes.

In terms of testing the wrong patient, not every woman who is a member of a breast ovarian cancer family who develops breast or ovarian cancer will carry a mutation. Non-carriers in these families remain at the population risk, and it is possible that we are testing a patient with a sporadic case of breast or ovarian cancer.

In terms of doing the wrong test, as has been described in other chapters, not all genetic tests find all mutations. For example, full gene sequencing can miss total exon deletions, and protein truncation can miss mutations in exons other than 11.

A mutation discovered that is not clearly deleterious raises similar issues. If no mutation, or a mutation of unknown significance, is found in the affected patient, further investigation is in order before embarking on prophylactic surgery.

In the Jewish woman, the issues are different. It can be assumed that most of the hereditary families have one of the 3 defined mutations. If a woman does not have one of these 3 mutations, and if the more suspicious side of her family is found to carry one of these mutations, then she is unlikely to be above the population risk. However, due to the high background frequency of these mutations, a woman considering prophylactic surgery should be tested for all three mutations, even if one mutation has already been detected in her family.

6. CONCLUSION

In summary, if a woman is considering prophylactic surgery, she should be encouraged to have genetic testing. If the testing conclusively shows she does not carry a deleterious mutation, an attempt should be made to dissuade her from her decision. She is at no more risk than the general population, and prophylactic surgery is not indicated at that risk level. If the testing conclusively shows she does carry a deleterious mutation, then prophylactic surgery should be considered and discussed in the context of the information presented here. If the testing is inconclusive, the risk estimate based on pedigree analysis combined with the likelihood of a false negative test should be used to determine the appropriate course of action

Currently, we believe prophylactic oophorectomy is superior to intensive screening, due to the inadequacy of ovarian screening and the purported efficacy of prophylactic oophorectomy. On the other hand, the relative efficacy of screening, and the impending improvements in screening, chemoprevention and treatment make prophylactic mastectomy a close alternative to intensive screening.

When faced with a woman who carries a BRCA1 or BRCA2 mutation, we discuss the pros and cons of screening, chemoprevention, and prophylactic surgery. Prophylactic oophorectomy is for now, and will remain for the foreseeable future, the preferred alternative. Prophylactic mastectomy is reasonable at this time, though its superiority over screening is less dramatic. In the future, we can look forward to prophylactic mastectomy becoming obsolete.

REFERENCES

1. Easton DF, Ford D, Bishop DT: Breast and ovarian cancer incidence in BRCA1-mutation carriers. Am J Hum Genet 56:265–71, 1995
2. Ford D, Easton DF, Bishop DT, et al: Risks of cancer in BRCA1-mutation carriers. Lancet 343:692–695, 1994
3. Ford D, Easton DF: The genetics of breast and ovarian cancer. Br J Cancer 72:805–812, 1995

4. Easton DF, Bishop DT, Ford D, et al: Genetic linkage analysis in familial breast and ovarian cancer. Am J Hum Genet 52:678–701, 1993
5. Burke W, Daly M, Garber J, et al: Recommendations for follow-up care of individuals with an inherited predisposition to cancer. BRCA1 and BRCA2. JAMA 277:997–1003, 1997
6. Struewing JP, Hartge P, Wacholder S, et al: The risk of cancer associated with specific mutations of BRCA1 and BRCA2 among Ashkenazi Jews. N Engl J Med 336:1401–1408, 1997
7. Fiorica JV, Roberts WS: Screening for ovarian cancer. Cancer Control 3:120–129, 1996
8. Hankinson SE, Colditz, GA, Hunter JJ, et al: A quantitative assessment of oral contraceptive use and risk of ovarian cancer. Obstet Gynecol 80:708, 1992
9. Weber AM, Hewett WJ, Gajewski WH, et al: Serous carcinoma of the peritoneum after oophorectomy. Obstetrics and Gynecology 80:(3) Part 2, Sept, 1992
10. Struewing JP, Tucker MA, Lynch HT, et al: Prophylactic oophorectomy in inherited breast/ovarian cancer families. J Natl Cancer Inst Monogr 17:33–35, 1995
11. Iselius L, Wilking N: Screening for familial cancer, in Weber W, Mulvihill JJ, Narod S (Eds): Familial Cancer Management. CRC Press, New York, pp 75–76
12. National Institutes of Health Consensus Development Conference Statement: Breast Cancer Screening for Women Ages 40–49, January 21–23, 1997. National Institutes of Health Consensus Development Panel. J Natl Cancer Inst 89(14):1015–26, 1997
13. Landis SH, Murray T, Bolden S, et al: Cancer statistics, 1998. CA Cancer J Clin 48:6–29, 1998
14. Spratt JS, Meyer JS, Spratt JA. Rates of growth of human solid neoplasms: Part I. Journal of Surgical Oncology 60:137–146, 1995
15. Spratt JS, Meyer JS, Spratt JA. Rates of growth of human neoplasms: Part II. Journal of Surgical Oncology 61:68–83, 1996
16. Personal communication Barbara Smith
17. Foulkes WD, Wong N, Brunet JS, et al: Germ-line mutation is an adverse prognostic factor in Ashkenazi jewish women with breast cancer. Clinical Cancer Research 3:2465–2469, 1997
18. Verhoog LC, Brekelmans CTM, Seynaeve C, et al: Survival and tumour characteristics of breast-cancer patients with germline mutations of BRCA1. Lancet 351:316–321, 1998
19. Johannson OT, Ranstam J, Borg A, et al: Survival of BRCA1 breast and ovarian cancer patients: a population-based study form southern Sweden. J Clin Oncol 16:397–404, 1998
20. Crook T, Crossland S, Crompton MR, et al: p53 mutations in BRCA1-associated familial breast cancer [letter] Lancet 350(9078):638–639, 1997
21. Breast cancer Linkage Consortium. Pathology of familial breast cancer: differences between breast cancers in cariers of BRCA1 and BRCA2 mutations and sporadic cases. Lancet 349:1505–1510, 1997
22. Lerman C: Few BRCA1 carriers take recommended precautions. Oncology News 7, No.2:1, 1998
23. Holleb AI, Montgomery R, Farrow JH: The hazard of incomplete simple mastectomy. Surg Gynec & Obst 121:819, 1965
24. Ziegler LD, Kroll SS: Primary breast cancer after prophylactic mastectomy. Am J Clin Oncol 14:451–454, 1991
25. Goodnight JE Jr, Quagliana JM, Morton DL: Failure of subcutaneous mastectomy to prevent the development of breast cancer. J Surg Oncol 26:198–201, 1984
26. Bowers DG, Radlauer CB: Breast cancer after prophylactic subcutaneous mastectomies and reconstruction with silastic prostheses. Plast Reconstr Surg 44:541, 1969
27. Mendez-Fernandez MA, Henly WS, Geis RC: Paget's disease of the breast after subcutaneous mastectomy and reconstruction with a silicone prosthesis. Plast Reconstr Surg 65(5):683–685, 1980
28. Eldar S, Meguid MM, Beatty JD: Cancer of the breast after prophylactic subcutaneous mastectomy. Am J Surg 148:692–693, 1984
29. Jameson MB, Braatvedt GD, Probert JC, et al: Metastatic breast cancer 42 years after bilateral subcutaneous mastectomies. Clin Oncol (R Coll Radiol) 9(2):119–121, 1997
30. Humphrey LJ: Subcutaneous mastectomy is not a prophylaxis against carcinoma of the breast: Opinion or knowledge? Am J Surg 145:311–321, 1983
31. Pennisi VR, Capozi A: Subcutaneous mastectomy data: A final statistical analysis of 1500 patients. Aesth Plast Surg 13:15–21, 1989
32. Woods JE, Meland NB: Conservative management in full thickness nipple-areolar necrosis after subcutaneous mastectomy. Plastic and reconstructive Surgery 84:258–266, 1989
33. Slade C, Lawrence: Subcutaneous mastectomy; Acute complications and long-term follow-up. Plastic and Reconstructive Surgery 73(1):84–88, 1984
34. Fredericks S: A 10 year experience with subcutaneous mastectomy. Clin Plast Surg 2:347–357, 1975

35. Amaaki T, Yasumura K, Kami T, et al: Prophylactic subcutaneous total glandectomy for mammary cystic disease, with immediate primary breast reconstruction. Ann Plast Surg 3:420–424, 1979
36. Hartmann L, Jenkins R, Schaid D, et al: Prophylactic mastectomy (PM): Preliminary retrospective cohort analysis. Proc Of the Am Assoc for Cancer Research 38:168, 1997
37. Mackarem G, Roche CA, Silverman ML, Hughes KS: Brief clinical report: The development of new, primary non-invasive carcinoma of the breast 29 years after bilateral radical mastectomy. The Breast Journal (in press)
38. Gabriel SE, Woods JE, O'Fallon WM, et al: Complications leading to surgery after breast implantation, New Eng Jour Med 336:677–682, 1997
39. Bostwick J: Breast reconstruction following mastectomy. CA Cancer J Clin 45:289–304, 1995
40. Slade CL: Subcutaneous mastectomy: Acute complications and long term follow-up. Plast Reconstr Surg 73:84–88, 1984
41. Horton CE, Dascombe WH: Total mastectomy: indications and techniques. Clin Plast Surg 15:677–687, 1988
42. Jarrett JR: Prophylactic mastectomy, in Marsh JL, B.C. Decker BC (ed): Current Therapy in Plastic and Reconstructive Surgery, Toronto, pp 64–70, 1989
43. Jarrett JR, Cutler, RG, Teal DF: Aesthetic refinements in prophylactic subcutaneous mastectomy with submuscular reconstruction. Plast Reconstr Surg 69:625–631, 1982
44. Bostwick J, Jones G: Why I choose autogenous tissue in breast reconstruction. Clin Plast Surg 21:165–175, 1994
45. Elliott LF: Options for donor sites for autogenous tissue breast reconstruction. Clin Plast Surg 21:177–189, 1994
46. Hartrampf CR, Scheflen M, Black PW: Breast reconstruction following mastectomy with a transverse abdominal island flap, anatomic and clinical observations. Plast Reconstr Surg 69:216, 1982
47. Beasley ME: The pedicled TRAM as preference for immediate autogenous tissue breast reconstruction. Clin Plast Surg 21:191–205, 1994
48. Bucky LP, May JW: Synthetic mesh: Its use in abdominal wall reconstruction after the TRAM. Clin Plast Surg 21:273–277, 1994
49. Mizgala CL, Hartrampf CR, Bennett GK, Abdominal function after pedicled TRAM flap surgery. Clin Plast Surg 21:255–272, 1994
50. Schusterman MA, Kroll SS, Miller MJ, et al: The free rectus abdominis musculoral contraceptivesutaneous flap for breast reconstruction: one centers experience with 211 consecutive cases. Ann Plast Surg 32:234–242, 1994
51. Watterson PA, Bostwick J, Hester TR, et al: TRAM flap anatomy correlated with a 10 year clinical experience with 556 patients. Plast Reconstr Surg 95:1185–1193, 1995
52. Leibman AJ, Stylbo TM, Bostwick J: Mammography of the postreconstruction breast. Plast Reconstr Surg 99:698–704, 1997
53. Noone RB, Frazier TG, Noone GC, et al: Recurrance of breast carcinoma following immediate reconstruction: a 12 year review. Plast Reconstr Surg 93:96, 1994
54. Slavin SA, Love SM, Goldwyn RM: Recurrent breast cancer following immediate reconstruction with myoral contraceptivesutaneous flaps. Plast Reconstr Surg 93:1191, 1994
55. Yamamoto Y, Nohira K, Sugihara T, et al: Superiority of the microvascularly augmented flap: Analysis of 50 TRAM flaps for breast reconstruction. Plast Reconstr Surg 97:79–83, 1996
56. Grotting JC, Urist MM, Maddox WA, et al: Conventional TRAM flap versus free microsurgical TRAM flap for immediate breast reconstruction. Plast Reconstr Surg 83:828, 1989
57. Banic A, Boeckx W, Greulich M, et al: Late results of breast reconstruction with free TRAM flaps: a prospective multicenter study. Plast Reconstr Surg 95:1195–1204, 1995
58. Kroll SS: Invited discussion, re: Banic, et. al., Plast Reconstr Surg 95:1205–1206, 1995
59. Shaw WW: Invited discussion, re: Shusterman, et al., Ann Plast Surg 32:241–242, 1994
60. Gross TP, Schlesselman JJ: The estimated effect of oral contraceptive use on the cumulative risk of epithelial ovarian cancer. Obstet Gynecol 83:419, 1994
61. Stadel RW, Rubin PA, Webster LA, et al: Oral contraceptives and breast cancer in young women. Lancet 2(8462):970–973, 1985
62. Hankinson SE, Colditz GA, Hunter JJ, et al: A quantitative assessment of oral contraceptive use and risk of ovarian cancer. Obstet Gynecol 80:708, 1992
63. Jacobs I, Bast R: The CA125 associated antigen: A review of the literature. Hum Reprod 4:1–12, 1989
64. Carlson KJ, Skates SJ, et al: Screening for ovarian cancer. Ann Intern Med 121:124–132, 1994
65. DePriest PD, van Nagell JR, Gallion H, et al: Ovarian cancer screening in symptomatic post-menopausal women. Gynecol Oncol 51:205, 1993

66. Struewing JP, Watson P, Easton DF, Ponder BAJ, Lynch HT, Tucher MA. Prophylactic oophorectomy in inherited breast/ovarian cancer families. J Natl Cancer I Monographs 17:33–35, 1995
67. Weber AM, Hewett WJ, Gajewski WH, Curry SL: Serous carcinoma of the peritoneum after oophorectomy. Obstetrics and Gynecology 80:(3) Part 2, 1992
68. American College of Obstetricians and Gynecologists. Prophylactic Oophorectomy. ACOG Criteria Set number 2. Washington, D.C.: ACOG, 1994
69. Colditz GA, Stampfor MJ, Willett WC, et al: Prospective study of estrogen replacement therapy and risk of breast cancer in postmenopausal women. JAMA 264:2648–2653, 1990

9

CHEMOPREVENTION AND HERITABLE CANCER RISK

Victor G. Vogel

Director, Comprehensive Breast Program
Professor of Medicine and Epidemiology
University of Pittsburgh Cancer Institute Magee-Womens Hospital
300 Halket Street
Room 3524
Pittsburgh, PA 15213

Chemoprevention can be defined as the use of specific natural or synthetic chemical agents to reverse, suppress, or prevent the progression of premalignant lesions to invasive carcinoma.[1,2,3] Our basic understanding of human carcinogenesis indicates that the process proceeds through multiple discernible stages of molecular and cellular alterations that provide the basis and scientific rationale for clinical cancer chemoprevention. There are, however, a number of unique features of the clinical discipline of primary cancer prevention. First, is the issue of the "target population." Cancer is a rare disease among individuals who are at usual risk. It is clear, however, that individuals with a family history of the disease, with or without an identified predisposing genetic mutation, constitute a unique target population for primary preventive interventions. It is difficult, though, to determine whether these individuals should be considered "patients," "subjects," or "participants." Labeling healthy individuals as patients carries the potentially negative connotations of illness in all of the behavioral metaphors associated with illness. The creation of new classes of the asymptomatic sick (e.g., considering gene carriers as ill), and the medicalization of conditions for which there may not be a medical solution, have important implications for the predisposed individual's sense of self identity, health beliefs, and behaviors, and specific social institutions such as health insurance and employment.

Second, is the issue of allowable toxicity from a putative chemopreventive agent. While cancer patients and their physicians may tolerate significant toxicity, or even

Email: vogelv@msx.upmc.edu, Office: 412-692-2620, Fax: 412-692-2610, Contact person: Agnes C. Zachoszcz

Cancer Genetics for the Clinician, edited by Shaw.
Kluwer Academic / Plenum Publishers, New York, 1999.

death, as a result of therapy, it is unlikely that patients who do not yet have malignancy, even if they are at substantially increased risk of developing cancer, will find serious toxicity acceptable. The challenge then in chemoprevention clinical trials is to find agents that are both effective and safe.

Finally, the duration of treatment must be considered. Our current understanding of carcinogenesis is that it is a chronic process that must be suppressed with chronic drug administration. It is not possible at the present time to administer a single dose of a preventive agent and reverse the tendency for development of malignancy permanently. Each chronic suppressive approach requires daily administration of an active agent and creates the need for the healthy individual to remain in contact with the health care system throughout prolonged periods of drug administration. This can be a difficult burden for active, mobile, healthy subjects who are employed and dealing with other demanding life issues, as well as cancer prevention.

In this chapter, we shall review the preclinical, basic science data that points us to several potentially active agents for the prevention of inheritable breast cancer. We shall use breast cancer as the model because of the wealth of understanding about breast carcinogenesis, its epidemiology, the important heritable syndromes, the availability of candidate chemoprevention agents, and the existence of several prospective, chemoprevention intervention trials for the primary prevention of breast cancer that are currently under way. We shall review issues of chemoprevention clinical trial design as they pertain to heritable cancer risk, and briefly discuss some of the issues related to the costs and ethics of conducting prospective primary prevention trials.

MAMMARY GLAND DEVELOPMENT AND THE BIOLOGY OF PREVENTION

The mammary gland is one of the few organs that is not fully developed at birth,[4,5] and no other organ presents such dramatic changes in size, shape, and function as does the breast during growth, puberty, pregnancy, and lactation. Russo and Russo[4] have carefully described the developmental progression of the human breast and describe four distinct types of breast lobules. Type 1 lobules are the most undifferentiated ones; they are also called virginal lobules, because they are present in the immature female breast before menarche. Type 2 lobules evolve from the previous ones and have a more complex morphology, being composed of a higher number of ductular structures per lobule. Type 3 lobules are characterized by having an average of 80 ductules or alveoli per lobule; they are frequently seen in the breast of women under hormonal stimulation or during pregnancy. A fourth type of lobule, the type 4 lobule, has been described as being present during the lactational period. Study of the pathogenesis of human breast cancer indicates that the type 1 lobules are the site of origin of preneoplastic lesions such as atypical ductal hyperplasias, which evolve to ductal carcinoma in situ, progressing to invasive carcinoma. Although ductal breast cancer originates in type 1 lobules, or terminal ductal lobular units,[6] the epidemiological observation that nulliparous women exhibit a higher incidence of breast cancer than parous women indicates that type 1 lobules in these two groups of women might be biologically different or exhibit different susceptibility to carcinogenesis.[7,8,9] Parous women undergo lobular differentiation, whereas nulliparous women seldom reach the type 3 lobule stage.

Type 1, 2, and 3 lobules also exhibit different cell kinetic characteristics; type 1 and 2 lobules grow faster in vitro and have higher DNA labeling index and a shorter doubling time than type 3 lobules.[4,10,11] Correspondingly, the breasts of nulliparous women free of cancer and of nulliparous women with cancer have a similar architecture. The breast of parous women free of cancer have the lowest percentage of type 1 lobules, and a slightly higher percentage of type 2, and parous women who develop breast cancer have breasts that contain higher numbers of type 1 lobules.

The degree of breast development is of importance in the susceptibility to carcinogenesis and it has been suggested that parous women who develop breast cancer might exhibit a defective response to the differentiating effect of the hormones of pregnancy.[12] Breast tissue composed almost exclusively of type 3 lobules, exhibits a significantly lower number of doublings.[9] The proliferative activity of the breast varies depending upon the phase of the menstrual cycle: cell proliferative activity has been shown to be consistently lower in the follicular than in the secretory phase.[13,14,15] The use of cell proliferation as an intermediate endpoint for assessing the effect of chemopreventive agents requires determining the exact location of the cells in which proliferative activity is measured. The samples that reacted with the carcinogens were derived mainly from breast tissue containing type 1 or 2 lobules, alone or combined, and were derived from nulliparous women. The breast cells could be divided into two major groups; susceptible and nonsusceptible to carcinogens; the susceptible samples were affected by at least one carcinogen and were those derived from less differentiated breasts.[7,8]

THE ROLE OF HORMONES

Hormones, especially estrogens, have been linked to breast cancer[16,17] and their role has been attributed to their ability to stimulate cell proliferation, which in turn leads to accumulation of random genetic errors that result in neoplasia.[18] Epidemiologic studies indicate that estrogen-mediated events play a role in the development of breast cancer,[19,20] and support the hypothesis that intact ovarian function is required to develop breast cancer. Prior investigations also show that oophorectomy or radiation-induced ovarian ablation can reduce the incidence of breast cancer by up to 75%.[21,22]

These observations suggest that estrogen antagonists might play a role in the primary prevention of breast cancer by reducing the rate of cell division through administration of antihormones. Tamoxifen has shown to be species, tissue, and cell type specific.[23] In the pubertal rat, tamoxifen is capable of promoting full ductal development in the mammary gland.[24] In the mature cycling animal, tamoxifen acts as an antiestrogen causing atrophy of lobular structures.[25] In postmenopausal women, tamoxifen treatment results in up-regulation of the proportion of ductal cells expressing estrogen receptor.[26]

TAMOXIFEN

Tamoxifen is a triphenylethylene synthesized in 1966 as a potential fertility agent. The parent compound and the conjugates are excreted in the bile and undergo enterohepatic circulation. This recirculation and the high volume of distribution result in a terminal elimination half-life of four to seven days[23,27,28,29] and at least six different metabolites have been isolated from the bile. Demethylation to the active metabolite N-desmethyl tamoxifen is the principal metabolic pathway in humans. Maximum serum concentration of N-desmethyl tamoxifen is observed within 12 to 24 hours after dosing; its serum half-life is about 12 days.[30]

Tamoxifen can suppress the appearance of chemically induced breast tumors in laboratory animals.[31] Both DMBA and NMU induce hormone-responsive mammary tumors in rats, but spayed animals or animals treated with androgens rarely develop DMBA-induced mammary carcinomas.[32,33] Experimentally, chemical initiation by DMBA is followed by a period of promotion with estrogen, prolactin, and progesterone; tumors appear three to four months later. The simultaneous administration of a large dose of tamoxifen and DMBA to 50-day-old female Sprague-Dawley rats results in a dramatic reduction (<10% of control) in the number and type of palpable mammary tumors.[34,35] A second-dose regimen of tamoxifen administered 30 days after DMBA inhibits tumorigenesis for up to 120 days. In rats, ovariectomy or the injection of antiestrogens after carcinogen administration results in the appearance of very few mammary tumors.[36,37]

Administration of tamoxifen does not result in a dramatic increase in the proportion of animals that remain tumor-free, but a clear-cut dose-response relationship is observed in the number of mammary tumors that develop. When tamoxifen is given to rats one month after DMBA administration, there is a dose-related delay in the appearance of palpable mammary tumors. Eventually, however, all of the animals develop tumors, with some reduction in the tumor burden as compared to nontreated animals.[38,39] In contrast, the continuous administration of tamoxifen results in more than 90% of animals remaining tumor-free.[40] Retreatment following DMBA administration results in further inhibition of tumorigenesis.[35] Tamoxifen also produces a dose-related delay in the appearance of DMBA-induced tumors in animals that are not spayed[39] and continuous treatment with lower daily doses of tamoxifen suppresses the appearance of DMBA-induced tumors until therapy is withdrawn.[41] Tamoxifen, therefore, does not appear to produce a tumoricidal effect in animals but, because the drug has a long biologic half-life, it produces a tumoristatic effect until the drug is cleared.[39,42]

Several mechanisms of tamoxifen's ability to prevent or suppress breast carcinogenesis have been proposed. Tamoxifen may inhibit cell proliferation by:

(1) modulating the production of transforming growth factors (TGFα and TGFβ) that help regulate breast cancer cell proliferation, including proliferation of estrogen receptor-negative cell lines. Tamoxifen antagonizes estrogen-enhanced production of TGFα in estrogen receptor-positive cell lines, and it down-regulates TGFα levels in estrogen receptor-positive human breast carcinoma.[43] It is not yet known whether this mechanism of growth inhibition by tamoxifen plays a role in the primary prevention of breast cancer.

(2) binding to cytoplasmic antiestrogenic binding sites, increasing intracellular drug levels.[44]

(3) increasing sex-hormone-binding globulin (SHBG), which may decrease the availability of free estrogen for diffusion into tumor cells.[45]

(4) increasing levels of natural killer (NK) cells.[46]

(5) decreasing circulating insulin-like growth factor (IGF-I) which may, in turn, modify the endocrinologic regulation of breast cancer cell kinetics.[47,48] Serum IGF-I levels decline in women receiving tamoxifen.[49,50]

Not all effects of tamoxifen are beneficial. Prolonged administration shows suppression of natural killer cell activity, and this suppression may play some role in the inability of tamoxifen to prevent breast tumors with complete efficiency. Resistance to the inhibitory effects of tamoxifen is also possible through several alterative mechanisms:[51] (1) through the production and localized accumulation of an estrogenic metabolite(s) of tamoxifen; (2) through the loss of estrogen receptor on precancerous or cancerous breast tissue; (3) through the production of mutated estrogen receptor that produces an estrogenic stimulus to cells when bound with estrogen; or (4) through altered subcellular factors and consequentially altered signal transduction. Any of these mechanisms or others not yet known could explain the failure of tamoxifen to prevent all newly emerging malignant breast clones.

The factors that determine hormone receptor status in human breast cancer are complex and far-ranging and include menopausal status, body weight, and complex endocrine interactions.[52] Postmenopausal breast cancer patients who receive tamoxifen demonstrate increases in both estrogen receptors (201%) and progesterone receptors (163%) measured using immunohistochemical techniques on fine needle aspiration from primary breast tumors over a period of 6 to 10 days.[52,53]

ADDITIONAL BENEFITS OF TAMOXIFEN

In addition to observed reductions in the odds of developing a second primary breast cancer, the treatment overview data demonstrate a 12% reduction in nonbreast cancer deaths, a 25% reduction in deaths from vascular disease, and a 9% reduction in other causes of death. A major proportion of the reduction in noncancer deaths is due to a reduction in cardiovascular disease mortality[54,55] and these results are due, in part, to decreases in LDL cholesterol observed as early as 2 months after the initiation of tamoxifen therapy. These reductions are followed at 6 months by either no change or an increase in HDL cholesterol, a fall in LDL cholesterol, and an increase in triglycerides.[56,57] Tamoxifen's estrogenic effect on the liver may lead to increased synthesis of very low-density lipoprotein cholesterol and increased triglyceride levels, decreased levels of apolipoprotein B synthesis, and increased levels of apolipoprotein A-1 synthesis, with resultant increased levels of HDL cholesterol.[58,59] Longitudinal observations of women at risk for heart disease are limited, but available data indicate that a 15% to 20% decrease in LDL cholesterol may result in a 6% to 20% decrease in coronary heart disease.[60,61]

The effect of tamoxifen on the development of atherosclerotic cardiovascular disease may also relate to its antithrombotic properties. Postmenopausal women taking tamoxifen show an average drop of only 10% in antithrombin III levels during therapy, while fibrinogen levels decline 16% or more.[62] Population studies demonstrate a relationship between fibrinogen levels, myocardial infarction, and stroke, with lower fibrinogen levels associated with lower cardiovascular risk.[63,64] Concerns about the durability of these effects arise from studies of former users of tamoxifen that show reversal of the increases in HDL cholesterol at the cessation of tamoxifen therapy.[65] A final assessment of the effect of tamoxifen on the risk of morbidity and mortality from cardiovascular disease in healthy women awaits completion of ongoing studies.

In addition to these beneficial effects on the apparent rates of developing cardiovascular disease, tamoxifen appears to have beneficial effects on bones as well.

Tamoxifen preserves bone mineral density in postmenopausal women,[66,67] presumably because of its estrogenic effect on osteoclasts, which slows bone resorption. Experimental data in vitro showing that tamoxifen blocks bone resorption induced by parathyroid hormone, prostaglandin E2, and 1,25-dihydroxy vitamin D3 support these clinical observations of benefit.[68] Of some concern is the observation that tamoxifen may reduce bone mineral density in premenopausal women by 1.9% annually while increasing bone density in postmenopausal women by 1.8%.[69] Prospective, randomized studies of women taking tamoxifen for the primary prevention of breast cancer will clarify this issue.

TOXICITY ASSOCIATED WITH TAMOXIFEN

Tamoxifen therapy is associated with a variety of symptomatic toxicities including gynecological symptoms (particularly hot flashes and vaginal discharge in perimenopausal women).[70] Early reports of an increased risk of thrombotic events were not confirmed in subsequent prospective trials with prolonged periods of observation,[71] and no hepatic neoplasms have been reported in women taking the usually prescribed 20 mg daily despite preliminary reports of hepatic neoplasms in women taking 40 mg daily.[72] Isolated reports of an increased incidence of gastrointestinal neoplasms occurring in women exposed to tamoxifen[73] were not confirmed in the overview analysis that showed a reduction in all second primary malignancies except endometrial cancer among women taking tamoxifen for the adjuvant treatment of breast cancer.[74] Similar negative conclusions were also reached when early reports of ocular toxicity associated with tamoxifen were investigated with properly conducted prospective investigations.

A well-established consequence of tamoxifen therapy is an increased incidence of endometrial carcinoma. In a randomized trial from Sweden that used 40 mg of tamoxifen daily, the incidence of uterine tumors (both endometrial carcinomas and uterine sarcomas) was 6.5-fold higher in the women who received tamoxifen than in those who received placebo, and the cumulative frequency of uterine tumors was 0.4% in the control group, 0.9% in women who received tamoxifen for 2 years, and 5.5% in women treated with tamoxifen for 5 years.[72,75] In another trial using tamoxifen 30 mg daily for 48 weeks, the incidence ratio for endometrial carcinomas was 1.9, with a cumulative incidence after 10 years of 0.3% and 1.0% in the patients receiving placebo and tamoxifen, respectively.[76,77]

Additional data are available from the National Surgical Adjuvant Breast and Bowel Project (NSABP) trial B-14, that was designed to evaluate tamoxifen as adjuvant therapy for breast cancer. The study included 1419 women randomly assigned to receive tamoxifen, 1220 women who entered the study on tamoxifen after randomization closed, and 1424 women randomly assigned to receive placebo (control patients). After an average time on study between 5 and 8 years, two patients in the placebo group and 24 in the tamoxifen group developed endometrial carcinoma.[78] A number of women in both groups had used estrogen replacement therapy for various periods of time, and the relative contribution of the estrogen therapy to the risk of endometrial carcinoma in these women is unknown. The hazard rate in the placebo group was 0.2 per 1000 women compared with 1.6 per 1000 women in the tamoxifen group (relative risk = 7.5). Occurrences of endometrial carcinoma in the placebo group subsequent to the initial publication of the study have lowered the estimated relative risk to approximately 4.0. Endometrial sampling and abdominal or vaginal ultrasound examination of the endometrium before and during tamoxifen therapy are currently being investigated for their ability to detect early malignancy and to lower the chance of dying of endometrial cancer after exposure to tamoxifen.

Breast cancer patients enrolled in clinical trials may be different in many ways from healthy women in the population who might use tamoxifen for primary prevention of breast cancer. Population-based studies of breast cancer patients who have used tamoxifen for less than two years show a 50% reduction in the risk of contralateral breast cancer and no increase in the risk of either ovarian or endometrial cancer.[79] Such studies also show a twofold risk of endometrial cancer with cumulative tamoxifen doses greater than 15 grams (i.e., 2 years of 20 mg daily).[80] The effect of prolonged administration of tamoxifen to healthy women can only be addressed in a clinical trial.

CLINICAL TRIALS OF TAMOXIFEN AS ADJUVANT THERAPY FOR BREAST CANCER

The most compelling evidence for the chemopreventive or chemosuppressive actions of tamoxifen in breast cancer derives from observations on the occurrence of second primary breast tumors on women participating in clinical trials of adjuvant therapy. An unexpected but important observation from these trials is the reduction in the incidence of contralateral breast cancer in the patients receiving tamoxifen. The largest of these trials is NSABP protocol B-14, which began in 1982 and randomized 2892 women to either placebo or tamoxifen twice a day for at least 5 years.[81] Although distinction between secondary, primary cancers and metastatic lesions of the contralateral breast is not always possible, it has previously been demonstrated that most are second malignancies.[82] Women taking tamoxifen adjuvant therapy in the B-14 trial experienced approximately one third fewer second primary breast tumors as women taking placebo (2.4% vs 1.6%).

A comprehensive assessment of the ability of tamoxifen to prevent second primary breast tumors is found in the overview of the world's literature on tamoxifen as adjuvant therapy for breast cancer,[74] where there are more than 18,000 women for whom information about contralateral second primary breast cancers is available. At the time of the publication, there were 42 reported randomized comparisons of tamoxifen and placebo. Among the 9135 women who received placebo in these trials, 184 (2.0%) developed contralateral second primary breast cancers compared with 122 (1.3%) second breast cancers among 9128 women who received tamoxifen adjuvant therapy for a median of 2 years. The 35% relative reduction in the risk (2.0–1.3/2.0) or 39% reduction in the actuarial odds of a second primary breast cancer varied with the duration of tamoxifen adjuvant therapy. Among those women who received less than two years of adjuvant therapy, the reduction on the odds was only 26%, compared with 37% among those women with exactly two years of therapy and 56% for the women who received more than two years of adjuvant tamoxifen therapy.

RETINOIDS

More that 1500 derivatives of vitamin A called retinoids have been synthesized, and extensive laboratory and clinical investigations have been carried out using retinoids for the prevention of carcinogenesis. Rat mammary cancers can be induced either by 7,12-dimethylbenz [a] anthracene (DMBA) or N-methyl-N-nitrosourea (MNU), and retinoids increase the latency of first tumor appearance in the rat model. Minor alterations in basic retinoid structures significantly alter the activity of the molecule. The chemopreventive effect of retinoids in breast cancer suggests that breast cancer cells may express retinoic acid receptors, and may be the biomolecular basis for the increased ability of retinoids to inhibit breast cancer cell growth.[83] Retinoids effectively alter the growth of hormone-independent cell populations. Whether retinoids preferentially suppress the growth of hormone-independent cell populations, reverse the neoplastic potential of these cells, or induce terminal differentiation of these cells is not yet known.

Retinyl acetate and the synthetic retinoid N-(4-hydroxyphenyl)-retinamide (4-HPR, fenretinide) are effective inhibitors of chemically induced breast cancer in rats.[84] Fenretinide reduces the incidence and time to appearance of these tumors, and doses up to 200 mg daily with a 3-day drug holiday monthly can be administered chronically to humans without significant toxicity. The effect of fenretinide is enhanced in rats by oophorectomy, but the drug does not affect circulating levels of estradiol, testosterone, dihydroepiandrosterone sulfate, prolactin, luteinizing hormone, follicle-stimulating hormone, or SHBG.

Retinoids induce the synthesis of transforming growth factor-β, a growth factor that negatively modulates cancer growth, and they lower the levels of insulin-like growth factor-I, a potent mitogen for transformed breast epithelium, in both breast cancer cell lines and breast cancer patients.[85]

Retinoids other than 4-HPR have activity in preventing breast cancer in animal carcinogenesis experiments. The retinoid 9-cis-retinoic acid has affinity for both the RXR and RAR families of retinoid receptors, and it is effective in reducing tumor incidence in a rat MNU carcinogenesis model.[86] The combination of 9-cis retinoic acid and tamoxifen is more effective than the retinoid alone, suggesting that the combination may allow reduction in tamoxifen dose to reduce tamoxifen-related side effects while maintaining chemopreventive effectiveness.

TAMOXIFEN AND FENRETINIDE

Animal studies show that 4-HPR can enhance the tumor suppressive action of tamoxifen[87,88] and suggest a more efficient action of combined 4-HPR and tamoxifen administration compared to the action of either agent alone.[89] In female rats, 4-HPR and bilateral oophorectomy inhibit mammary cancer induction synergistically. In virgin rats, exposure to 4-HPR or tamoxifen alone reduces mammary cancer multiplicity and increases the time to development of mammary tumors compared with controls. Combined administration of tamoxifen and 4-HPR results in enhanced inhibition of mammary carcinogenesis and causes a significant reduction in tumor-related mortality.[88] This suggests that retinoid administration may provide a means to increase the efficacy of hormonal manipulation in breast cancer prevention. Furthermore, the data suggest that the preventive activity of 4-HPR is not mediated through an effect on estrogen synthesis, release, or activity. Ovarian factors may modulate retinoid activity in mammary tissue in the rat in that the effect of 4-HPR plus tamoxifen is different than the effect of 4-HPR and ovariectomy.

CLINICAL TRIALS IN CHEMOPREVENTION OF BREAST

The Breast Cancer Prevention Trial

Because the lifetime probability of developing breast cancer is large among women with heritable cancer risk as well as among women with other known epidemiological risk factors for breast cancer, there is considerable interest in identifying agents that can reduce this risk by employing the mechanism of prospective clinical trials. The National Cancer Institute, in collaboration with the NSABP, a large clinical trials cooperative group, launched the Breast Cancer Prevention Trial (BCPT) in 1992 to evaluate the ability of tamoxifen to prevent breast cancer in women at increased risk.[70] Women eligible for the trial were either older than 60 years at entry, were age 35 or older with a breast biopsy showing lobular carcinoma *in situ*, or were between the ages of 35 and 59 years with an estimated annual risk for developing breast cancer equal to that of a 60 year-old woman. Risk was estimated using the model developed by Gail and his colleagues[90] that was validated by Bondy,[91] Spiegelman,[92] and their colleagues. This model considers current age, ages at menarche and first live birth, number of first-degree relatives with breast cancer, and the number of breast biopsies ever done. A previous diagnosis of atypical hyperplasia doubles the estimated risk, and there are interaction terms for age and the number of breast biopsies, and for family history and the age at first live birth. Hormone replacement therapy for menopausal symptoms was not permitted during the trial, although former users of replacement therapy were eligible to participate after stopping hormones for 90 days.

The BCPT enrolled 13,388 women at more than 300 clinical sites in the United States and Canada through 1997, and was stopped by its data monitoring committee in early 1998 because of an observed benefit. Preliminary results were provided to participants in the trial and to the study's principal investigators in early April 1998 prior to publication of the study's results. Among the participants, 40% were between the ages 35–49 at enrollment; 30%, between 50 and 59 years; and 30%, 60 years or older. Mean follow-up time through March 1998 was 3.5 years, and 57% of participants were followed for 4 or more years. Among 6707 women receiving placebo in the trial there were 154 invasive breast cancers and 59 non-invasive breast cancers compared with 85 invasive and 31 non-invasive breast cancers among 6681 women taking tamoxifen. The 5-year cumulative hazard rate for invasive breast cancer in the placebo group was 32 per 1000 while it was only 17.9 per 1000 among the women taking tamoxifen. Overall, this represents a 45% reduction in the risk of invasive breast cancer among the women taking tamoxifen, and all age groups benefited. The benefit was greater, however, in the older group of women (age > 60 years at entry); they experienced a 53% reduction in the incidence of breast cancer, compared to women aged 49 years or younger, in whom only a 35% reduction was observed. Non-invasive breast cancers were also reduced by tamoxifen with 59 incident cases of ductal carcinoma *in situ* (DCIS) observed in the placebo group but only 31 cases of DCIS observed in the tamoxifen group.

The results of the BCPT have been published,[93] but no data are yet available regarding the efficacy of tamoxifen among women with heritable risk for breast cancer. In the entire participant group, 30% had no first-degree relatives with breast cancer, 55% had only one affected relative, and 15% had two or more affected relatives. Because all of these women have heritable risk for developing breast cancer, and some have high probabilities of harboring mutations in breast cancer susceptibility genes, the trial investigators will perform genetic testing in all cases of breast cancer and in selected controls to determine the efficacy of tamoxifen in preventing breast cancer in carriers of mutations in either the *BRCA1* or *BRCA2* genes.

Tamoxifen is a drug with both estrogen agonist and estrogen antagonist properties.[93] Reflecting this fact is the observation in BCPT that there was a significant reduction in hip fractures and a non-significant reduction in the number of fractures of the wrist and spine. Also consistent with the estrogenic properties of tamoxifen was a fourfold increase in the risk of endometrial carcinoma as well as a 41% increase in thrombotic events in postmenopausal women, including fatal and non-fatal stroke, transient ischemic attacks, pulmonary emboli, and deep venous thrombi. There was no difference between the treatment groups in the number of ischemic heart disease events observed, possibly due to the fact that less than one-third of trial participants were older than 60 years. Consistent with tamoxifen's estrogen antagonist role, on the other hand, is the observation that 24% of subjects taking tamoxifen discontinued therapy due to side effects that included hot flashes and gynecological symptoms.

TAMOXIFEN: MECHANISM OF ACTION IN HERITABLE BREAST CANCER

The use of tamoxifen for the primary prevention of breast cancer is now approved in the United States. The results of the BCPT are encouraging, especially because all age groups derived benefit. Critics of the trial argued at its inception that an antiestrogen could not benefit premenopausal women due to their endogenous high-estrogen environment. The empirical observation of reduction of breast cancer incidence among younger women in the trial raises interesting questions about the mechanisms of action of tamoxifen and similar antiestrogens. It is not yet known whether antiestrogens, or any chemoprevention drug, can prevent the development of malignancy in women with heritable risk. It does appear, however, that *BRCA1* acts, in part, as a tumor suppressor gene. This is suggested by the observation that reduction in *BRCA1* expression *in vitro* results in accelerated growth of breast and ovarian cell lines while over-expression of *BRCA1* results in inhibited growth.[94,95] The murine homologue of *BRCA1* is expressed at highest levels in rapidly proliferating cells such as the breast during puberty and pregnancy, and expression of *BRCA1* is regulated in a cell cycle-dependent fashion with peak mRNA protein produced at the G1/S transition. *BRCA1* also serves as a substrate for certain cyclin-dependent kinases.

It is known, too, that estradiol induces *BRCA1* through an increase in DNA synthesis suggesting that *BRCA1* may serve as a negative modulator of estradiol-induced growth.[96] The kinetics and magnitude of this induction are different from the estradiol gene pS2 in that *de novo* protein synthesis is required, but resemble the growth induced by either insulin-like growth factor 1 (IGF-1) or epidermal growth factor (EGF). *BRCA1* genomic fragments near the 5′ end fail to respond to estradiol when transfected into breast cancer cell lines. Like *BRCA1*, *BRCA2* expression in the breast is induced during puberty and pregnancy and following treatment with estradiol and progesterone. In multiple fetal and adult tissues, the temporal expression of *BRCA2* mRNA is indistinguishable from *BRCA1*,[94,97] and it appears that both *BRCA1* and *BRCA2* expression may be regulated by similar pathways. Expression of both genes is differentially regulated by hormones during the development of specific target tissues, but the up-regulation of mRNA expression in the breast by ovarian steroid hormones is greater for *BRCA1* than for *BRCA2*. Together, these data suggest that in women who carry mutations in either BRCA1 or 2 that predispose to the development of malignancy, the absence of the negative regulatory role of intact *BRCA1* and *BRCA2* molecules may still be abrogated by the negative modulation of estradiol and other estrogens and by selective estrogen response modulators such as tamoxifen and raloxifene. Additional clinical and laboratory studies will address this fascinating preventive hypothesis.

Other Agents

Several investigators have conducted a pilot trial of ovarian steroid suppression using leuprolide acetate depot as the gonadotropin releasing hormone agonist along with replacement doses of conjugated estrogen and medroxyprogesterone acetate to eliminate the hypoestrogenic side effects of the gonadotropin-releasing hormone agonist.[98] Symptoms with this regimen are tolerable, but loss of bone density in the lumbar spine necessitates addition of an androgen to the regimen. Favorable changes in mammographic density have been reported with this regimen, but it is not known whether this approach will result in the predicted lowering of the risk of breast cancer. It is certainly too early to apply this prevention strategy outside the context of a clinical trial.

A prospective clinical trial is being conducted in Italy to investigate the ability of 4-HPR to reduce the incidence of second primary breast cancers in women with a first breast cancer.[99] Eligible women are 35 to 65 years old with T1 or T2 primary breast cancers, negative axillary lymph nodes, and no evidence of distant disease who did not receive either adjuvant endocrine therapy or chemotherapy. The results of that study will be important for many obvious reasons, as is the observation in rats that tamoxifen and 4-HPR result in enhanced inhibition of mammary carcinogenesis and reduction in tumor-related mortality.[89] If both retinoids and tamoxifen are shown individually to prevent breast cancer in women, additional clinical trials of combination therapy will be warranted.

Retinoids also hold great promise as primary preventive agents. A clinical trial to prevent second breast malignancies is being conducted in Italy using the synthetic retinoid 4-hydroxy phenylretinamide (4-HPR).[100] Eligible women are those with stage 1 or 2 invasive breast cancer. After they completed primary and adjuvant therapy for their breast cancer, 2972 women were randomly assigned to receive either 4-HPR at a dose of 200 mg per day or placebo. A three-day drug holiday was given monthly to prevent night blindness. The primary outcome of interest was the development of second contralateral primary breast malignancies. Preliminary data with a median follow-up of 65 months are shown in Table 1. It is of interest that a benefit was observed only for premenopausal women in the preliminary analyses, but results of additional observation time are pending. Final results should be available shortly. The benefit, if one exists, in women with heritable cancer risks has not been reported.

The next large-scale trial for primary prevention of breast cancer in the United States will compare tamoxifen with the second-generation selective estrogen response modulator (SERM) raloxifene. The trial, which began in 1999, is projected to require 22,000 postmenopausal women. Plans for an evaluation of the effect of raloxifene or other SERMs on heritable cancer risk have not been announced.

Table 1. Incidence of Second Primary Breast Cancers in a Randomized Clinical Trial of 4-Hydroxy Phenylretinamide (4-HPR) in Italian Women with Stage 1 or 2 Breast Cancer

Menopausal Status	Follow-up Period	Number of Second Primary Breast Cancers Treatment Group 4-HPR	Control	Total Number	Hazard Rate (95% Confidence Interval)
	Active therapy plus observation post-therapy				
Premenopause		19	33	52	0.59 (0.33–1.04)
Postmenopause		28	18	46	1.62 (0.87–3.01)
	Active therapy only				
Premenopause		12	26	38	0.53
Postmenopause		15	14	39	1.16

From Veronesi U, DePaolo G, Costa A. In: The Proceedings of the Ninth International Congress on Breast Diseases, Houston, Texas, 1996, p. 118.

ETHICAL ISSUES IN CLINICAL CHEMOPREVENTION TRIALS

Chemoprevention is not yet the standard of care in managing heritable risk for malignancy. The standard will be defined gradually as clinical trials such as those described above are completed. Despite a long and rich history in biomedical ethics, the normative assumptions associated with clinical trials in chemoprevention have not yet been defined.[101] The associated issues are complicated because these trials occur at the intersection between disease management and health promotion. There are competing interests between the clinical research that is chemoprevention and values of both investigators as they relate to the risks and benefits of the trial. Participants are not typical patients; rather, they are healthy research subjects. Treatment or cure is one goal among many, and the interests of physician researchers may conflict with subjects' interests. This may be an issue of even greater weight when the subjects in the trial have heritable cancer risks.

In chemoprevention clinical trials, risks will be incurred by individuals, but benefits will be accrued in the aggregate, not individually. Furthermore, the risk/benefit equations in these trials have not been well defined. It seems evident that non-medical values must be weighed equally with medical values, and that individuals differ in the priorities they assign to avoiding a particular disease or to the disutility they attribute to being ill. Further complicating the assessment of risks and benefits is the reality that the subjects often have no therapeutic relationship with the investigator conducting the chemoprevention research. Particularly germane to trials involving subjects with heritable cancer risk is the recognition that recruiting family members as trial participants raises issues of confidentiality for index cases. Finally, prior to the identification of effective agents for the prevention of malignancy, there were substantial ethical issues related to the use of placebos in chemoprevention clinical trials. With several potent chemoprevention agents now available, future trials are obligated to compare new

Table 2. "Preventive Ethics" Strategies in Chemoprevention Clinical Trials

- Inform subjects in stages of increasingly detailed information
- Do not record initial offers of participation in prevention clinical trials in the medical record
- Inform prospective participants about psychological, economic, and health-related risks of participating in the trial
- Inform subjects of the dual roles of the physician-researcher who is both a care provider and an investigator with global goals that may differ from personal care interests of the subjects
- Advise subjects of new developments as they arise in the course of the trial through a process of renewed consent forms or written advisories
- Counsel subjects that they may decide to leave the trial without adverse consequences
- Enlist an independent data monitoring board comprised of individuals with no scientific, personal, or commercial interest in the trial's outcome to examine the data periodically

adapted from Vogel VG, Parker LS. Ethical issues of chemoprevention clinical trials. Cancer Control 4:142–149, 1997. Used by permission.

agents to drugs with known efficacy. An interim preventive ethics strategy is outlined in Table 2. Clinicians and counselors who manage subjects with heritable cancer risk can anticipate rapid and multiple developments in this field as additional agents are evaluated in prospective clinical trials.

CLINICAL CHEMOPREVENTION TRIAL DESIGN ISSUES IN HERITABLE BREAST CANCER

The initiation of a trial design to prevent breast cancer in women with heritable risk must be preceded by a clear statement of the objectives and endpoint of the trial. The trial must be feasible based on the availability of a suitable drug, and the ability to identify and recruit subjects who are eligible for the trial. This is challenging among women who are mobile over a period of time. The timing of such a trial is crucial. For example, now that raloxifene has been approved by the Food and Drug Administration for the prevention of osteoporosis, it may be difficult to enroll subjects who are at risk of breast cancer into a prospective trial to assess the ability of raloxifene to prevent breast cancer because eligible subjects may not be willing to be randomly assigned to an agent other than raloxifene in such a trial. If eligible subjects realize that they can receive raloxifene under the pretense of preventing osteoporosis, a thorough evaluation of the drug's ability to prevent breast cancer may not be possible. The duration of such a trial must also be considered. Even among women with heritable risk for breast cancer, the breast cancer incidence rate is only about 1 to 2 cases per hundred women per year. In order to adequately evaluate the ability of a chemopreventive agent to prevent breast cancer, and to adequately evaluate toxicity, the trial will probably continue for five years or longer. This requirement places burdens on both subjects and investigators—or patients and their physicians—once acceptable agents for primary chemoprevention become widely available. Chemoprevention clinical trials also raise issues of generalizability because it is likely that subjects who volunteer to participate may have risk profiles that are different from subjects at usual risk, even those subjects with usual heritable risk.

All of these considerations raise the need for endpoints other than the development of invasive malignancy, but such endpoints have not been identified and validated

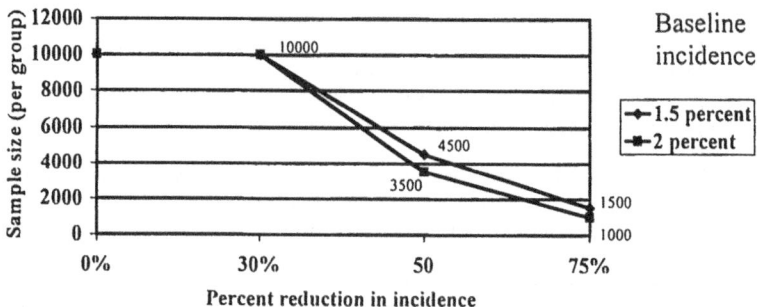

Figure 1. Sample size for a chemoprevention clinical trial of hereditary breast cancer.

for the important heritable cancer syndromes. Finally, there are issues of sample size to be considered. Figure 1 shows an example of a hypothetical chemoprevention clinical trial among women with heritable cancer risk. Two assumptions are shown in the figure. The upper line shows the sample size requirement if invasive breast cancer develops among 1.5 percent of the subjects at risk each year. The lower line shows the sample size requirements if the event rate is 2 percent of the subjects per year. The horizontal axis shows 3 different possibilities for the agent under study to reduce the risk of developing invasive breast cancer, varying from 25 percent to 75 percent, with power held constant at 0.80. The figure clearly shows that the major determinant of the sample size in such a prospective trial is not the event rate, but rather the ability of the agent to reduce the incidence of invasive breast cancer. It is obvious that a highly effective agent will be demonstrated to be effective with substantially fewer subjects in a prospective clinical trial.

LIMITATIONS OF PRIMARY PREVENTION IN INDIVIDUALS WITH HERITABLE CANCER RISK

Evaluating candidate agents for the primary prevention of malignancy is a challenge. The available interventions remain somewhat empirical, because the functional role of the genes is not yet fully understood. In addition, the details of the mechanism of action of the agents remain to be fully described. It is conceivable that these actions may be mutation-specific, and that different agents will be required for different inherited mutations. Importantly, the long-term toxicity of the available agents is not fully described, although a number of trials are under way to provide this important information. Finally, the optimal evaluation of candidate primary prevention agents is dependent upon genetic testing, a procedure that is not yet in widespread use because of the complex, ethical, legal, and social implications of the testing described elsewhere in this book. Ongoing and future investigations will better define both the ideal agents and the proper design of clinical trials for their investigation.

REFERENCES

1. Sporn MB, Dunlop NM, Newton DL, et al.: Prevention of chemical carcinogenesis by vitamin A and its synthetic analogs (retinoids). Fed Proc 35:1332–1338, 1976

2. Lippman SM, Benner SE, Hong WK: Cancer chemoprevention. J Clin Oncol 12:851–873, 1994
3. Lippman SM, Hong WK, Benner SE: The chemoprevention of cancer, in Greenwald P, Kramer BS, Weed DL (eds): Cancer Prevention and Control. New York, Marcel Dekker, pp 329–352, 1995
4. Russo J, Russo IH: Development of the human mammary gland, in Neville MD, Daniel C (eds): The Mammary Gland. New York, Plenum Publishing Inc, pp 67–93, 1987
5. Vorher H: The Breast. New York, Academic Press, pp 1–18, 1974
6. Russo IH, Koszalka M, Russo J: Human chorionic gonadotropin and rat mammary cancer prevention. J Natl Cancer Inst 82:1286–1289, 1990
7. Russo IH, Russo J: Hormone prevention of mammary carcinogenesis: a new approach in anticancer research. Anticancer Res 8:1247–1264, 1988
8. Russo J, Reina D, Frederick J, et al: Expression of phenotypical changes by human breast epithelial cells treated with carcinogens in vitro. Cancer Res 48:2837–2857, 1988
9. Russo J, Mills MJ, Moussalli MJ, et al: Influence of human breast development of the growth properties of primary cultures. In Vitro Cell Dev Biol 25:643–649, 1989
10. Russo J, Russo IH: Biological and molecular bases of mammary carcinogenesis. Lab Invest 57:112–137, 1987
11. Russo IH, Calaf G, Russo J: Hormones and proliferative activity in breast tissue, in Stoll BA (ed): Approaches to Breast Cancer Prevention. Dordrecht, Kluwer Academic Publishers, pp 35–51, 1990
12. Russo IH, Russo J: Chorionic gonadotropin: a tumoristatic and preventive agent in breast cancer, in Teicher BA (ed): Drug Resistance in Oncology. New York, Marcel Dekker, Inc, pp 537–560, 1992
13. Longacre TA, Bartow SA: A correlative morphologic study of human breast and endometrium in the menstrual cycle. Am J Surg Pathol 10:382–393, 1986
14. Potten CS, Watson RJ, Williams CT, et al: The effect of age and menstrual cycle upon proliferative activity of the normal human breast. Br J Cancer 58:163–168, 1988
15. Anderson TJ, Battersby S, Kiing RJ, et al: Oral contraceptive use influences breast proliferation. Hum Pathol 20:1139–1144, 1989
16. Henderson BE, Ross RK, Pike MC, et al: Endogenous hormones as a major factor in human cancer. Cancer Res 42:3232–3239, 1982
17. Russo J, Russo IH: Toward a physiological approach to breast cancer prevention. Cancer Epidemiol Biomarkers Prev 3:353–364, 1994
18. Henderson BE, Ross RK, Pike MC: Hormonal chemoprevention of cancer in women. Science 259:633–638, 1993
19. Kelsey JL: A review of the epidemiology of human breast cancer. Epidemiol Rev 1:74–109, 1979
20. Petrakis NL, Ernster VL, King MC: Breast, in Schottenfeld D, Fraumeni JF, Jr (eds): Cancer Epidemiology and Prevention. Philadelphia, W B Saunders, p 855–870, 1982
21. Hirayama T, Wynder E: Study of epidemiology of cancer of the breast: influence of hysterectomy. Cancer 15:28–38, 1962
22. Mac Mahon B: Breast cancer in relation to nursing and menopausal history. J Natl Cancer Inst 24:733–753, 1960
23. Furr BJ, Jordan VC: The pharmacology and clinical uses of tamoxifen. Pharmacol Ther 25:127–205, 1984
24. Nicholson RI, Gotting KE, Gee J, et al: Actions of oestrogens and anti-oestrogens on rat mammary gland development: relevance to breast cancer prevention. Journal of Steroid Biochemistry 30:95–103, 1988
25. Gotze S, Nishino Y, Neumann F: Anti-oestrogenic effects of tamoxifen on mammary gland and hypophysis in female rats. Acta Endocrinol [Copenhagen] 105:360–370, 1984
26. Walker KJ, Price-Thomas JM, Candlish W, et al: Influence of the antiestrogen tamoxifen on normal breast tissue. Br J Cancer 64:764–768, 1991
27. Buckley MM, Goa KL: Tamoxifen: A reappraisal of its pharmacodynamic and pharmacokinetic properties, and therapeutic use. Drugs 37:4591–4490, 1989
28. Jordan VC, Murphy CS: Endocrine pharmacology of antiestrogens as antitumor agents. Endocr Rev 11:578–610, 1990
29. Herrlinger C, Braunfels N, Fine E, et al: Pharmacokinetics and bioavailability of tamoxifen in healthy volunteers. Int J Pharmacol Ther Toxicol 30:487–489, 1992
30. Adam HK: Pharmacokinetic studies with Nolvadex. Reviews on endocrine-related cancer [suppl] 9:131–143, 1981
31. Jordan VC: Chemosuppression of breast cancer with long-term tamoxifen therapy. Prev Med 20:3–14, 1991

32. Briziarelli G: Effects of dosage and time of administration of testosterone propionate on 7,12-dimethylbenzanthracene mammary carcinogenesis in the rat. Z Krebsforsch Klin Onkol 66:517–522, 1965

33. Terenius L: Effect of anti-estrogens on initiation of mammary cancer in the female rat. Eur J Cancer 7:65–70, 1971

34. Jordan VC: Antitumor activity of the antiestrogen ICI 46,474 (tamoxifen) in the dimethylbenzanthracene (DMBA)-induced rat mammary carcinoma model. Journal of Steroid Biochemistry 5:354, 1974

35. Jordan VC: Effect of tamoxifen (ICI 46,474) on initiation and growth of DMBA-induced rat mammary carcinomata. Eur J Cancer 12:419–424, 1976

36. Dao TL: The role of ovarian hormones in initiating the induction of mammary cancer in rats by polynuclear hydrocarbons. Cancer Res 22:973–981, 1962

37. Tsai TLS, Katzenellenbogan BS: Antagonism of development and growth of 7,12-dimethylbenz(a)anthracene-induced rate mammary tumors by the antiestrogen U23,469 and effects on estrogen and progesterone receptors. Cancer Res 37:1537–1543, 1977

38. Jordan VC, Dix CJ, Allen KE: The effectiveness of long-term tamoxifen treatment in a laboratory model for adjuvant hormone therapy of breast cancer, in Jones SE, Slamon SE (eds): Adjuvant therapy of cancer II. New York, Gruen and Stratton, pp 19–26, 1979

39. Jordan VC, Allen KE: Evaluation of the antitumor activity of the nonsteroid antioestrogen monohydroxytanoxifen in the DMBA-induced rat mammary carcinoma model. Eur J Cancer 16:239–251, 1980

40. Jordan VC, Allen KE, Dix CJ: Pharmacology of tamoxifen in laboratory animals. Cancer Treat Res 64:745–759, 1980

41. Robinson SP, Mauel DA, Jordan VC: Antitumor actions of toremifene in the 7,12-dimethylbenzanthracene (DMBA)-induced rat mammary tumor model. Eur J Cancer Clin Oncol 24:1817–1821, 1988

42. Robinson SP, Jordan VC: Reversal of the antitumor effects of tamoxifen by progesterone in the 7,12-dimethylbenzanthracene-induced rat mammary carcinoma model. Cancer Res 47:5386–5390, 1987

43. Noguchi S, Motomura K, Inaji H, et al: Up-regulation of estrogen receptor by tamoxifen in human breast cancer. Cancer 71:1266–1272, 1993

44. Murphy LC, Sutherland RL: Antitumor activity of clomiphene analogs in vitro: relationship to affinity for the estrogen receptor and another high affinity antiestrogen-binding site. J Clin Endocrinol Metab 57:373–379, 1983

45. Jordan VC, Fritz NF, Tormey DC: Long term adjuvant therapy with tamoxifen: effects on sex hormone binding globulin and antithrombin III. Cancer Res 47:4517–4519, 1987

46. Berry J, Green BJ, Matheson DS: Modulation of natural killer cell activity by tamoxifen in state I postmenopausal breast cancer. Eur J Cancer Clin Oncol 23:517–520, 1987

47. Colletti:

48. Pollak MN, Huymk HT, Lefebre SP: Tamoxifen reduces serum insulin-like growth factor I (IGF-I). Breast Cancer Res Treat 22:91–100, 1992

49. Lonning PE, Hall K, Aakvaag A, et al: Influence of tamoxifen on plasma levels of insulin-like growth factor B and insulin-like growth factor binding protein I in breast cancer patients. Cancer Res 52:4719–4723, 1992

50. Friedl A, Jordan VC, Pollack M: Suppression of serum insulin-like growth factor-1 levels in breast cancer patients during adjuvant tamoxifen therapy. Eur J Cancer 29A:1368–1372, 1993

51. Morrow M, Jordan VC: Molecular mechanisms of resistance to tamoxifen therapy in breast cancer. Arch Surg 128:1187–1191, 1993

52. Giuffrida D, Lupo L, La Porta GA, et al: Relation between steroid receptor status and body weight in breast cancer patients. Eur J Cancer 28:112–115, 1992

53. Noguchi S, Motomura K, Inaji H, et al: Down regulation of transforming growth factor-α by tamoxifen in human breast cancer. Cancer 72:131–136, 1993

54. Wattenberg LW: Chemoprevention of cancer. Cancer Res 45:1–8, 1985

55. Welsh CW, Brown CK, Goodrich-Smith M, et al: Synergistic effect of chronic prolactin suppression and retinoid treatment in the prophylaxis of N-methyl-N-nitrosourea-induced mammary tumorigenesis in female Sprague-Dawley rats. Cancer Res 40:3095–3099, 1980

56. Willet WC, Hunter DJ, Stampfer MJ, et al: Dietary fat and fiber in relation to the risk of breast cancer: an eight-year follow-up. JAMA 268:2037–2044, 1992

57. Ziegler RG, Hoover RN, Nomura AMY, et al: Relative weight, weight change, height, and breast cancer risk in Asian-American women. J Natl Cancer Inst 88:650–660, 1996
58. Windler E, Kovanen PT, Chao YS, et al: The estradiol stimulated lipoprotein receptor of rat liver: a binding site that mediates uptake of rat lipoproteins containing apoproteins B and E. J Biol Chem 255:10464–10471, 1980
59. Stacls B, Anwer J, Chan L, et al: Influence of development, estrogens, and food intake on apolipoprotein A-I, A-III, and E in RNA in rat liver and intestine. J Lipid Res 30:1137–1147, 1989
60. Bush T, Fried LP, Barrett-Connor E: Cholesterol, lipoprotein, and coronary heart disease in women. Clin Chem 34:60–70, 1988
61. Yusuf SA, Wittes J, Friedman L: Overview of results of randomized clinical trials in heart disease. II. Unstable angina, heart failure, primary prevention with aspirin and risk factor modification. JAMA 260:2259–2263, 1988
62. Love RR, Wiebe DA, Newcomb PA, et al: Effects of tamoxifen on cardiovascular risk factors in postmenopausal women. Ann Intern Med 115:860–864, 1991
63. Kannel WB, Wolf PA, Castelli WP, et al: Fibrinogen and risk of cardiovascular disease. JAMA 258:1183–1186, 1987
64. Hoffman CJ, Miller RH, Lawson WE, et al: Elevation of factor VII activity and mass in young adults at risk of ischemic heart disease. J Am Coll Cardiol 14:941–946, 1989
65. Cuzick J, Allen D, Baum M, et al: Long-term effects of tamoxifen–Biological Effects of Tamoxifen Working Party. Eur J Cancer 29:15–21, 1993
66. Love RR, Mazess RB, Borden HS, et al: Effects of tamoxifen on bone mineral density in postmenopausal women with breast cancer. N Engl J Med 326:852–856, 1992
67. Kristensen B, Ejlertsen B, Dalgaard P, et al: Tamoxifen and bone metabolism in post-menopausal low-risk breast cancer patients: a randomized study. J Clin Oncol 12:992–997, 1994
68. Stewart PJ, Stern PH: Effects of the antiestrogens tamoxifen and clomiphene on bone resorption in vitro. Endocrinology 118:125–131, 1986
69. Powles TJ, Hickish TF, Kanis JA, et al: Tamoxifen preserves bone mineral density in post-menopausal women but causes loss of bone density in premenopausal women. Proceedings of the American Society of Clinical Oncology, p 165
70. Nayfield SG, Karp JE, Ford LG, et al: Potential role of tamoxifen in prevention of breast cancer. J Natl Cancer Inst 83:1450–1459, 1991
71. Rutqvist LE, Mattson A: Cardiac and thromboembolic morbidity among postmenopausal women with early-stage breast cancer in a randomized trial of adjuvant tamoxifen. J Natl Cancer Inst 85:1398–1406, 1993
72. Fornander T, Rutvqvist LE, Cedermark B, et al: Adjuvant tamoxifen in early breast cancer: occurrence of new primary cancers. Lancet 1:117–120, 1989
73. Rutqvist LE, Johansson H, Signomklao T, et al: Adjuvant tamoxifen therapy for early stage breast cancer and second primary malignancy. J Natl Cancer Inst 87:645–651, 1995
74. Early Breast Cancer Trialists' Collaborative Group. Systemic treatment of early breast cancer hormonal, cytotoxic, or immune therapy. Lancet 339:1–15, 1992
75. Fornander T, Hellstrom AC, Moberger B: Descriptive clinicopathological study of 17 patients with endometrial cancer during or after adjuvant tamoxifen in early breast cancer. J Natl Cancer Inst 85:1850–1855, 1993
76. Andersson M, Storm HH, Mouridsen HT: Carcinogenic effects of adjuvant tamoxifen treatment and radiotherapy for early breast cancer. Acta Oncol 31:259–263, 1992
77. Andersson M, Storm HH, Mouridsen HT: Incidence of new primary cancers after adjuvant tamoxifen therapy and radiotherapy for early breast cancer. J Natl Cancer Inst 83:1013–1017, 1991
78. Fisher B, Costantino JP, Redmond CK, et al: Endometrial cancer in tamoxifen-treated breast cancer patients: findings from the National Surgical Adjuvant Breast and Bowel Project (NSABP) B-14. J Natl Cancer Inst 86:527–537, 1994
79. Cook LS, Weiss NS, Schwartz SM, et al: Population-based study of tamoxifen therapy and subsequent ovarian, endometrial, and breast cancer. J Natl Cancer Inst 87:1359–1364, 1995
80. van Leeuwen FE, Benraadt J, Coebergh JW, et al: Risk of endometrial cancer after tamoxifen treatment of breast cancer. Lancet 343:448–452, 1994
81. Fisher B, Costantino J, Redmond C, et al: A randomized clinical trial evaluating tamoxifen in patients with node-negative breast cancer who have estrogen receptor-positive tumors. N Engl J Med 320:479–484, 1989

82. Fisher ER, Fisher B, Sass R, et al: Pathological findings from the National Surgical Adjuvant Breast Project (Protocol no. 4). XI bilateral breast cancer. Cancer 54:3002–3011, 1984

83. Roman SD, Clarke CL, Hall RE, et al: Expression and regulation of retinoic acid receptors in human breast cancer cells. Cancer Res 52:2236–2242, 1992

84. Vogel VG, Lippman SM, Boyd N: Is breast cancer preventable? Can J Oncol 1:28–37, 1991

85. Torrisi R, Pensa F, Orengo MA, et al: The synthetic retinoid fenretinide lowers plasma insulin-like growth factor I levels in breast cancer patients. Cancer Res 53:4769–4771, 1993

86. Anzaro MA, Byeu SW, Smith JM, et al: Prevention of breast cancer in the rat with 9-cis-retinoic acid as a single agent and in combination with tamoxifen. Cancer Res 54:4614–4617, 1994

87. Secreto G, Costa A, Recchione C, et al: The synthetic retinoid Fenretinide does not effect circulating hormone concentrations. Breast Cancer Res Treat 12:315–316, 1988

88. McCormick DL, Moon RC: Retinoid-tamoxifen interaction in mammary cancer chemoprevention. Carcinogenesis 7:193–196, 1986

89. Ratco TA, Detrisac CJ, Dinger NM, et al: Chemopreventive efficacy of combined retinoid and tamoxifen treatment following surgical excision of a primary cancer in female rats. Cancer Res 48:4472–4476, 1989

90. Gail MH, Brinton LA, Byar DP, et al: Projecting individualized probabilities of developing breast cancer for white females who are being examined annually. J Natl Cancer Inst 81:1879–1886, 1989

91. Bondy ML, Lustbader ED, Halabi S, et al: Validation of a breast cancer risk assessment model in women with a positive family history. J Natl Cancer Inst 86:620–625, 1994

92. Spiegelman D, Colditz GA, Hunter D, et al: Validation of the Gail et al. model predicting individual breast cancer risk. J Natl Cancer Inst 86:600–607, 1994

93. Fisher B, Costantino JP, Wickerham DL, et al: Tamoxifen for prevention of breast cancer: Report of the National Surgical Adjuvant Breast and Bowel Project P-1 Study. J Natl Cancer Inst 90:1371–1388, 1998

94. Rajan JV, Marquis ST, Gardner HP, et al: Developmental expression of BRCA2 colocalizes with BRCA1 and is associated with proliferation and differentiation in multiple tissues. Dev Biol 184:385–401, 1997

95. Lane TF, Deng C, Elson A, et al: Expression of BRCA1 is associated with terminal differentiation of ectodermally and mesodermally derived tissues in mice. Dev Biol 9:2712–2722, 1995

96. Marks JR, Huper G, Vaughn JP, et al: BRCA1 expression is not directly responsive to estrogen. Oncogene 14:115–121, 1997

97. Marquis ST, Rajan JV, Wynshaw-Boris A, et al: The developmental pattern of BRCA1 expression implies a role in differentiation of the breast and other tissues. Nat Genet 11:17–26, 1995

98. Spicer DV, Pike MC: Breast cancer prevention through modulation of endogenous hormones. Breast Cancer Res Treat 28:179–193, 1993

99. Costa A, Formelli F, Chiesa F, et al: Prospects of chemoprevention of human cancers with the synthetic retinoid fenretinide. Cancer Res 54:2032s–2037s, 1994

100. Veronesi U, DePalo G, Costa A, et al: Chemoprevention of breast cancer with fenretinide. IARC Scienficic Publications 136:87–94, 1996

101. Vogel VG, Parker LP: Ethical issues of chemoprevention clinical trials. Cancer Contr 4:142–149, 1997

10

GENETICS OF COLORECTAL CANCER

An Updated Review

Henry T. Lynch,* Jane F. Lynch,* Trudy G. Shaw,*
and Thomas C. Smyrk#

*Department of Preventive Medicine
  Creighton University School of Medicine
  2500 California Plaza, Omaha, Nebraska 68178
#Department of Pathology
  University of Nebraska Medical Center
  4350 Dewey Avenue, Omaha, Nebraska 68105

1. INTRODUCTION

The annual incidence of colorectal cancer (CRC) in the United States is approximately 131,600.[1] A positive family history is the most common risk factor for hereditary colon cancer (CRC).[2] If one accepts the most conservative estimate that 10% of CRC is hereditary, more than 13,000 of these CRC cases will have a hereditary etiology. The majority of hereditary CRC cases will be hereditary nonpolyposis colorectal cancer (HNPCC), although the exact frequency is not known. Estimates range from a low of about 2% to a high of 10–15% of the total CRC burden. The rare hereditary CRC disorders, such as familial adenomatous polyposis (FAP) and Peutz-Jeghers syndrome (PJS), account for less than 1% of all cases. Table 1 describes hereditary disorders that predispose to CRC. Advancing knowledge may aid in additional molecular genetic diagnoses for hereditary forms of cancer.

When an individual has one or more first-degree relatives with CRC, there will be a 2-to-3-fold empirical increased risk for this disease. This is referred to as "*familial* CRC".[3,4] The risk may increase if certain parameters known to associate with hereditary cancer are present. Factors that should be included as part of the family history assessment are early age of onset, multiple primary cancers with distinctive patterns of tumor combinations within syndromes, i.e. periampullary carcinoma and desmoid tumors in FAP, and variable extra-cancer phenotypic findings, i.e. mucocutaneous lesions in PJS. Finding Mendelian segregation of these clinical features in a family will

Cancer Genetics for the Clinician, edited by Shaw.
Kluwer Academic / Plenum Publishers, New York, 1999.

Table 1. Differential Diagnosis of Hereditary Colorectal Cancer

Hereditary Form of Colorectal Cancer (CRC)	Inheritance Pattern/Germline Mutation	Polyps	Cancer	Non-Cancer Features
Familial Adenomatous Polyposis (FAP)	AD; *APC* gene at chromosome 5q, distal to 5′	Adenomatous, often start in distal colon/rectum; usually >100; adenomas may occur in small bowel; gastric polyps common, usually fundic gland polyps	CRC, average age onset 39; many cases teens and twenties; cancer of small bowel; stomach (particularly in Japan), papillary thyroid cancer, periampullary carcinoma, sarcoma, brain tumor	Gardner's variant-epidermoid cysts of skin, osteomas of mandible, congenital hypertrophy of the retinal pigment epithelium. Desmoid tumors (intraabdominal) do not metastasize but may kill by direct extension; desmoids may be initiated by surgery (dissected surfaces); adrenal adenomas
Attenuated Familial Adenomatous Polyposis Coli (AFAP)	AD; *APC* gene at chromosome 5q, proximal to 5′	Ordinary adenomas but also flat adenomas with proximal colonic predominance; may be few (5–10), sometimes >100	CRC with average age onset at 50; occasional periampullary carcinoma	Fundic gland polyps in stomach; adenomas in duodenum
Turcot's Syndrome	AD; both FAP and HNPCC variants	Florid colonic adenomas, 50 to >100	CRC and central nervous system, particularly brain tumors. In *APC* (FAP families) cerebellar medulloblastomas. In *hMLH1* and *hPMS2* (HNPCC families) glioblastoma multiforme	Rare examples of multiple *café-au-lait* spots and pigmented nevi but not clear if truly integral to the syndrome
Ashkenazi Jewish I1307K mutation	AD; *APC* gene I1307K mutation	Occasional adenomatous colonic polyps	CRC, "young" but average age of onset not known	None known
Juvenile Polyposis Coli	AD; protein tyrosine phosphate gene (*PTEN*)	Diffuse hamartomatous, (may have adenomatous component) of colon, but may occur in small bowel and stomach	CRC	Children may manifest diarrhea (may be severe)

Screening	Surgical Management and/or Prophylaxis	Presymptomatic DNA Testing	Genetic Counseling
Baseline flexible sigmoidoscopy age 10–12; flexible sigmoidoscopy annually thereafter, for *APC* germline positive. If at risk but not tested for *APC*, same strategy. If eventually found to be *APC* negative, then baseline flexible sigmoidoscopy at age 15–20; if negative, no further screening. Upper endoscopy every 1–3 years starting when colonic polyps first appear. Screen remaining rectal segment after surgical prophylaxis	Prophylactic subtotal colectomy with low ileorectal anastomosis when phenotype (florid polyposis) identified; may consider rectal mucosectomy with ileal pouch anal anastomosis if too many rectal polyps to manage or if compliance for rectal segment follow-up is poor. Consider sulindac chemoprevention (while) reducing polyps, cancer may still occur)	Test for *APC* germline mutation as early as age 10–12	Initiate pre-teens, include parents
Colonoscopy and upper endoscopy, initiate at age 20 and annually for *APC* germline positive patients or every 2 years if at genetic risk but not tested for *APC*	Prophylactic subtotal colectomy if too many polyps to manage; consider chemo-preventive sulindac	Test for *APC* germline mutation at age 20	Initiate at age 20, include parents
Baseline flexible sigmoidoscopy age 10 to 12 and annual flexible sigmoidoscopy thereafter; consider CAT scan or MRI of brain	Prophylactic subtotal colectomy if colonic polyps present, as in FAP. In HNPCC variant, colonoscopy	Two DNA variants: 1) *APC* gene with predominance of cerebellar medulloblastoma. 2) *hMLH1* or *hPMS2*, with predominance of glioblastoma multiforme	Initiate age 10–12, include parents
Full colonoscopy, start at age 30–35 in gene carriers	Standard CRC surgery	Ashkenazi *APC* mutation	Start at age 25
Initiate colonoscopy age 10–12	Prophylactic subtotal colectomy when phenotype present with too many polyps to manage	Tyrosine phosphate gene (*PTEN*)	Initiate preteens, include parents

(continued)

Table 1. (*Continued*)

Hereditary Form of Colorectal Cancer (CRC)	Inheritance Pattern/Germline Mutation	Polyps	Cancer	Non-Cancer Features
Puetz-Jeghers Syndrome	AD; gene encoding serine threonine kinase (STK11) on chromosome 19p13.3	Peutz-Jeghers polyps (may have adenomatous features) in stomach, small bowel, and colon	Stomach, small bowel, colon, sex cord tumors of ovary and testes	Mucocutaneous melanin pigmentation
Discrete Colonic Adenomatous Polyps and CRC of Burt	AD; may be similar to some familial CRC	Occasional (never florid) adenomatous colonic polyps	CRC, average age in accord with population expectations	None known
Hereditary Nonpolyposis Colorectal Cancer (HNPCC)	AD; germline mutations of any of the mismatch repair genes: *hMSH2* at chromosome 2p; *hMLH1* at chromosome 3p; *hPMS1* at chromosome 2q; *hPMS2* at chromosome 7q	Occasional colonic adenomas which are on average larger, more villous, and at younger age than general population. Colonic polyps no more frequent than general population	CRC most common with proximal predominance, an excess of synchronous and metachronous CRC. Others include cancer of the endometrium, ovary, small bowel, stomach, and transitional cell carcinoma of ureter and renal pelvis. Average age of cancer onset is 44; may show rapid progression from adenoma to CRC	Muir-Torre syndrome variant shows cancer features of HNPCC but includes sebaceous adenomas, sebaceous epitheliomas, basal cell epitheliomas with sebaceous differentiation, meibomian gland carcinomas and sebaceous carcinomas; single or multiple keratoacanthomas
Familial CRC	Empirical risk 3 fold increase for CRC in patients with one or more first-degree relatives with CRC; likely multifactorial and/or low penetrant genes	In accord with population expectations	CRC, comparable to general population for age of onset and colonic location	None
Familial Ulcerative Colitis and Crohn's Disease	Unknown; possible AD in some families; polygenic also likely	Pseudopolyps (non-adenomatous)	CRC, lymphoma of GI tract	Arthritis, pyoderma gangrenosum, annular erythemas, and vascular thromboses, sclerosing cholangitis

Legend for Abbreviations.
AD—Autosomal Dominant.
CRC—Colorectal Cancer.
IBD—Inflammatory Bowel Disease.
Adapted with permission from Lynch et al., *Eur J Cancer 31A*:1039–1046, 1995.

Screening	Surgical Management and/or Prophylaxis	Presymptomatic DNA Testing	Genetic Counseling
Baseline colonoscopy and upper endoscopy, initiate age 20; flexible sigmoidoscopy annually thereafter	Consider prophylactic subtotal colectomy if too many polyps to manage and if mixed adenomatous features	Serine threonine kinase (STK11) on chromosome 19p13.3	Initiate teens, include parents
Initiate baseline flexible sigmoidoscopy at age 40 and every 3 years thereafter	Standard CRC surgical approach	None known	Initiate at age 25–30
Colonoscopy, initiate age 20–25, annually for germline mutation carriers; every other year when mutation studies are lacking; endometrial aspiration biopsy at the same time as colonoscopy	Subtotal colectomy for initial CRC; consider option of prophylactic subtotal colectomy for germline carriers; consider prophylactic total abdominal hysterectomy and bilateral salpingo-oophorectomy for patients with initial CRC who have completed their families	Test for germline mutations no earlier than age 18–20	Initiate at age 18, prior to any consideration for gene testing
Baseline flexible sigmoidoscopy at age 35, repeat every 3 years; if two first-degree relatives affected or one less than age 50 years, risk is 4–6 fold increased and full colonoscopy every 3–5 years is indicated	Standard surgical procedure for CRC	None	Initiate at age 30–35
Colonoscopy, annual in patients with chronic pancolitis of 8 or more years duration; check for high-grade dysplasia colonic mucosa	Subtotal colectomy for CRC; consider prophylactic subtotal colectomy for patients with persistent high-grade dysplasia of colonic mucosa; proctocolectomy if IBD mandates	None	Initiate at age 18–20

point heavily to a hereditary cancer syndrome. A syndrome diagnosis might then be confirmed beyond any doubt through molecular genetic finding of a culprit germ-line mutation.

This report will elucidate the role of primary genetic factors in CRC. Selected hereditary CRC prone disorders, inclusive of FAP, PJS, familial juvenile polyposis coli (FJP), and HNPCC will be described. Particular attention will be given to the molecular genetics of these disorders and their role in diagnosis and genetic counseling.

2. FAMILIAL ADENOMATOUS POLYPOSIS (FAP)

Bulow[5] has traced the history of FAP to a report in 1861 by Luschka[6] that "may have been FAP." However, the first definite example of a patient with multiple colonic polyposis was published in 1881 by Sklifasowski.[7] The first "familial" example was that of a brother and sister with FAP reported by Cripps[8] in 1882. Examples of CRC occurring in patients with FAP were reported by Smith in 1887.[9] Discussion of the histologic findings of the changes from adenoma to adenocarcinoma was first described by Handford.[10] Finally, Lockhart-Mummery[11] was the first to express the concern that the hereditary factor was not for cancer per se in this disease but, rather, for the presence of multiple adenomas because of their tendency to undergo malignant transformation. This report was in context with findings in the histories from 3 families and has formed the basis for the now-renowned St. Mark's Hospital Polyposis Registry in London, England. Much has been learned about FAP since these early historical accounts.

The principal diagnostic phenotypic feature of FAP is the presence of multiple colonic adenomas. Their pathology findings are consistent with tubular adenomas, although tubulovillous, villous, or hyperplastic colonic lesions may be present. Prophylactic proctocolectomy or subtotal colectomy with annual sigmoidoscopic examination follow-up of the remaining rectal-sigmoid segment is the primary cancer preventive approach to this disorder. Upper endoscopy with a side viewing duodenoscope for gastric and duodenal adenomas is recommended on a periodic basis, given the prominence of periampullary adenomas with an increased risk for periampullary carcinoma. In addition to CRC, integral cancers in FAP include papillary thyroid carcinoma, carcinoma of the stomach, small bowel, pancreas, adrenal cortex, and brain. Unfortunately, desmoid tumors may also occur. Desmoids may be precipitated by surgical intervention, as in prophylactic colectomy,[12] and is an example of genotypic predisposition and an environmental stimulus (surgical trauma) interacting with a genotypic predisposition.[13]

The responsible germ-line mutation (*APC* gene) for FAP has been identified on chromosome 5q.[14,15]

3. ATTENUATED FAMILIAL ADENOMATOUS POLYPOSIS (AFAP)

A variant of FAP characterized by a generally milder phenotype, aptly termed attenuated familial adenomatous polyposis (AFAP), has been described.[16] AFAP is characterized by fewer colonic adenomas, usually only several but in rare cases as many as 50 to 100, most of which are located in the *proximal* colon. Upper gastrointestinal lesions, particularly fundic gland polyps and duodenal adenomas, frequently are present. The colonic adenomas are often flat as opposed to polypoid. Colon cancer will occur in most patients with AFAP, but the age of onset is late (average age 55) as compared to its FAP counterpart where the average age of onset is 39. The *APC* gene is mutated in AFAP. Importantly, intragenic mutations proximal to 5' appear to be responsible for the more subtle phenotype, when compared to its more classical FAP variant where the intragenic mutations are distal to 5'.[17]

The clinical significance of AFAP is still emerging, given the fact that the disorder has only been recognized in the past several years.[16] Given the extreme difficulty in its clinical diagnosis, due in a major way to the subtle features of its colonic phenotype, the frequency of AFAP remains unknown. For example, when an individual patient has several adenomas, particularly located proximal to the splenic flexure, one might appropriately wonder whether that patient might manifest AFAP. If that individual has one or more first-degree relatives who also manifest occasional colonic adenomas, and CRC was diagnosed at an average age of 55, the confidence in the possibility of AFAP will be strengthened. Extension of that particular pedigree may shed further light on its diagnosis which can conceivably be confirmed through identification of one of AFAP's intragenic mutation sites within the large *APC* gene. Unfortunately, a patient with several colonic adenomas in the proximal colon rarely receives a genetic workup in the clinical practice setting. Thus, it is extremely unlikely that a true estimate of the frequency of AFAP will be attained short of an extensive research program.

4. PEUTZ-JEGHERS SYNDROME (PJS)

PJS is a rarely occurring, autosomal dominantly inherited cancer-associated genodermatosis. Its phenotype involves multiple mucocutaneous melanocytic macules of the oral and peri-oral cavity, gastrointestinal hamartomatous polyps which may occur throughout the gastrointestinal tract, and an increased frequency of neoplasms involving the gastrointestinal tract, inclusive of the duodenum, colorectum, and a distinctive ovarian tumor of sex cord-stromal origin (i.e., sex cord tumor with annular tubules).[18]

PJS is thought to have a frequency about one-tenth as common as FAP.[19] Hamartomatous polyps are most often present in the small bowel and are only slightly less common in the stomach and colon. They may range from a few to dozens. Giardiello and colleagues[20] observed that cancer in patients with PJS was 18 times greater than expected in the general population (p < 0.0001).

PJS has recently been mapped to a locus on chromosome 19p13.3.[21,22] Olschwang et al.[23] analyzed 20 PJS families. The majority were found to be consistent with a PJS gene on chromosome 19p13.3, but 3 of the families were unlinked. Interestingly, these authors could not find any obvious clinical, pathological, or ethnic differences between the 19p13.3-linked and the unlinked families. They concluded that, "There appears, therefore, to be a major PJS locus on chromosome 19p13.3 and the possibility exists of a minor locus (or loci) elsewhere."

Mehenni et al.[24] performed a genome-wide linkage analysis employing DNA polymorphisms from 6 PJS families from the United States, India, and Portugal. They were able to localize the PJS gene to 19p13.3 around the marker D19S886 in accord with prior reports for its location. However, these authors also identified markers on 19q13.4 which showed significant evidence for linkage. Specifically, ". . . D19S880 resulted in a maximum LOD score of 3.8 at θ = .13. Most of this positive linkage was contributed by a single family, PJS07. These results confirm the mapping of a common PJS locus on 19p13.3 but also suggest the existence, in a minority of families, of a potential second PJS locus, on 19q13.3. Positional cloning and characterization of the PJS mutations will clarify the genetics of the syndrome and the implication of the gene(s) in the predisposition to neoplasias."

Lynch et al.[18] suggest that screening of patients at risk for PJS should begin in the second decade and should include fecal occult blood testing and flexible sigmoidoscopy. Surveillance of the upper and lower gastrointestinal tract should occur every three years. "Gastric, duodenal and colonic polyps should be removed endoscopically. If surgical intervention is necessary, intraoperative endoscopy with polypectomy may prevent the development of a short bowel syndrome."[18]

5. FAMILIAL JUVENILE POLYPOSIS COLI (FJP)

Sporadic juvenile hamartomatous polyps of the colon are not uncommon (manifested in perhaps 1% of children). These sporadic polyps do not appear to have an increased risk of CRC.[25] Conversely, the familial variant of juvenile polyposis *does* have significant colonic cancer consequences for affected individuals. The diagnosis may be difficult since an affected individual in the familial variant may have only a few juvenile polyps while, on the other hand, sporadic, innocuous juvenile polyps may be multiple. It may be particularly difficult to rule out FAP when biopsy samples are taken of only one or two colonic polyps and they happen to contain dysplastic areas. Hence, when patients harbor multiple colonic polyps it will be prudent to sample many of the polyps.[18]

Lynch et al.[26] discuss the protein tyrosine phosphatase and tensin homologue (PTEN), and note that it is a tumor suppressor of glioblastoma, breast cancer, prostate cancer, and malignant melanoma and is located on chromosome 10q23. PTEN is responsible for Cowden disease (CD) and juvenile polyposis. Somatic mutations of PTEN occur in several differing tumors, particularly glioblastomas. These authors studied PTEN from constitutional DNA in 25 families, and PTEN mutations were identified in all 5 of the families with breast cancer and CD. A single family with FJP and 1 in 4 families with breast and thyroid tumors also showed PTEN. These authors noted that in the single family with breast and thyroid cancer the signs of CD were subtle and the diagnosis was established only in the context of mutational analysis. *PTEN* mutations were not detected in 13 families at high risk of breast and/or ovarian cancer. These authors concluded that, "Germ-line PTEN mutations predispose to breast cancer in association with CD, although the signs of CD may be subtle."

6. HNPCC (LYNCH SYNDROME)

6.1. Historical Background

In 1895 the renowned pathologist Aldred Warthin learned that his seamstress was depressed because she was convinced, based on her family history, that she would one day die from cancer of the female organs or bowels. Indeed, as she had predicted, she died of endometrial carcinoma at a young age. This malignancy, in addition to colorectal cancer, was found to occur repeatedly in her kindred, now known as Warthin's Family G, which he published in 1913.[27] Gastric carcinoma was also a predominant lesion in Warthin's initial descriptions of the kindred.[28,29] Over the decades, gastric carcinoma has become less common in Family G, paralleling its decline in the general population.[30]

The significance of Family G's aggregation of colonic, gastric, and endometrial carcinoma was not fully appreciated until two extended kindreds were described under the appellation of Cancer Family Syndrome (CFS).[31] One of the CFS families (Family N), was ascertained in 1961. The proband had been in delirium tremens. When asked why he drank, he stated that he did so because he was going to die of cancer since ". . . everyone in the family dies of cancer,"[31] a sentiment strikingly similar to that of Warthin's seamstress.

Subsequently, a series of international studies documented the existence of cancer families in countries around the world, including England,[32] New Zealand,[33] the Netherlands,[34] Italy,[35,36] Israel,[37] and Finland.[38] The Finnish group, having access to a population-based cancer registry, was able to demonstrate that the syndrome was not rare in that country.[39] During this phase of international recognition, the term HNPCC came into use[34] and it has also been referred to as Lynch syndrome I and II.[40]

HNPCC is characterized by the following criteria: Lynch syndrome I shows an autosomal dominant inherited predilection to carcinoma of the colon with a proximal colonic predominance ($\approx$70% proximal to the splenic flexure), an excess of synchronous and metachronous cancers ($\approx$30% frequency of metachronous cancer within 10 years of initial colon cancer in patients who had limited surgical resection such as hemicolectomy or segmental resection), and improved survival from CRC when compared to carefully stage-matched historical controls;[41-46] Lynch syndrome II shows these identical natural history features of CRC but in addition includes extracolonic cancers, foremost of which is endometrial carcinoma, followed by carcinoma of the ovary, stomach, small bowel, hepatobiliary tract, transitional cell carcinoma of the ureter and renal pelvis,[47] as well as sebaceous adenomas, sebaceous carcinomas, and multiple keratoacanthomas in the Muir-Torre syndrome variant.[48-50] Carcinoma of the pancreas appears to occur in excess in selected HNPCC families. Brain tumors, particularly glioblastoma multiforme, appear in HNPCC Turcot's-like families in association with multiple colonic adenomas.[51] The cutaneous signs which characterize the Muir-Torre syndrome and the multiple colonic adenomas in the Turcot's-like variant of HNPCC represent, so far as we know, are the only premonitory signs of cancer susceptibility for HNPCC. Therefore, prior to the recent discoveries regarding the genetic basis for HNPCC, the clinician had to make a diagnosis based exclusively on a detailed family history of his or her patient.

6.2. Molecular Genetics and the Lynch Syndrome

DNA mismatch repair (MMR) genes that have been identified as being mutated in HNPCC include *hMSH2*,[52] *hMLH1*,[53] *hPMS1*,[33] *hPMS2*[54] and *hMSH6/GTBP*.[54,55] Collectively, these genes are now believed to account for $\approx$50–70% of all families with HNPCC.

Identification of the molecular genetic basis for HNPCC enables the identification of individuals who inherited a germ-line mutation in one of the several genes responsible for repairing DNA mismatches. Consequently, gene carriers could benefit from the most current surveillance and management strategies which are responsive to HNPCC's natural history.

The genetic basis for HNPCC was first documented by Peltomäki et al.,[56] who used a panel of microsatellite markers that covered the entire genome and matched the HNPCC gene to 2p15–16 in two families. Almost immediately thereafter, Lindblom et al.[57] employed a combined approach with microsatellite markers and restriction fragment length polymorphisms to link cancer occurrences in HNPCC with mutations on chromosome 3p. Subsequently, DNA microsatellites provided a critical clue regarding the nature of the genetic defect in HNPCC.

Ionov et al.[58] and Thibodeau et al.[59] found that certain sporadic CRC tumors featured microsatellite instability and the length of the microsatellites varied between tumor DNA and non-tumor DNA from the same patient.

Tomlinson et al.[60] identified 50 patients who were under the age of 45 years and who had nonpolyposis CRC without a family history of CRC or any other HNPCC cancer. Only 6% of these patients showed germ-line HNPCC variants at the *hMSH2* or *hMLH1* loci. They considered that these variants possibly represented new or low penetrance mutations or even polymorphisms, or that possibly a portion of their sample could have an inherited predisposition to CRC that is not a result of HNPCC mutations or known polyposis syndromes. Their results seriously question the value of mass population genetic screening programs for HNPCC employing current technology.

Peltomäki et al.[61] and Aaltonen et al.[62] found that most CRCs from HNPCC patients harbored microsatellite instability. They used the term "replication error positive" (RER+) to describe these tumors. Subsequently, Strand et al.[63] suggested that the HNPCC gene might be a human homolog of DNA mismatch repair genes that had been described in yeast and bacteria. Fishel et al.[52] cloned the *hMSH2* gene, localized it to chromosome 2p21–22, and almost concurrently Leach et al.[53] reported similar findings. About a year later, two groups reported the cloning of the mutL homolog (*hMLH1*) on chromosome 3p21.[64,65] Eight other mutL homologs (*hPMS1*)[33] and mutS homolog (*GTBP*)[54,55] have since been identified. Thus, genes identified up to that point in HNPCC were *hMSH2* at 2p21–22, *hMLH1* at 3p21, *hPMS1* at 2p31–33, and *hPMS2* at 7p22. These genes are believed to account for about 40–70% of all HNPCC families.

Viel et al.[66] studied the mismatch repair (MMR) genes *hMSH2* and *hMLH1* in an attempt to determine the relevance of these two genes in an Italian HNPCC population. They performed mutational analysis on a set of 17 HNPCC families, all of whom fulfilled the Amsterdam criteria. The *hMSH2* gene mutation was found in two of the families, while the *hMLH1* mutation was found in five of the families. The investigators noted that all of the mutations were characterized by DNA sequencing which appeared to involve different molecular mechanisms inclusive of short in-frame and out-of-frame deletions, splicing errors, and nonsense mutations. They concluded that in the Italian population at least 41% of the HNPCC families were linked to *hMSH2* and *hMLH1* mutations.

Liu et al.[67] examined the prevalence of genetic instability in CRCs in relation to age among patients without HNPCC. They found that the majority of patients who were ≤35 years of age manifested genetic instability (58% of 31 patients), in contrast to patients >35 years of age (12% of 158 patients, p < 0.0001). Interestingly, of 12 patients ≤35 with instability who were examined for alterations of mismatch repair genes, 5 harbored germ-line mutations. These investigators concluded that the patho-genetic mechanisms contributing to tumor development in young CRC patients differ from older patients, whether or not they are afflicted with HNPCC. In addition, while 5 of the 12 evaluated young patients with RER tumors had germ-line mutations of a mismatch repair gene, it is noteworthy that patients >35 with RER cancers only rarely showed germ-line mutations of MMR genes. Specifically, Liu et al.[68] found that none of 8 patients over 35 who showed RER cancers harbored a germ-line mutation of an MMR gene. These findings have important implications for one day elucidating the pathogenetic mechanisms which contribute to CRC. In addition, the results suggest that youthful patients with CRC, particularly those under age 35, have a strong probability of harboring a germ-line MMR gene mutation and thereby are candidates for inten-sive family study and genetic counseling.

Miyaki et al.[69] found that *hMSH6/GTBP* is essential for mismatch repair, a conclusion supported by Palombo et al.[55] as well as Fuji and Shimada.[70] Miyaki et al.[69] wished to determine whether or not mutations in *hMSH6* were implicated in HNPCC. They studied five Japanese HNPCC families wherein germ-line mutations of *hMSH2* or *hMLH1* were not detected. They identified the *hMSH6* germ-line mutation in one of these families, thereby suggesting that *hMSH6* mutations can cause HNPCC. They concluded that in that particular HNPCC family the germ-line mutation could account for patients with colonic, endometrial, ovarian, and pancreatic cancers which were similar to other typical HNPCC families. Interestingly, their particular family did not fulfill the Amsterdam criteria. Rather, it showed a predominance of endometrial and ovarian carcinomas, in contrast to the predominance of colorectal car-cinomas in families with *hMSH2* and *hMLH1* germ-line mutations. The mean age for carcinoma in their family was 58 years, which they noted was much later than the mean age of 41 in HNPCC families with germ-line mutations of *hMSH2* or *hMLH1*. They, therefore, suggested that the effect of germ-line mutations in *hMSH6* on cancer patho-genesis may differ from that of *hMSH2* and *hMLH1* mutations. They suggested that germ-line mutations of *hMSH6* will require more extensive clinical evaluation in HNPCC patients.

Akiyama et al.[71] also described a germ-line mutation of the *hMSH6/GTBP* gene in an atypical HNPCC kindred from Japan. The proband was 62 years of age and manifested carcinoma of the rectum and two colonic adenomas. The family history of gastrointestinal tumors did not fulfill the Amsterdam HNPCC criteria. Germ-line mutations of *hMSH2, hMSH3*, and *hMLH1*, were not detected in the patient. However, somatic mutations of *hMSH6* were observed in three colorectal tumors of the patient, findings that were consistent with two-hit inactivation. Microsatellite instabilities at mononucleotide repeats were present in each of these three tumors, suggesting that *hMSH6* was the culprit mutation for cancer occurrence in this atypical HNPCC kindred.

Peltomäki and Vasen[72] analyzed 126 predisposing HNPCC mutations which were gathered as part of the International Collaborative Group on HNPCC's database of DNA mismatch repair gene mutations and polymorphisms. Findings disclosed that, "A majority of the mutations affected either the Mut L homologue (MLH) 1 (n = 75) or the Mut S homologue (MSH) 2 (n = 48) and were quite evenly distributed, with some clustering in MSH2 exon 12 and MLH1 exon 16. Most MSH2 mutations consisted of frameshift (60%) or nonsense changes (23%), whereas MLH1 was mainly affected by frameshift (40%) or missense alterations (31%). . . . Of the families studied (n = 202),

82% met the Amsterdam criteria and 15% did not; the general mutation profile was similar in both groups." It was concluded that construction of mutation profiles will aid in the elucidation of diagnostic strategies in HNPCC.

Wijnen et al.[73] studied HNPCC families that showed clear-cut familial clustering of CRC but did not fulfill the Amsterdam criteria. They screened for *hMSH2* and *hMLH1* mutations in one set of HNPCC families that complied with the Amsterdam criteria and a second set where at least one of the criteria was not satisfied. They found *hMSH2* and *hMLH1* mutations in 49% of the kindreds that fulfilled the Amsterdam criteria, but only 8% of the families in which the criteria were not fulfilled showed a disease-causing mutation. They concluded that their findings emphasized the practical value of the Amsterdam criteria and this did provide a valid clinical subdivision between families based upon their chance of carrying an *hMSH2* or *hMLH1* mutation.

6.3. Cancer Risk by Mutation Analysis in HNPCC

Vasen et al.[74] assessed the age-specific cancer risk by mutation analysis in 19 families with *hMSH2* or *hMLH1* germ-line mutations. They found that the lifetime risk of CRC was the same in both groups of gene carriers (80%), but endometrial carcinoma was greater in *hMSH2* mutation carriers when compared to *hMLH1* mutation carriers (61% vs 42%), although the difference was not statistically significant. They observed an extremely high risk of small bowel cancer (relative risk of >100) in carriers of either gene. Importantly, transitional cell carcinoma of the ureter and renal pelvis showed a significantly increased relative risk (75.3), of the stomach (relative risk of 19.3) and of the ovaries (relative risk of 8.0), only in the carriers of *hMSH2*.

Lin et al.[75] in a study similar to that of Vasen et al.[74] investigated 67 members of *hMLH1* kindreds, 45 members of *hMSH2* kindreds, and 1189 members of the general CRC population, where they compared synchronous and metachronous colon cancer rates, tumor stage, extracolonic cancer incidence, and survival. Colon cancer site distribution showed a disparity of rectal cancers (8% *hMLH1* vs 28% *hMSH2*, p = 0.01) based on genotypes. Overall synchronous CRC rates were 7.4%, 6.7%, and 2.4%, for *hMLH1*, *hMSH2*, and the general population respectively (p = 0.016). Annual metachronous CRC rates were 2.1%, 1.7%, and 0.33% for *hMLH1*, *hMSH2*, and the general population respectively (p = 0.041). CRC stage at presentation was statistically significantly lower in HNPCC as opposed to the controls (p = 0.0028).[75] As in the case of Vasen et al.,[74] extracolonic cancers were noted in 33% of *hMSH2* patients, compared to 12% of *hMLH1* patients and 7.3% in the general population with CRC (p < 0.001). Finally, combined *hMLH1* and *hMSH2* 10-year survival was 68.7% compared to 47.8% for the general CRC population (p = 0.009 stage stratified, hazard ratio 0.57).[75]

Beck et al.[76] studied 10 families where the pedigrees were suggestive of HNPCC but wherein the Amsterdam criteria were not fulfilled. Each of the 10 kindreds was evaluated for germ-line mutations in *hMSH2* and *hMLH1*. Mutations were identified in 6 of the families, 3 missense, 1 nonsense, 1 frameshift, and 1 putative splice-site mutation. Three of the mutations were in *hMSH2* and 3 in *hMLH1*. These investigators concluded that all families with a pedigree suggestive of HNPCC should be referred for genetic study, even if the Amsterdam criteria are not fulfilled. Furthermore, gene carrier status enables targeted surveillance inclusive of the possibility of early surgical intervention and has the potential of being curative.

6.4. Extremely Early Onset CRC—DNA Testing Implications

Certain patients with extremely early onset CRC may be considered candidates for HNPCC germ-line testing. In one such family, a 20-year-old male with rectal carcinoma and liver metastases but with a negative family history among all of his first-degree relatives underwent DNA testing (Patrick M. Lynch, J.D., M.D, personal communication). He was found to have a single base-pair deletion in codon 705 of the *hMSH2* gene. Since he already manifested metastatic cancer, this finding had no bearing on his immediate management. His father was age 55, his mother 54, and his two brothers were ages 26 and 28, all of whom were cancer free. However, his 26-year-old brother, at baseline colonoscopy, had a 1.5 cm adenoma. HNPCC DNA testing was performed on each of these individuals at which time the patient's two brothers and his father were found to be carriers of the *hMSH2* mutation. The paternal grandmother, age 87, was said to have had breast cancer at age 40. However, review of her medical records disclosed that at age 40 she underwent a hysterectomy at which time early adenocarcinoma of the endometrium was diagnosed. The identification of this germ-line mutation in the family now enables highly targeted colonoscopic evaluation of the respective family members in the interest of cancer prevention.

This case shows the value of germ-line testing given the exceptional circumstance of markedly early age of onset CRC in an otherwise "negative" family history. The penetrance of the deleterious gene is about 85% while the average age of CRC is 44. Thus, the patient's affected father, age 55, is still at inordinately high risk for developing CRC since he is only about a decade above the average age of CRC onset. He also may show reduced penetrance of the gene mutation and never develop cancer.

Liu et al.[68] has shown that screening initially for evidence of microsatellite instability in CRC led to the identification of germ-line HNPCC mutations in about one-fourth of patients below age 35 regardless of their cancer family history.

6.5. Genotype-Phenotype Differences

Genetic and clinical (phenotypic) heterogeneity is an important issue in HNPCC. Hamilton et al.[51] identified families considered to have Turcot's syndrome, which is characterized by multiple colonic adenomas, CRC, and central nervous system (CNS) malignancies. Most of the Turcot's syndrome kindreds showed *APC* germ-line mutations typical of FAP. The CNS malignancies were predominantly cerebellar medulloblastomas. Glioblastomas were present in patients who otherwise appeared to have FAP but who were found to harbor HNPCC germ-line mutations (*hMLH1* and *hPMS2*).

Muir-Torre syndrome is characterized by multiple visceral adenocarcinomas, early age of onset, relatively good survival, and multiple sebaceous neoplasia and keratoacanthomas.[77,78] This phenotype's connection to HNPCC was first described by Lynch et al.[48,79] and, more recently, it has been shown to involve mutations of the same genes which predispose to HNPCC.[80]

6.6. Workshops on Pathology, Genetics, and RER in HNPCC

A National Cancer Institute workshop (under the direction of the Early Detection Branch, held November 11–12, 1996) dealt with "The Intersection of Pathology and Genetics in the Hereditary Nonpolyposis Colorectal Cancer (HNPCC) Syndrome." The purpose was to clarify the role of genetics in the pathology of HNPCC.[81]

Germ-line mutations involving *hMSH2*, *hMLH1*, *hPMS1*, *hPMS2*, and *hMSH6/GTBP*, which have been identified in HNPCC affected individuals,[71,82] were discussed. There was full agreement that genomic instability is a fundamental property of tumor cells. In HNPCC, the malfunction of the DNA mismatch repair system was found to result in the accumulation of mutations at simple repetitive sequences referred to as microsatellites, and contribute to the replication error (RER) phenotype, also referred to as microsatellite instability (MIN).

At a subsequent NCI workshop (December 8–9, 1997),[83] the terminology for microsatellite instability was changed and is now defined as MSI-high and MSI-low. MSI-high is characterized by the presence of instability in two microsatellites out of a panel of five, or 30–40% unstable microsatellites in bigger panels. MSI-low is characterized by one or no unstable microsatellites in a panel of five, or <30–40% in a bigger band. The suggested first panel of markers is: BAT25, BAT26, D2S123, Mfd15 (d17s250), APC (d5s346). An additional panel of 30 suggested markers will be published subsequently. It was recommended that immunohistochemistry be performed concurrently with MSI testing. The Bethesda Guidelines[81] were suggested as being pertinent for the performance of MSI/immunohistochemical testing. These guidelines for testing of colorectal tumors for microsatellite instability are as follows: 1) Individuals with cancer in families that meet the Amsterdam Criteria; 2) Individuals with two HNPCC-related cancers, including synchronous and metachronous CRCs or associated extracolonic cancers; 3) Individuals with CRC and a first-degree relative with CRC and/or HNPCC-related extracolonic cancer and/or a colorectal adenoma (one of the cancers diagnosed at <45 years of age, and the adenoma diagnosed at <40 years of age; 4) Individuals with CRC or endometrial cancer diagnosed at age <45 years; 5) Individuals with right-sided CRC with an undifferentiated pattern (solid/cribiform: poorly differentiated or undifferentiated carcinoma composed of irregular, solid sheets of large eosinophilic cells and containing small gland-like spaces) on histopathology diagnosed at <45 years of age; 6) Individuals with signet-ring-cell-type CRC (composed of >50% signet cells) diagnosed at age <45 years; 7) Individuals with adenomas diagnosed at <40 years of age.

A special histology known as "undifferentiated medullary" or "solid-cribiform" carcinoma has recently been identified in CRCs from HNPCC. This histology is uncommon in the general population, but is characteristic of colon cancers with microsatellite instability.

Finally, Jeremy Jass, M.D., a pathologist from Australia, reported a new finding in HNPCC colorectal cancer pathology, namely he identified the presence of tumor infiltrating lymphocytes (TILs) in addition to a Crohn's-like reaction and peritumoral lymphocytic infiltration (inflammatory cells surrounding the border of the colon tumor). The significance of these TILs remains elusive. One suggestion is that they could be partially responsible for the known survival advantage in HNPCC colon cancers[43,44] (discussed below).

6.7. Adenomas and Accelerated Carcinogenesis in HNPCC

In HNPCC, the evolution of colorectal adenoma to carcinoma occurs over a period of only 2–3 years,[84] compared to general population estimates of 8–10 years.[85] Jass et al.[86] described a patient from an HNPCC family who developed 2 CRCs and multiple polyps within 4 years of a negative colonoscopic examination.

Jass[84] considers focal neoplastic changes to be a frequent occurrence within the colorectum. Of the hundreds of microadenomas that might be present within an individual's colorectum, only one or two over that individual's lifetime will develop into a clinically diagnosable colonic adenoma. In turn, only a small fraction of adenomas will ultimately progress to cancer. The risk that any individual microadenoma will complete its natural history and ultimately evolve into a carcinoma is markedly variable and dependent upon the particular clinical context in which it is present. Thus in FAP, where hundreds or even thousands of colonic adenomas may be present, the risk of malignant transformation in an individual adenoma is very low. This is in contrast to HNPCC where the risk that a given adenoma will progress to overt malignancy is inordinately high, despite the presence of only occasional adenomas (no more than occur in the general population). Subsequently, Jass has suggested that the mutator effect was, ". . . more evident at the step of adenoma progression than initiation. . . . This opened the possibility of cancer control through dietary or chemopreventive blockade of the early steps of neoplasia."[87] Trials of chemopreventive agents, inclusive of NSAIDs and COX-2 inhibitors, are being considered in the interest of suppressing colonic adenomas and thereby preventing CRC.[88,89]

6.8. Guidelines for CRC Screening in HNPCC

A multidisciplinary expert panel provided specific recommendations for screening and surveillance in people at average risk and at high risk for CRC.[85] It was recommended that patients with a family history of CRC suggestive of HNPCC receive genetic counseling and consider genetic testing. They should be offered an examination of the entire colon every 1–2 years, starting between 20 and 30 years of age, and then annually after the age of 40 years. The panel indicated that colonoscopy is more accurate than barium enema for small polyps, but both may test clinically important regions.

HNPCC patients presenting with CRC and potential for cure require no less than a subtotal colectomy. The rectal colonic segment must then be evaluated annually. Rodriguez-Bigas et al.[90] analyzed the incidence of rectal cancer in patients with HNPCC after an abdominal colectomy. They identified the risk of developing rectal cancer to be about 3% every 3 years following abdominal colectomy, for the first 12 years (12% in 12 years) following abdominal colectomy. They concluded that aggressive surveillance of the rectum is mandatory following abdominal colectomy.

Lynch[91] proposed that there is a role for prophylactic subtotal colectomy among HNPCC germ-line mutation carriers. Church,[92] when considering that the lifetime colon cancer risk in HNPCC mutation carriers is 80–85%, states that prophylactic colectomy becomes an acceptable procedure. Clearly, patients will require careful genetic counseling regarding this issue.

The need for uterine endometrial screening[93] is demonstrated by the finding of Dunlop et al.[42] that female HNPCC mutation carriers have a 42% risk of uterine cancer. It is notable that this endometrial cancer risk exceeded that for CRC in these women.

6.9. DNA-Based Genetic Counseling and HNPCC

Genetic testing should not be performed randomly. Rather, DNA testing for HNPCC should be performed only on families in which there is a strong likelihood that the syndrome is present.[94] DNA testing should be restricted to consenting individuals who are above age 18 and who are first-degree relatives of HNPCC syndrome affecteds in the direct genetic lineage. When they have been fully informed about the advantages and disadvantages of genetic testing, and after signed consent, blood can be drawn for DNA studies.

6.10. Survival Advantage

Patients with CRC in HNPCC show better survival than age and stage matched comparison groups.[43-46] Myrhoj et al.[95] studied 108 Danish HNPCC patients and compared them with 870 individuals with sporadic CRC. They found more synchronous CRCs (7% vs 1%), more metachronous CRCs after 10 years (29% vs 5%), and more localized carcinomas (62% vs 39%). Of keen interest was the finding of a significantly higher crude cumulative 5-year survival (56% vs 30%). They found the metastatic tendency from CRC in HNPCC patients to be less than that for patients with sporadic CRC. Why do HNPCC patients with CRC show improved survival? Although the answer remains elusive, we suspect that a different immunologic response to cancer may be responsible. Finally, Watson et al.[43] in a case-control study of HNPCC showed statistically significant survival advantage for HNPCC at every CRC stage.

6.11. Mismatch Repair and Chemotherapy Resistance

Maintaining fidelity of genomic stability is dependant upon the proper functioning of DNA replication, repair, and recombination processes. Herein, mismatch repair (MMR) plays a crucial role in the correction of those replicative mismatches that escape DNA polymerase proofreading. Fink et al.,[96] in describing the role of MMR in oncogenesis, also discuss how loss of MMR activity may be important in evoking resistance to those chemotherapeutic agents which have been used in the treatment of CRC. Herein, the loss of MMR and its consequence of drug resistance appear to relate directly to the impairment of the ability of the cell to detect DNA damage and thereby ". . . activate apoptosis and indirectly by increasing the mutation rate throughout the genome. The MMR proteins are involved in mediating the activation of cell cycle checkpoints and apoptosis in response to DNA damage." Herein, Fink et al.[96] note that MMR deficient cells are resistant to the methylating agents procarbazine and temozolomide, the alkylating agent busulfan, the platinum-containing drugs cisplatin and carboplatin, the antimetabolite 6-thioguanine, and the topoisomerase II inhibitors etoposide and doxorubicin.

7. CONCLUSION

In conclusion, much has been learned about hereditary CRC thanks in a major way to the veritably exponential advances in molecular genetics during the past decade. Now that the 21st century is in sight, we fervently hope for better control of this all too deadly disease.

REFERENCES

1. Landis SH, Murray T, Bolden S, et al: Cancer statistics, 1998. CA: a Cancer Journal for Clinicians 48:6–29, 1998

2. Zwick A, Munir M, Ryan CK, et al: Gastric adenocarcinoma and dysplasia in fundic gland polyps of a patient with attenuated adenomatous polyposis coli. Gastroenterology 113:659–663, 1997
3. Fuchs C, Giovannucci E, Colditz G, et al: A prospective study of family history and the risk of colorectal cancer. N Engl J Med 331:1669–1674, 1994
4. St. John JB, McDermott FT, Hopper JL, et al: Cancer risk in relatives of patients with common colorectal cancer. Ann Intern Med 118:785–790, 1993
5. Bulow S: Familial polyposis coli. Dan Med Bull 34:1–15, 1987
6. Luschka H: Ueber polypose Vegetationen der gesammten Dickdarmschleimhaut. Arch Path Anat Phys Klin Med 20:133–142, 1861
7. Sklifasowski NW: Polyadenoma tractus intestinalis. Vrac 4:55–57, 1881
8. Cripps WH: Two cases of disseminated polyps of the rectum. Trans Path Soc London 165–168, 1882
9. Smith T: Three cases of multiple polypi of the lower bowel occurring in one family. St Bartholomew's Hosp Rep 23:225–229, 1887
10. Handford H: Disseminated polypi of the large intestine becoming malignant: strictures (malignant adenoma) of the rectum and of the splenic flexure of the colon; secondary growths in the liver. Trans Path Soc London 41:133–137, 1890
11. Lockhart-Mummery P: Cancer and heredity. Lancet i:427–429, 1925
12. Lynch HT, Fitzgibbons R, Jr, Chong S, et al: Use of doxorubicin and dacarbazine for the management of unresectable intra-abdominal desmoid tumors in Gardner's syndrome. Dis Colon Rectum 37:260–267, 1994
13. Lynch HT, Fitzgibbons R, Jr: Surgery, desmoid tumors and familial adenomatous polyposis: case report and literature review. Am J Gastroenterol 91:2598–2601, 1996
14. Groden J, Thliveris A, Samowitz W, et al: Identification and characterization of the familial adenomatous polyposis coli gene. Cell 66:589–600, 1991
15. Kinzler KW, Nilbert MC, Su L-K, et al: Identification of FAP locus genes from chromosome 5q21. Science 253:661–665, 1991
16. Lynch HT, Smyrk T, McGinn T, et al: Attenuated familial adenomatous polyposis (AFAP): a phenotypically and genotypically distinctive variant of FAP. Cancer 76:2427–2433, 1995
17. Spirio L, Olschwang S, Groden J, et al: Alleles of the APC gene: an attenuated form of familial polyposis. Cell 75:951–957, 1993
18. Lynch HT, Smyrk T, Lynch J: Wanebo HJ, editors. Surgery for Gastrointestinal Cancer: A Multidisciplinary Approach. Philadelphia: Lippincott-Raven Publishers, 1997, 59–86
19. Burt RW, Bishop DT, Cannon LA, et al: Dominant inheritance of adenomatous colonic polyps and colorectal cancer. N Engl J Med 312:1540–1544, 1985
20. Giardiello FM, Welsh SB, Hamilton SR, et al: Increased risk of cancer in the Peutz-Jeghers syndrome. N Engl J Med 316:1511–1514, 1987
21. Jenne DE, Reimann H, Nezu J, et al: Peutz-Jeghers syndrome is caused by mutations in a novel serine threonine kinase. Nat Genet 18:38–44, 1998
22. Hemminki A, Tomlinson I, Markie D, et al: Localization of a susceptibility locus for Peutz-Jeghers syndrome to 19p using comparative genomic hybridization and targeted linkage analysis. Nature Genet 15:87–90, 1997
23. Olschwang S, Markie D, Seal S, et al: Peutz-Jeghers disease: most, but not all, families are compatible with linkage to 19p13.3. J Med Genet 35:42–44, 1998
24. Mehenni H, Blouin J-L, Radhakrishna U, et al: Peutz-Jeghers syndrome: confirmation of linkage to chromosome 19p13.3 and identification of a potential second locus, on 19q13.4. Am J Hum Genet 61:1327–1334, 1997
25. Lynch HT, Smyrk T, Lynch J, et al: Genetic counseling in an extended attenuated familial adenomatous polyposis kindred. Am J Gastroenterol 91:455–459, 1996
26. Lynch ED, Ostermeyer EA, Lee MK, et al: Inherited mutations in PTEN that are associated with breast cancer, Cowden disease, and juvenile polyposis. Am J Hum Genet 61:1254–1260, 1997
27. Warthin AS: Heredity with reference to carcinoma. Arch Intern Med 12:546–555, 1913
28. Warthin AS: The further study of a cancer family. J Cancer Res 9:279–286, 1925
29. Warthin AS: Heredity of carcinoma in man. Ann Int Med 4:681–696, 1931
30. Lynch HT, Krush AJ: Cancer family "G" revisited: 1895–1970. Cancer 27:1505–1511, 1971
31. Lynch HT, Shaw MW, Magnuson CW, et al: Hereditary factors in cancer: study of two large midwestern kindreds. Arch Intern Med 117:206–212, 1966
32. Itoh H, Houlston RS, Harocopos C, et al: Risk of cancer death in first-degree relatives of patients with

hereditary nonpolyposis cancer syndrome (Lynch Type II): a study of 130 kindreds in the United Kingdom. Br J Surg 77:1367–1370, 1990

33. Jass JR, Stewart SM, Schroeder D, et al: Screening for hereditary nonpolyposis colorectal cancer in New Zealand. Eur J Gastroenterol Hepatol 4:523–527, 1992
34. Vasen HF, Hartog Jager FCA, Menko FH, et al: Screening for hereditary nonpolyposis colorectal cancer: a study of 22 kindreds in the Netherlands. Am J Med 86:278–281, 1989
35. Ponz de Leon M, Sassatelli R, Sacchetti C, et al: Familial aggregation of tumors in the three year experience of a population-based colorectal cancer registry. Cancer Res 49:4344–4348, 1989
36. Cristofaro G, Lynch HT, Caruso ML, et al: New phenotypic aspects in a family with Lynch syndrome II. Cancer 60:51–58, 1987
37. Abusamra H, Maximova S, Bar-Meir S, et al: Cancer family syndrome of Lynch. Am J Med 83:981–981, 1987
38. Mecklin J-P, Jarvinen HJ, Peltokallio P: Cancer family syndrome: genetic analysis of 22 Finnish kindreds. Gastroenterology 30:328–333, 1986
39. Mecklin JP: Frequency of hereditary colorectal carcinoma. Gastroenterology 93:1021–1025, 1987
40. Boland CR, Troncale FJ: Familial colonic cancer without antecedent polyposis. Ann Intern Med 100:700–701, 1984
41. Lynch HT, Smyrk T: Hereditary nonpolyposis colorectal cancer (Lynch syndrome): an updated review. Cancer 78:1149–1167, 1996
42. Lynch HT, Smyrk T, Lynch J: An update of HNPCC (Lynch syndrome). Cancer Genet Cytogenet 93:84–99, 1997
43. Watson P, Lin K, Rodriguez-Bigas MA, et al: Colorectal carcinoma survival in hereditary nonpolyposis colorectal cancer family members. Cancer 83:259–266, 1998
44. Sankila R, Aaltonen LA, Jarvinen HJ, et al: Better survival rates in patients with MLH1-associated hereditary colorectal cancer. Gastroenterology 110:682–687, 1996
45. Lynch HT, Albano W, Recabaren J, et al: Prolonged survival as a component of hereditary breast and nonpolyposis colon cancer. Med Hypoth 7:1201–1209, 1981
46. Albano WA, Recabaren JA, Lynch HT, et al: Natural history of hereditary cancer of the breast and colon. Cancer 50:360–363, 1982
47. Watson P, Lynch HT: Extracolonic cancer in hereditary nonpolyposis colorectal cancer. Cancer 71:677–685, 1993
48. Lynch HT, Fusaro RM, Roberts L, et al: Muir-Torre syndrome in several members of a family with a variant of the cancer family syndrome. Br J Dermatol 113:295–301, 1985
49. Lynch HT, Lynch PM, Pester JA, et al: Lynch HT, Fusaro RM, editors. Cancer-associated Genodermatoses. New York: Van Nostrand Reinhold, 1982, 366–393
50. Lynch HT, Fusaro RM: Muir-Torre Syndrome: heterogeneity, natural history, diagnosis, and management. Problems in General Surgery 10:1–14, 1993
51. Hamilton SR, Liu B, Parsons RE, et al: The molecular basis of Turcot's syndrome. N Engl J Med 332:839–847, 1995
52. Fishel R, Lescoe MK, Rao MRS, et al: The human mutator gene homolog MSH2 and its association with hereditary nonpolyposis colon cancer. Cell 75:1027–1038, 1993
53. Leach FS, Nicolaides NC, Papadopoulos N, et al: Mutations of a mutS homolog in hereditary nonpolyposis colorectal cancer. Cell 75:1215–1225, 1993
54. Nicolaides NC, Papadopoulos N, Liu B, et al: Mutations of two PMS homologues in hereditary nonpolyposis colon cancer. Nature 371:75–80, 1994
55. Palombo F, Gillinari P, Iaccarino I, et al: GTBP, a 160-kilodalton protein essential for mismatch-binding activity in human cells. Science 268:1912–1914, 1995
56. Peltomaki P, Aaltonen L, Sistonen P, et al: Genetic mapping of a locus predisposing to human colorectal cancer. Science 260:810–812, 1993
57. Lindblom A, Tannergard P, Werelius B, et al: Genetic mapping of a second locus predisposing to hereditary nonpolyposis colorectal cancer. Nature Genet 5:279–282, 1993
58. Ionov YM, Peinado MA, Malkhosyan S, et al: Ubiquitous somatic mutations in simple repeated sequences reveal a new mechanism for colonic carcinogenesis. Nature 363:558–561, 1993
59. Thibodeau SN, Bren G, Schaid D: Microsatellite instability in cancer of the proximal colon. Science 260:816–819, 1993
60. Tomlinson IPM, Beck NE, Homfray T, et al: Germline HNPCC gene variants have little influence on the risk for sporadic colorectal cancer. J Med Genet 34:39–42, 1997
61. Peltomaki P, Lothe RA, Aaltonen LA, et al: Microsatellite instability is associated with tumors that

characterize the hereditary nonpolyposis colorectal carcinoma syndrome. Cancer Res 53:5853–5855, 1993

62. Aaltonen LA, Peltomaki P, Leach FS, et al: Clues to the pathogenesis of familial colorectal cancer. Science 260:812–816, 1993

63. Strand M, Prolla TA, Liskay RM, et al: Destabilization of tracts of simple repetitive DNA in yeast by mutations affecting DNA mismatch repair. Nature 365:274–276, 1993

64. Bronner CE, Baker SM, Morrison PT, et al: Mutation in the DNA mismatch repair gene homologue hMLH1 is associated with hereditary nonpolyposis colon cancer. Nature 368:258–261, 1994

65. Papadopoulos N, Nicolaides NC, Wei Y-F, et al: Mutation of a mutL homolog in hereditary colon cancer. Science 263:1625–1629, 1994

66. Viel A, Genuardi M, Capozzi E, et al: Characterization of *MSH2* and *MLH1* mutations in Italian families with hereditary nonpolyposis colorectal cancer. Genes Chromosomes Cancer 18:8–18, 1997

67. Liu B, Farrington SM, Petersen GM, et al: Genetic instability occurs in the majority of young patients with colorectal cancer. Nature Med 1:348–352, 1995

68. Liu B, Nicolaides NC, Markowitz S, et al: Mismatch repair gene defects in sporadic colorectal cancers with microsatellite instability. Nature Genet 9:48–55, 1995

69. Miyaki M, Konishi M, Tanaka K, et al: Germline mutation of *MSH6* as the cause of hereditary nonpolyposis colorectal cancer. Nat Genet 17:271–272, 1997

70. Fujii H, Shimada T: Isolation and characterization of cDNA clones derived from the divergently transcribed gene in the region upstream from the human dihydrofolate reductase gene. J Biol Chem 264:10057–10064, 1989

71. Akiyama Y, Sato H, Yamada T, et al: Germ-line mutation of the *hMSH6/GTBP* gene in an atypical hereditary nonpolyposis colorectal cancer kindred. Cancer Res 57:3920–3923, 1997

72. Peltomäki P, Vasen HFA, International Collaborative Group on Hereditary Nonpolyposis Colorectal Cancer: Mutations predisposing to hereditary nonpolyposis colorectal cancer: database and results of a collaborative study. Gastroenterology 113:1146–1158, 1997

73. Wijnen J, Khan PM, Vasen H, et al: Hereditary nonpolyposis colorectal cancer families not complying with the Amsterdam criteria show extremely low frequency of mismatch-repair-gene mutations. Am J Hum Genet 61:329–335, 1997

74. Vasen HFA, Wijnen JT, Menko FH, et al: Cancer risk in families with hereditary nonpolyposis colorectal cancer diagnosed by mutation analysis. Gastroenterology 110:1020–1027, 1996

75. Lin KM, Shashidharan M, Ternent CA, et al: Colorectal and extracolonic cancer variations in MLH1/MSH2 hereditary nonpolyposis colorectal cancer kindreds and the general population. Dis Colon Rectum 41:428–433, 1998

76. Beck NE, Tomlinson IPM, Homfray T, et al: Genetic testing is important in families with a history suggestive of hereditary non-polyposis colorectal cancer even if the Amsterdam criteria are not fulfilled. Br J Surg 84:233–237, 1997

77. Muir EG, Bell AJ, Barlow KA: Multiple primary carcinomata of the colon, duodenum, and larynx associated with keratoacanthomata of the face. Br J Surg 54:191–195, 1966

78. Torre D: Multiple sebaceous tumors. Arch Dermatol 98:549–551, 1968

79. Lynch HT, Lynch PM, Pester J, et al: The cancer family syndrome: rare cutaneous phenotypic linkage of Torre's syndrome. Arch Intern Med 141:607–611, 1981

80. Hall NR, Murday VA, Chapman P, et al: Genetic linkage in Muir-Torre syndrome to the same chromosomal region as cancer family syndrome. Eur J Cancer 30A:180–182, 1994

81. Rodriguez-Bigas MA, Boland CR, Hamilton SR, et al: A National Cancer Institute workshop on hereditary nonpolyposis colorectal cancer syndrome: meeting highlights and Bethesda Guidelines. J Natl Cancer Inst 89:1758–1762, 1997

82. Liu B, Parsons R, Papadopoulos N, et al: Analysis of mismatch repair genes in hereditary nonpolyposis colorectal cancer patients. Nat Med 2:169–174, 1996

83. International Workshop on Microsatellite Instability and RER Phenotypes in Cancer Detection and Familial Predisposition Meeting. National Cancer Institute; 1997; Bethesda, MD. 1997

84. Jass JR: Colorectal adenoma progression and genetic change: is there a link? Ann Med 27:301–306, 1995

85. Winawer SJ, Fletcher RH, Miller L, et al: Colorectal cancer screening: clinical guidelines and rationale. Gastroenterology 112:594–642, 1997

86. Jass JR, Cottier DS, Pokos V, et al: Mixed epithelial polyps in association with hereditary nonpolyposis colorectal cancer providing an alternative pathway of cancer histogenesis. Pathology 29:28–33, 1997

87. Jass JR: Familial cancer: histopathological perspectives. J Clin Pathol 50:892–895, 1997
88. Sheng GG, Shao J, Sheng H, et al: A selective cyclooxygenase 2 inhibitor suppresses the growth of H-*ras*-transformed rat intestinal epithelial cells. Gastroenterology 113:1883–1891, 1997
89. Elder DJE, Paraskeva C: NSAIDs to prevent colorectal cancer: a question of sensitivity. Gastroenterology 113:1999–2003, 1997
90. Rodriguez-Bigas MA, Vasen HFA, Pekka-Mecklin J, et al: Rectal cancer risk in hereditary nonpolyposis colorectal cancer after abdominal colectomy. Ann Surg 225:202–207, 1997
91. Lynch HT: Is there a role for prophylactic subtotal colectomy among hereditary nonpolyposis colorectal cancer germline mutation carriers? Dis Colon Rectum 39:109–110, 1996
92. Church JM: Prophylactic colectomy in patients with hereditary nonpolyposis colorectal cancer. Ann Med 28:479–482, 1996
93. Lynch HT, Cavalieri RJ, Lynch JF, et al: Gynecologic cancer clues to Lynch syndrome II diagnosis: a family report. Gynecologic Oncol 44:198–203, 1992
94. Lynch HT, Fusaro RM, Lemon SJ, et al: Survey of cancer genetics: genetic testing implications. Cancer 80(suppl):523–532, 1997
95. Myrhoj T, Bisgaard ML, Bernstein I, et al: Hereditary non-polyposis colorectal cancer: clinical features and survival: results from the Danish HNPCC Register. Scand J Gastroenterol 32:572–576, 1997
96. Fink D, Aebi S, Howell SB: The role of DNA mismatch repair in drug resistance. Clin Cancer Res 4:1–6, 1998

11

INSURANCE ISSUES IN GENETIC TESTING FOR CANCER

Maimon M. Cohen and Karen R. Eanet

The Harvey Institute for Human Genetics
Greater Baltimore Medical Center
Baltimore, Maryland 21204

1. INTRODUCTION

Advances in genomic technology have given rise to new approaches in the gathering and use of genetic information. DNA-based testing may not only enable early detection of a genetically-determined condition, but can also assess an individual's predisposition to develop disease. The power of disease-specific testing lies in its predictive nature, but genetic information can also be inferred from the medical history (not predictive, but useful in assessing genetic risk) or by observing the phenotype or clinical picture. Recently, developments in medical information sciences have spurred public concern over the control and use of genetic information, particularly that derived from genetic tests. At the same time, a growing awareness of the potential for conflict among private, governmental, and commercial interests has raised concern over maintaining the confidentiality of such information and preventing "genetic discrimination" while preserving access to these data for treatment, research, and reimbursement.

2. SETTING THE SCENE

Given the predictive nature of information resulting from genetic tests, the current ferment over "genetic discrimination" on the part of insurers and employers has had two opposing outcomes: it has made the public aware of progress in the detection of disease-associated gene mutations and risk assessment while simultaneously limiting the access to these services by those in greatest need of them.

Most insurance products are designed to provide financial protection against unexpected loss by the insurer. Therefore, insurance underwriters must conduct fiscally responsible risk assessment of applicants using a variety of information sources. The evaluation of risk factors is known as "risk selection and classification" or, more commonly, underwriting. Medical underwriting is the process by which insurance companies determine whether a group, family, or individual represents an acceptable risk to the company. A fundamental principle of insurance is equity—that is, those with similar risks are charged the same amount. The higher the risk, the greater the premium. Those with lower risks pay reduced premiums. Risk determination is based on type and size of the proposed contract and the financial, health, lifestyle, and other characteristics of the applicant(s). This composite picture is compared with those of other applicants to determine if more or fewer claims than the average will be generated. On the basis of such comparisons, risks are classified as "preferred", "standard", "substandard", or "declined". Applications are declined or considered substandard when early and/or considerable claims can be expected based on the information examined.

2.1. Types of Policies

It is important to distinguish the type of policy sought (individual, small group, or large group) since the evaluation process differs for each of them. Individual policies are underwritten using factors such as age, height, weight, medical and occupational history, and lifestyle (i.e., hobbies and sports activities).[1] Group underwriting is based on the characteristics of the group—number of individuals, age and sex distribution, prior claims, types of occupations included—and coverage is usually issued through an employer without regard to health status.[2] Group plans frequently restrict benefits for pre-existing conditions, either totally or for a defined period.[3] The risk assessment procedure for small groups (usually less than 25 individuals) is similar to that of individual policies.[4] Small groups do not have the advantage of "spreading risks" among large numbers, and the premium rates for such groups consequently rely on the health status of individual members, their occupational histories, the number of part-time employees, etc. Large groups (usually more than 500 members) are generally healthy people who are actively working. Therefore, there is both greater stability of the risk pool and greater reliability in risk prediction, resulting in increased ability to distribute the risk equitably among the group.

2.2. Rating Systems

Two of the primary approaches used by underwriters to determine premium rates are "community rating" and "experience rating". Community rating bases group premiums on the average cost of all insured persons within a defined geographical region. Experience rating, on the other hand, bases premiums on the recent claims history of the group under consideration. Employer groups are usually healthier than geographic community groups, which include those not able to work. Experience rating therefore results in lower rates to employers and has become the standard underwriting method for most firms.

According to the Health Insurance Association of America,[5] medical underwriting is based on some or all of the following information sources: the application itself, medical or paramedical exam, physician's statement, agent's statement, hospital records, inspection reports, and the files of the Medical Information Bureau (MIB). The MIB maintains medical information files on more than 15 million individuals and, upon request, provides this information to 750 participating insurance companies in North America. Data from the applications of every individual who seeks life, health, or disability coverage is entered into the MIB. The MIB's regulations prohibit use of these data in underwriting, but it is not known whether these rules are observed or are even enforceable.[6]

2.3. Adverse Selection (Antiselection)

If insurance purchasing decisions were made at random, it would be impossible to calculate the premiums to cover the risk of each individual in a given group. Adverse selection is defined as "the actions of individuals, acting for themselves or for others, who are motivated directly or indirectly to take advantage of the risk calculation system".[7] Adverse selection can occur when individuals applying for health insurance have more information about their risks than the underwriting company. The obvious concern of insurance companies is that applicants who know that they are at higher risk, but do not disclose this fact, will purchase coverage at lower premiums which will not cover their loss claims. If adverse selection was widespread, it would threaten the solvency of the company. Its impact may be far greater than the actual number of applicants involved because such individuals may: (1) buy more insurance than the average policy-holder; (2) submit claims earlier than expected; or (3) selectively purchase coverage (e.g., life insurance if early death is anticipated or long-term care insurance if non life-threatening disability is anticipated).

Adverse selection is particularly worrisome to insurance companies whose policies pay benefits directly to the policy holder rather than to a beneficiary. Consider, for example, the hypothetical applicant whose risk for hereditary breast cancer or colorectal cancer has been demonstated by genetic testing and who purchases a large lump-sum payment policy without revealing the test results. The company would be obligated to pay the applicant's claim at the time of diagnosis, even though the test outcome might lead to increased medical surveillance, detection of the disease at an early stage, and a "cure" for the policyholder. Some insurers argue that widespread adverse selection could increase premiums to the point that "healthy" individuals (i.e., those without adverse test results) would seek more affordable coverage elsewhere or be driven out of the insurance market entirely. This scenario would result in an upward spiral of premium increases to cover the higher average risk of the remaining policyholders, leading ultimately to completely unaffordable rates.[4,8,9]

2.4. Current Underwriting Practices for Genetic Testing

Recent figures indicate that nearly 85% of Americans have third-party health insurance coverage[4,5,10] through a variety of commercial, non-profit, managed care (HMO), self-insurance, and public plans (Medicaid, Medicare, and Social Security). Some 40 million individuals remain uninsured. The wide disparity of coverage for specific conditions, procedures, and tests is nowhere more obvious than in regard to genetic tests and the use of the information derived from them. In the past, conventional diagnostic techniques have resulted in the limiting of insurance or denial of claims for a few individuals because of the small number and relative rarity of inherited conditions for which test procedures were available. The flood of new gene-based tests, associated with an ever-increasing number of genetic diseases, has already become a priority issue among medical underwriters for individual coverage, and will undoubtedly impact the small- and large-group markets as well. The growing trend of employers to "self-insure" allows them the latitude to change plan benefits at will in order to reduce costs, so that entire categories of conditions (e.g., inherited diseases and the tests which detect them) may not be included.

The determination of which tests, conditions, and limits of coverage are to be included in insurance products varies greatly among providers of such services. In "predictive genetic testing", the issue is even more complex than with the more straight-forward diagnostic tests. The transition of an investigative procedure to a clinical tool (i.e., a genetic test) has been chronicled by *The Task Force on Genetic Testing* convened by the NIH-US Department of Energy Working Group on Legal, Ethical, and Social Implications of Human Genome Research.[11,12] When dealing with DNA-based tests, the difference between screening tools and diagnostic outcomes becomes blurred and the two approaches tend to merge. Great care is needed in interpreting these test results. The statistical validity of a test as diagnostic tool (its sensitivity, specificity, and predictive value) may be an accepted fact when disease is manifest. However, as a prognosticator of disease, genetic tests remain indeterminate relative to any single individual. This inexactitude arises from the variation of expression and penetrance of different mutations within a specific gene, evoking a host of biological, environmental, and cultural interactions. Until a much larger body of data is amassed (including clinical outcomes), these tests remain an indicator of increased risk but not the absolute determiner of a disease condition. For example, there is currently a lack of successful interventions and treatment protocols based on the results of BRCA testing for inherited breast cancer susceptibility. Although the current imprecision of genetic testing is paramount in insurers' policies concerning coverage for genetic testing, the issue is still under active debate. Dr. J.A. Lowden (Crown Life Insurance of Canada and a member of the Genetic Testing Task Force) expressed this concern in a presentation to the annual meeting of the Canadian Medical Officers Association:

"We must learn to underwrite genetic disease. We must do so realizing that our knowledge of the impact of a specific mutation on the long-term health or survival of an individual is somewhat uncertain".[13]

Varying approaches to coverage for genetic testing have been adopted by insurance providers. Kaiser Permanente has developed internal clinical practice guidelines for genetic testing and counseling for inherited breast and ovarian cancer. Plan members who meet established inclusion criteria are covered for these services.[14] Dr. Anne Mengehetti (Blue Cross/Blue Shield of Massachusetts) has stated that insurance plans must move beyond the clear-cut cases "where you know if you have the genes you'll get the cancer" to those genetic tests with less obvious benefits. At present, Massachusetts Blue Cross/Blue Shield covers only those genetic tests whose results impact on clinical management.[15] Tests which show a distinct benefit in a defined group (e.g., testing for mutations in the RET proto-oncogene in medullary thyroid cancer) are covered. Other providers look to the professional organizations and colleges for direction as to the suitability of new technologies, treatment modalities, and medical programs. Although most insurers have in-house groups which also consider these issues, standard-of-care statements by organized medicine are of utmost importance.

3. AN INTRIGUING PARADOX

Almost 50 health insurers across the country cover costs of the laboratory components of genetic testing for breast cancer. Paradoxically, genetic counseling is an entirely different issue. Several groups and organizations have already stated the importance of patient education through pre- and post-test genetic counseling, recommending that it be considered an integral component of the testing process.[16-19] As stated above, the results of gene-based testing can be complex or non-informative, and those tested may need support to deal with the information received. One of the insurance industry's reservations about the underwriting of genetic tests is its inability to provide appropriate genetic counseling, which is now suggested by the above groups as inseparable from testing. However, in spite of covering the laboratory component of genetic testing, many health insurance plans do not cover genetic counseling. Lack of coverage for counseling discourages a significant number of interested persons from considering genetic testing and has resulted in a *de facto* barrier to such services.

In order to evaluate this barrier, we conducted an informal e-mail survey of the National Society of Genetic Counselors Cancer Special Interest Group. The responses mirrored our own experience and re-confirmed the findings of a more comprehensive survey of billing practices for cancer risk assessment.[20] Of the 22 responses we received, nine were from cancer centers operating under research protocols in which no financial obligation to either the patient or the insurance carrier was incurred. Ten respondents were billing via a physician's signature for genetic counseling provided by a master's degree-level, trained genetic counselor. The remaining three centers were either collecting fees at the time of service or sending bills directly to the patients (no physician's signature).

Most of the respondents who billed insurance companies for genetic counseling were unaware of the level of reimbursement, suggesting that more attention needs to be paid to this issue by genetic professionals. When asked what mechanism, if any, was used to alleviate the financial problems faced by their patients, some counselors admitted to "forgetting" to send bills for financially strained patients. Others were applying (with limited success) for small service grants from private sources to cover some or all of the the cost of genetic counseling for cancer risk assessment. Still others took advantage of a patient's appointment with another health professional to provide risk assessment counseling, and no separate bill for genetic counseling was submitted.

According to the results of our survey, cancer risk assessment programs which bill for genetic counseling are seeing an average of 2–3 patients/week (range 7–0.5 patients/week), a rate similar to that noted by Bernhardt et al.[20] The majority of patients counseled (75%) are referred from physicians, as opposed to self-referred (25%). Several respondents mentioned that this is a relatively new pattern reversal, due to greater physician awareness of the genetic basis of cancer and the availability of genetic counseling services. An estimated 40% of initial inquiries for cancer risk assessment refused counseling when apprised of the cost. One respondent stated that even though state funding is available to pay testing fees for uninsured individuals, 95% of those eligible turn down testing and/or counseling. While payment was the major issue, perceived discriminatory behavior on the part of insurance carriers was also mentioned as an additional barrier to genetic counseling for cancer risk assessment.

Although our sample is small, two major assertions can be made: (1) genetic counseling is not being adequately covered by health insurance plans, seriously affecting access to these services and perhaps partially explaining the small number of individuals utilizing genetic cancer risk assessment; (2) the perceived or actual threat of health insurance discrimination due to documentation of a family history of cancer is a very real barrier to the provision of services.

These informal but telling results attest to an obvious and important paradox. Since inherited breast cancer accounts for, at best, 10% of the breast cancer population, careful pedigree analysis and genetic counseling would most likely eliminate 90% of those interested in genetic testing as inappropriate candidates for this testing. Genetic counseling is an extremely efficient gateway to testing services and, if properly exploited, would minimize subsequent costs. However, despite the recommendations of various governmental, professional, and consumer groups that pre- and post-test counseling be an integral part of the process,[16-19] why is this service not covered? An average counseling fee of approximately $150/session pales in comparison to costs for total sequencing and screening of both breast cancer genes, which exceeds $2000 per case. Moreover, if interested parties cannot enter the process through pre-test counseling, their need for testing cannot be assessed properly. In the words of Dr. Meneghetti of Massachusetts Blue Cross/Blue Shield, genetic counseling is "far more important than the particular laboratory test offered. Even with proper counseling and appropriate reasons for going forward with testing, approximately 50% of patients decide against it".[15] Given a probable 10% "yield" of those deemed appropriate for further testing (with its more than ten-fold increase in cost), it would seem fiscally astute for the industry to cover the cost of counseling without restriction. Such a policy would also serve to ameliorate the perception among both patients and professionals that insurance companies have erected a barrier to patients' access to genetic testing. Furthermore, for those found to be mutation carriers, earlier disease detection and intervention would most likely lead to decreased costs of medical management. Therefore, we suggest that insurers carefully re-examine their policies regarding genetic counseling and testing, evaluating the use of these educational and diagnostic tools as a long-term preventive strategy.

4. ABUSE OF GENETIC INFORMATION

4.1. "Genetic Discrimination"

Since the mid 1980's, "genetic discrimination" has been considered a possible by-product of the genetic revolution. Apparent cases of such discrimination in health insurance coverage and employment seem to increase as more disease-associated genes are discovered and diagnostic tests are developed. Genetic discrimination has been defined as

"... discrimination against an individual or against members of that individual's family solely because of real or perceived differences from the normal genome of that individual. Genetic discrimination is distinguished from discrimination based on disabilities caused by altered genes by excluding, from the former category, those instances of discrimination against an individual who at the time of the discriminatory act was affected by the genetic disease."[21]

In other words, genetic discrimination can only occur against normal, apparently healthy individuals who may have a predisposition to develop a disease in the future, or have affected children.

Analysis of the published documentation on genetic discrimination[22] yields some interesting observations. The original publication by Billings et al.[21] surveyed more than 1000 geneticists and related professionals, soliciting examples of "genetic discrimination". Since these individuals had professional interactions with a large population of patients and families who might be targets for discriminatory practices, it is surprising that of the 42 responses received, only 29 met the study's inclusion criteria. From these 29 responses, a total of 39 cases was ascertained. Of these, 32 cases involved health insurance and seven involved employment discrimination, principally concerning the issuance of new insurance coverage or renewed coverage because of employment changes. Despite the seemingly insignificant response to the survey (39 cases from among, perhaps, hundreds or thousands of possible families at risk), the case scenarios in this paper drew national attention to the "problem".

Surveys of insurance industry representatives (state commissioners and medical directors of life insurance companies) indicated that few were using available genetic tests and that interest in this approach was dependent upon specific test availability and the coverage desired.[23,24] Actuarial data on genetic conditions for underwriting policies was sorely lacking, and genetic testing was not perceived as a problem in applicant rating. Respondents to these surveys felt that regulators had a right to request genetic tests, but a surprisingly small number of formal complaints against discriminatory practices had been lodged.[25] It is of interest that 10 years earlier, similar responses were obtained in a survey of employment practices among 500 of the largest U.S. industrial companies: of 366 responses, only 6% had used genetic testing and only 16% had some interest in future testing.

The largest published survey of this type involved 27,700 questionnaires sent to "individuals at risk to develop a genetic condition and parents of children with specific genetic conditions".[26] There was a 3.3% response rate (917 respondents), of whom 50% (455) claimed some experience with genetic discrimination. The vast majority of these were "positive" cases for Huntington disease. Only 1.7% of the respondents indicated evidence of discrimination on the basis of genetic information. A similar approach to consumers associated with the Alliance of Genetic Support Groups resulted in 332 interviews, in which 22% claimed denial of health insurance coverage because of a genetic condition.[27] However, because these interviewees were asked about "prejudicial actions" based on much broader criteria than those of the original definition of "genetic discrimination", there is a basic definitional difference underlying the premise of this survey. More significant, perhaps, is the fact that 78% of those interviewed reported no problems in obtaining health insurance.

Despite the paucity of "hard data", the perception exists among the media (both print and electronic) that there is a serious risk of discrimination based on genetic information. These sentiments have been verified by a series of public opinion polls during the last decade[28] (Table 1), and have raised sufficient apprehension over the issue that nationwide legislative efforts to provide protection for such abuses are underway.

4.2. Legislative Efforts to Protect Genetic Information

It is becoming apparent that virtually all diseases have some genetic component and that every individual carries several (possibly deleterious) mutations. Since we have entered a period in which genetic testing is becoming increasingly integral to clinical practice, eventually all medical information (barring, perhaps, incidents of trauma) will be genetically relevant. Therefore, it will become almost impossible to distinguish between genetic and non-genetic information in the medical record. The current approach of multiple legislative efforts, each addressing individual aspects of the much broader problem, may be counterproductive. Protection of both the privacy and use of all medical information should be the desired goal.

Table 1. National Public Opinion Polls on Genetic Testing[28]

Date		Results	Source
1986	66%	genetic engineering would improve life	Harris Poll
1989	66%	genetic screening will do more harm than good	Gallup/Columbia Univ.
1992	90%	against genetic testing in pre-employment process	
	60%	against genetic testing even when employee safety involved	
	75%	for employees having exclusive control of access to records "attitudes to genetic screening in workforce . . . are overwhelmingly negative"	National Opinion Research Center
1992	38%	stop genetic testing until primary issue resolved	Harris/March of Dimes
1993	91%	opposed use of genetic information to reduce health benefits	
	86%	opposed use of genetic information in underwriting decisions	
	63%	in favor of testing designed to ascertain special risks to employees (susceptibilities)	Harris/Westin
	85%	against refusal to hire based on late-manifesting diseases	
	88%	against testing to determine predispositions (carriers)	
1994	<85%	very concerned or somewhat concerned that insurers or employers might have access to genetic information	Harris
1995	63%	would not be tested if health insurers or employers had access to reports	
	85%	felt employers should be prohibited from obtaining information about genetic conditions, risks, and predisposition	National Center for Genome Resources (unpublished)

4.2.1. Federal Level. Various levels of governmental controls exist for the insurance industry. Although the McCowan-Ferguson Act (1974) transferred the primary regulatory control of insurance companies to the states, several federal laws still affect certain insurance practices:

(1) *The Consolidated Omnibus Budget Reconciliation Act of 1985 (COBRA)* requires employers to maintain employees' health insurance eligibility for a limited period of time, at the employee's expense, following termination of employment. (2) *The Health Maintenance Organization Act of 1973* established a department within the federal Department of Health and Human Services (DHHS) to regulate the activities of HMOs and set federal standards for rate-setting and underwriting. (3) *The Employee Retirement Income Security Act of 1974 (ERISA)* governs employer pension plans and covers a range of employer-provided benefits including health benefit plans. ERISA plans in self-insured organizations are exempt from state laws and regulations, and are allowed to alter or eliminate benefits for specific conditions at any time. (4) *The Americans with Disabilities Act (ADA)* protects persons with physical or mental impairments, or perceived impairments, from discrimination in employment, public transportation and accommodation, and telecommunications. However, it leaves regulation of insurance to the states. (5) *The Health Insurance Portability and Accountability Act of 1996 (HIPAA)* is the seminal federal law that represents the first step in protecting

Table 2. Federal Bills Introduced in the 105th Congress Pertaining to Individual Protection Based on Genetic Information and Testing

Bill Number	Title	Sponsor(s)
Health Insurance Discrimination		
HR305; S89	"The Genetic Information Nondiscrimination in Health Insurance Act"	Rep. L. Slaughter (D-NY) Sen. O. Snowe (R-ME)
HR2198	"The Genetic Privacy and Nondiscrimination Act of 1997"	Rep. C. Stearns (R-FL)
HR328	"The Genetic Information Health Insurance Nondiscrimination Act"	Rep. G. Solomon (R-NY)
Medical Privacy		
HR1815	"Medical Privacy in the Age of New Technologies Act"	Rep. J. McDermott (D-WA)
S422	"Genetic Confidentiality and Nondiscrimination Act of 1997"	Sen. P. Domenici (R-WA)
S193	"Human Research Subject Project Act"	Sen. J. Glenn (D-OH)
S2609	"The Health Care Privacy Protection Act"	Sen. R. Bennett (R-UT)
S1368	"Medical Information Privacy and Security Act"	Sen. P. Leahy (D-VT)
HR52	"The Fair Health Information Practice Act"	Rep. G. Condit (D-CA)
Employment Discrimination		
HR2275	"The Genetic Employment Protection Act of 1997"	Rep. N. Lowey (D-NY)
S1045	"The Genetic Justice Act of 1997"	Sen. T. Daschle (D-SD)
Cloning		
HR922; S368	"Human Cloning Research Prohibition Act"	Rep. V. Ehlers (R-MI) Sen. C. Bond (R-MO)

genetic information relative to health insurance. It pertains to group coverage and improves access to and portability of health insurance; clearly defines a pre-existing condition; and prohibits use of genetic test results for an exclusionary period. It also prohibits group health plans from conditioning member eligibility on information derived from genetic tests and pre-empts the ERISA exclusion from state regulations. However, it does not preclude the use of genetic information in premium-setting. This act sets August 31, 1999, as the deadline for Congress to deal with protecting the privacy of medical information.

A number of bills have been introduced (or re-introduced) in the 105th Congress and are currently under consideration. These bills assess insurance and employment discrimination; privacy and confidentiality protection; medical information security; and human cloning (Table 2). Most are single-purpose bills aimed at only one issue, but several are more globally crafted. There are, however, variations among them with regard to basic definitions of "genetic information", "genetic test", "medical information", and providers of various types which may ultimately lead to contradictory rulings and wreak havoc in their aggregate intent. Indeed, a common set of uniform definitions must be adopted at both the federal and state levels.

4.2.2. State Level. The states bear primary responsibility for regulating the insurance industry, but the current patchwork of statutes does not begin to provide a comprehensive solution to the perceived problem of genetic discrimination in health insurance. Initial attempts focused narrowly on genetic testing rather than its results or on the genetic information derived from medical records, physician exams, and family histories. North Carolina and Florida, in the early 1970's, were the first states to specifically cite genetic information, by prohibiting health insurers from refusing coverage or increasing premiums for carriers of the sickle cell trait. Maryland, in 1986, passed similar legislation, including additional conditions such as Tay-Sachs disease, but did not prohibit discriminatory use of genetic information based on "actuarial justification".

With the ever-increasing discovery rate of disease-associated genes and the almost coincident development of DNA-based tests for disease detection and predictive risk assessment, the amount of genetic information which is in need of protection has grown proportionately. As a result, the last decade has seen an explosion of state legislation in the health insurance sphere. Most of the earlier bills dealt with one or more of the following issues, prohibiting health insurers from:

- requiring or requesting that an individual (or family member) be tested;
- requiring or requesting test results, directly or indirectly;
- making coverage or benefits conditional on genetic testing;
- considering genetic testing or results in premium determination.

More recently, the release and transmission of genetic information, informed consent, and authorization for information release have assumed greater prominence. In 1996, more than a dozen state legislatures considered "genetic discrimination" bills. In 1997, legislatures in 44 states (Table 3) introduced more than 200 bills concentrating on the use of genetic information in four main areas: health insurance; employment; confidentiality and genetic testing; and control of genetic information.

Several of these statutes demonstrated deficiencies and shortcomings, which led to recommendations drafted by the National Action Plan for Breast Cancer (NAPBC) and endorsed by the National Advisory Council of the National Center for Human Genome Research,[29] designed to direct state and federal policy makers in drafting legislation:

a. Insurance providers should be prohibited from using genetic information, or an individual's request for genetic services, to deny or limit any coverage or establish eligibility, continuation, enrollment, or contribution requirements.
b. Insurance providers should be prohibited from establishing differential rates or premium payments based on genetic information or an individual's request for genetic services.
c. Insurance providers should be prohibited from requesting or requiring collection or disclosure of genetic information.
d. Insurance providers and other holders of genetic information should be prohibited from releasing genetic information without prior written authorization of the individual. Written authorization should be required for each disclosure and include to whom the disclosure would be made.

Although the current state bills have attempted to address these four areas (insurance, employment, testing, and confidentiality), there are still fundamental problems.

Table 3. State Bills Enacted in 1997 Pertaining to Individual Protection Based on Genetic Information and Testing

Genetic Testing/ Information	Insurance	Employment	Confidentiality
Alabama	Alabama	Arizona	Delaware
Arizona	Arizona	California	Hawaii
California	Connecticut	Illinois	Illinois
Colorado	Florida	North Carolina	Indiana
Florida	Illinois	Texas	Oregon
Georgia	Louisiana		
Louisiana	Nevada		
Maryland	New York		
Minnesota	North Carolina		
New Hampshire	Ohio		
New Jersey	Tennessee		
New Mexico	Texas		
New York	Virginia		
North Carolina			
Ohio			
Oregon			
Tennessee			
Virginia			
Wisconsin			

First, most statutes are narrowly focused, so that comprehensive legislation is lacking. Second, ERISA exempts self-insured plans from state insurance laws and regulations. Nationwide, almost half of those insured obtain coverage through such employer-derived self-insured plans, and this number will undoubtedly grow as more employers use self-funding to provide health benefits. Since the ERISA exemption pre-empts state law, it will be difficult to establish uniform regulation of genetic information in health insurance plans. Third, the NAPBC recommendations use certain terms which are not uniformly defined in existing law. There is a need for universally agreed-upon definitions of "genetic information", "genetic test", "genetic services", and "insurance provider" for uniform incorporation into all levels of legislation dealing with the use and protection of genetic information.

4.3. Impact on Research

The existing state measures have often been drafted solely for the protection of individuals from the discriminatory practices of insurers and employers, but the results are sometimes detrimental to both basic and clinical research. The following are areas which may impact negatively on access to and use of information in research.

4.3.1. Creation of a Property Right to Individual Genetic Information. It is becoming more difficult to distinguish genetic information from the general information in the medical record, which describes conditions, treatments, family histories, and test results. Few disagree that strong protection of patient-identifiable information should be in place to safeguard an individual's privacy. However, some of the state laws include a "property-right" to medical/genetic information, maintaining that the information belongs to the individual to whom it applies. Through this mechanism, a market may be created for such information, leading to a weakening of the protections being put in place. Ascribing ownership could also lead to disinclination on the part of potential research subjects to participate in experimental protocols: faced with perceived discrimination in employment or insurance, potential participants may be dissuaded from enrolling in clinical trials. Exercise of property rights allows research subjects not only to withdraw from research studies at any time (a privilege always available through IRB-approved protocols), but also to demand that their donated samples and the data derived from them, be destroyed. The results of such actions are self-evident to anyone familiar with experimental design and data analysis.

4.3.2. Expanded Requirements for Informed Consent. The model for informed consent has been radically changed, first by the AIDS experience and more recently by genetic testing. Previously, emphasis was focused on medical risks associated with the procedures involved in the protocol, which were usually minimal. The emphasis is now on disclosure and the possible psychological and societal consequences for the individual and family receiving information (i.e., test results). Many questions remain unanswered as to the validity of these inferred consequences.

The confidentiality of patient-identifiable information is protected by authorization procedures for its disclosure and research use. The responsibility for the establishment of such processes rests with the laboratory providing the primary (diagnostic) analysis of the specimen and with the Institutional Review Board (IRB) which approves the protocol and consent forms. Anonymization of data (removal of all patient identifiers and connections to any predispositions or conditions) can be easily achieved to ensure the preservation of epidemiological and outcomes research, which relies on historical data bases. However, some state bills (Maine, Delaware, New Mexico) require both informed consent for the original testing and supplemental agreements for every subsequent use of donated specimens. This, obviously, is a cumbersome system with negative impact. It should be possible to address the problem through a consent form which would provide assurance of complete anonymity and is worded to cover extended use of specimens donated for research, teaching, and quality control.

4.3.3. Restrictions on Use of Stored Tissue Samples. Tumor registries, newborn screening specimens, collections of mutant cell lines and abnormal karotypes, and other such repositories are important resources for basic and clinical research as well as optimizing patient care. Additional analysis of already-collected specimens—perhaps looking for extremely rare conditions—will be essential to understanding the genetic basis of disease. For population-based studies, anonymized data are suitable (perhaps preferable), and can be more easily achieved by use of these repositories. Agreements on how to handle additional research on repository samples have already been reached within the professional community. However, several state statutes (Delaware, Maine, Oregon) require mandatory destruction of such materials once the original testing has been completed, dooming these essential biological resources to eventual disappearance. Already-existing laws, regulations, and IRB practices covering research uses of donated specimens include provisions for confidentiality of identifiable material, making additional requirements irrelevant or restrictive.

In response to a provision in the HIPAA that Congress formulate standards for privacy and protection of individually identifiable health information, DHHS Secretary Donna E. Shalala[30] advanced five principles that should be addressed in crafting legislation: boundaries, security, consumer control, accountability, and public responsibility. Legislation based on these principles should:

- draw clear limits on who has access to health information;
- define the responsibilities of entities who possess health information to ensure that such information is protected from misuse and disclosure;
- establish patients' right to be advised as to how payers and providers will use their health information, to limit disclosure of health information in certain cases, to obtain a copy of their records, and to propose corrections in their records;
- authorize the disclosure of health information without explicit patient consent for use related to four national priority activities: audits and investigations of the health care system; public health tracking and medical emergencies; and health research and law enforcement activities.

5. GENETIC TESTING IN EMPLOYMENT

In the workplace, genetic testing may occur in two modalities: genetic screening and genetic monitoring. *Genetic screening* is obtaining genetic information about prospective employees or job applicants. The most common use of such information is to identify individuals affected by or predisposed to a given condition or those who may be susceptible or hypersusceptible to specific, possibly harmful, work environments. *Genetic monitoring* attempts to ascertain whether exposure to hazardous substances in the workplace is evoking "genetic changes" by monitoring somatic changes through cytogenetic or molecular means. The goal of genetic monitoring is to prevent or reduce the risk of disease arising from genetic damage. Its efficacy has yet to be proven, and its use in employment is difficult to justify.

As with health insurance coverage, these uses of genetic information have the potential for discriminatory practices: they could be used to deny employment to individuals regardless of their ability to fulfill the requirements of the job. This is particularly so in the case of the carriers of traits, who are asymptomatic and are not incapacitated or compromised relative to job demands. Existing protection against job discrimination is limited. There are no federal laws that directly and comprehensively protect the gathering or use of genetic information in the workplace. Title I of the Americans with Disabilities Act (ADA) does not explicitly address genetic information, but provides a modicum of protection for those affected with a visible phenotype, which is considered a disability. For those not visibly affected (i.e., asymptomatic carriers or those predisposed to late-onset disorders), protection is not clearly established. Attempting to redress this situation, the Equal Employment Opportunity Commission,[31] in 1995, issued an enforcement guideline. Adverse action on the basis of genetic information relating to illness, disease, or other disorders is prohibited since, as defined by the ADA, the individual involved is regarded as having a disability. This is only a policy guidance, not law. It is limited in scope and legal impact, and has yet to be tested in court. In addition, the ADA only prohibits an employer from requesting genetic information *prior* to extending a conditional offer of employment. Following such an offer (but before commencement of employment), the employer may obtain extensive medical or other information about the applicant.

As of October, 1997, 14 states had enacted laws to provide protection against various forms of genetic discrimination in the workplace. Given the substantial gaps in these laws, comprehensive federal legislation is needed to ensure that individuals are not denied employment based on genetic information, a view supported by the present administration. On January 20, 1998, Vice President Albert Gore, in an address to The Genome Action Coalition, stated, "the fear of genetic discrimination is prompting "Americans to avoid genetic tests that could literally save their lives." He also released a report entitled *Genetic Information and the Workplace*,[32] which proposes the following principles for anti-discrimination legislation:

- Employers should not require or request that employees or potential employees take a genetic test or provide genetic information as a condition of employment or benefits.
- Employers should not use genetic information to discriminate against, limit, segregate, or classify employees in a way that would deprive them of employment opportunities.
- Employers should not obtain or disclose genetic information about employees or potential employees under most circumstances.
- The use of genetic information and genetic testing should be permitted in some situations to ensure workplace safety and health and to preserve research opportunities if the employee has provided consent and if the information is maintained separately from personnel files, treated as a confidential medical record, and protected by applicable state and federal laws.

6. CONCLUSION

Genomic progress affects the entire spectrum of health care including diagnosis, possible therapy, and prediction of disease susceptibility. The ethical, legal, and social concerns that have been generated around these issues are important topics for discussion in both the professional and lay communities. Legislators and policy makers find themselves facing a multitude of conflicting interests and are attempting to balance the demands of consumers, investigators, health care providers, and insurers. Because genetic information is prone to potential abuse, genetic testing has become a lightening rod for a key political issue.

Among the many definitions of genetic information included in various pieces of legislation, perhaps the broadest is, "information about chromosomes, genes, gene products or inherited characteristics that may derive from an individual or blood-related family members, obtained for predictive purposes at the time when the individual to whom the information relates is asymptomatic for the disease in question." "Predictive purposes" is meant to include risk assessment of disease and/or the identification of carriers of disease-related mutations. Genetic information, so defined, can be obtained or inferred from many sources in family or individual medical histories and should not be limited to the results of genetic tests, which may have been restricted to DNA-based assays. Although pedigree analysis alone cannot usually predict which individual will develop a given condition, it can be used in risk assessment. The fact that biological relatives of an affected individual may also be at risk has changed the geneticist's definition of the "the patient" to encompass the extended, multi-generational family as well as the proband. This concept has serious implications for the protection of more than the privacy of the individual. It impacts on access to health care for the entire group.

It is becoming readily apparent that virtually all diseases have a genetic component and that we all carry several mutations. Genetic testing is rapidly demonstrating that all medical information will be genetically relevant, and it will be come increasingly difficult to separate "genetic" from "non-genetic" information in the medical record. Therefore, it is incumbent upon us to design appropriate protections for all such information in the context of fairness and utility.

REFERENCES

1. McGill DM, Holmes JS, Winberg JF: Selection and classification of risks (Part 1). In: *McGill's Life Insurance*. Graves EE, Hayes L, Eds. Bryn Mawr, PA, The American College, pp 435–451, 1994
2. Beam BT: Group life insurance. In: *McGill's Life Insurance*. Graves EE, Hayes L, Eds. Bryn Mawr, PA, The American College, pp 687–733, 1994
3. Light DW: The practice and ethics of risk-rated health insurance. JAMA 267:2503–2508, 1992
4. National Center for Human Genome Research. Genetic information and health insurance: report of the task force on genetic information and insurance. NIH Publication No. 93-3686. National Institutes of Health, Bethesda, MD, 1993
5. Health Insurance Association of American (HIAA). Individual Health Insurance, 1992
6. Ostrer H, et al: Insurance and genetic testing: where are we now? Am J Hum Genet 52:565–577, 1993
7. Society of Actuaries. Actuarial standard of practice #12 concerning risk classification. Section 2.1, 1989:1
8. Pokorski RJ: Use of genetic information by private insurers—genetic advances: The perspective of an insurance medical director. J Insur Medicine 2460–2468, 1992
9. Pokorski, RJ: Insurance underwriting in the genetic era. Cancer, supp 80:587–599, 1997
10. American Council of Life Insurance. *1994 Life Insurance Fact Book*. Washington, DC, 1994
11. Holtzman NA, et al: Predictive genetic testing: from basic research to clinical practice. Science 278:602–605, 1997
12. Task Force on Genetic Testing: Promoting Safe and Effective Testing in the United States, Final Report. Holtzman NA, Watson MS, Eds. National Institutes of Health, Bethesda, MD, 1997
13. Lowden JA: Underwriting lethal genetic diseases. Presented at the Annual Meeting of the Canadian Medical Officers Association, Montreal, Quebec, Canada. May 14, 1997
14. Reiss J: Personal communication, 1998
15. Report from the Field: Amid genetic advances, plans must wrestle with complex challenges. Medical Outcomes and Guidelines Alert, pp 5–8, November 6, 1997
16. Collins, FS, et al: National Action Plan on Breast Cancer, Position paper on hereditary susceptibility testing for breast cancer. Washington, DC, National Action Plan on Breast Cancer, March, 1966
17. Statement of the American Society on Clinical Oncology: Genetic testing for breast and ovarian cancer susceptibility. J Clin Oncol 14:1730–1736, 1996
18. Statement of the American Society of Human Genetics on Genetic testing for breast and ovarian cancer predisposition. Am J Hum Genet 55:i–iv, 1994
19. McKinnon WE, et al: Predisposition genetic testing for late-onset disorders in adults. A position paper of the National Society of Genetic Counselors. JAMA 278:1217–1220, 1997
20. Bernhardt B, Peshkin, B Kernel, Y: Billing and record keeping for familial cancer risk counseling (FCRC): A national survey. J Gen Couns 6:491–492, 1997
21. Billings PR, et al: Discrimination as a consequence of genetic testing. Am J Hum Genet 50:476–482, 1992
22. Reilly PR: Genetic discrimination. In: *Risk Regulation and Responsibility: Genetic Testing and the Age of Information*. Long C, Ed. AEI Press, Washington, DC. In Press
23. McEwen J, et al: A survey of state insurance commissioners concerning genetic testing and life insurance. Am J Hum Genet 51:785–792, 1992
24. McEwen J, et al: A survey of medical directors of life insurance companies concerning use of genetic information. Am J Hum Genet 53:33–45, 1993
25. Johnson JA: CRS Issue Brief. Genetic Screening. Congressional Research Service, The Library of Congress, pp I–15, 1991

26. Bird S, et al: Individual, family and societal dimensions of genetic discrimination case study analysis. Science and Engineering Ethics 2:71–78, 1996
27. Lapham V, et al: Genetic discrimination: perspectives of consumers. Science 274:621–624, 1996
28. Westin A: Report on national opinion surveys relating to genetic testing, screening, and uses of genetic information, with implications for a national survey focused on privacy issues and safeguards. ELSI Program (Part 2), U.S. Department of Energy, pp 1–22, 1994
29. Genetic Discrimination and Health Insurance: a Case Study on Breast Cancer. Workshop sponsored by the National Action Plan on Breast Cancer (NAPBC) and the NIH-DOE Working Group on the Ethical Legal, and Social Implications of Human Genome Research. Bethesda, MD, July 11, 1995
30. Shalala DE: Testimony before the U.S. Senate Committee on Labor and Human Resources. September 11, 1997
31. Equal Employment Opportunity Commission, Compliance Manual Volume 2, Section 902. Order 915.002, pp 902–945, 1995
32. Genetic Information and the Workplace. Department of Labor, Department of Health and Human Services, Equal Employment Opportunity Commission, Department of Justice. January 20, 1998

12

ETHICAL AND LEGAL ISSUES IN GENETIC TESTING FOR CANCER SUSCEPTIBILITY

Jeffrey R. Botkin

Professor of Pediatrics and
Medical Ethics
University of Utah
Primary Children's Medical Center
100 North Medical Drive
Salt Lake City, Utah 84113

Genetic testing for cancer susceptibility is new and therefore deserves the careful attention of physicians in order to assure that the tests are performed and interpreted in an appropriate fashion. On occasion, genetic testing for cancer susceptibility will present ethical dilemmas with which many clinicians will not be familiar. A brief case presentation will frame these issues for subsequent discussion.

I. CASE PRESENTATION

A 40 year old man, Ray, presents to his internist for a periodic checkup. The interval history is notable for recent family distress over the loss of Ray's aunt to ovarian cancer. A detailed family history reveals multiple cases of breast and ovarian cancer in Ray's maternal side of the family. Ray's other aunt is a breast cancer survivor. His mother is healthy. Ray has a brother, two sisters and two daughters ages 20 and 21, all of whom are healthy.

You discuss the possibility with Ray that his family may have a heritable mutation that increases the risk of breast and ovarian cancer in women and, possibly, prostate cancer in men. As it turns out, Ray is familiar with the possibility of genetic testing. Genetic testing had been offered to his aunts and mother. Prior to her death by ovarian cancer, his aunt was found to carry a BRCA1 mutation. Ray's mother and surviving aunt declined testing, apparently because they felt they could not handle the information after the difficult experience of their sister's death. They also are concerned about their insurance status.

Phone: (801) 588-3640, FAX: (801) 588-3642, e-mail: botkin@howard.med.utah.edu

Cancer Genetics for the Clinician, edited by Shaw.
Kluwer Academic / Plenum Publishers, New York, 1999.

After a discussion of the pros and cons, Ray indicates that he would like to proceed with genetic testing.

I.1. Question 1: What are your obligations as Ray's physician to Ray's mother? (Note that if Ray is mutation positive, that will indicate that his mother is mutation positive as well.)

Ray proceeds with testing and is found to be a mutation carrier for BRCA1. You discuss the implications for Ray's daughters. However, Ray has recently undergone a bitter divorce and communication with his former wife is limited and generally hostile. He also has a tenuous relationship with his daughters, both of whom tended to side with their mother in the divorce proceedings. Ray indicates that he does not plan to reveal his genetic test results to his former wife or children. He states that he may tell them someday when the relationships improve.

I.2. Question 2: As Ray's physician, what are your obligations to Ray's children? Should you contact them contrary Ray's wishes to inform them of their risk?

II. SPECIAL CONSIDERATIONS FOR GENETIC TESTING

A consideration of some of the broader issues involved in genetic testing will assist in placing these specific questions in their appropriate context. A question that has been receiving some debate in recent years is whether genetic testing is sufficiently different from other forms of testing to deserve special considerations. A small academic industry has developed to promulgate guidelines for testing protocols, genetic counseling, and informed consent. Are there really any significant differences between genetic testing and other forms of testing for which physicians are familiar? In short, what is all the fuss about genetics? Should we simply allow genetic testing to be integrated into clinical practice the way many other tests are gradually introduced as physicians become familiar with the technology?

The argument developed here is that genetic testing is different in some significant respects, but not entirely different.[1] Further there are some dangers in considering genetic testing as something special. The key differences worthy of attention by physicians are (1) the family implications of test results, (2) the increased predictive power of some genetic tests, (3) the psychosocial implications of testing, and (4) the limited responses available to reduce morbidity and mortality for mutation carriers.

The case presented illustrates the family implications of genetic testing. The results of one individual's test have direct implications for the genetic status of other family members, particularly first degree relatives—parents, children, and siblings. If Ray is mutation positive, his parent from the high risk kindred is an obligate carrier. Further, the risk of being a mutation carrier for his children increases to 50% as does the risk for his siblings. Even without genetic testing of these relatives directly, their risk of cancer has increased substantially over the risk in the general population.

The diagnosis of any disease or risk in one family member always has implications for others in the family. These implications may be emotional and financial, and include the time and effort necessary to support an ill relative. But these kinds of impacts do not impinge directly on the health status of relatives. Knowledge that your brother is ill from, or at substantial risk for, say, heart disease is different than knowledge that your brother is ill or at risk for a condition that you too are at risk for based on your genetic relationship. This direct implication is not unique to genetics. Family members with infectious disease may pose a direct risk to others—Hepatitis B and HIV being prime examples. Learning that one's spouse has HIV, for example, clearly has direct implications for the individual's own health.

So the claim cannot be made that genetics is unique in terms of the impact on others beyond the patient herself. HIV testing is probably the closest analogy to genetic testing for cancer susceptibility for each of the issues outlined here—family implications, predictive power of the test, and psychosocial implications. It is notable that HIV testing has been subject to significant scrutiny and special protocols since its inception more than ten years ago. Only recently have many clinics and hospitals begun to decrease the special precautions that have been instituted for HIV. So the fact that genetic testing is analogous to HIV testing in some respects reinforces the need to approach genetic testing with care.

The second distinction to be made for genetic testing is the predictive power of some tests. There is debate on the true risks of cancer for a BRCA1 mutation carrier and the risks may vary depending on the nature of the mutation as well the background genetic factors that may influence risk in any particular family. Nevertheless, the risk for breast cancer in some families is as high as 85% by age 70 years and for ovarian cancer is 60% by age 70 years. Physicians are familiar with predictive testing. Cholesterol testing and blood pressure measurement are two common forms of predictive testing, however, the magnitude of risk conferred by elevated cholesterol levels or blood pressure is substantially lower than genetic testing for BRCA1/2, HNPCC or p53 mutations. For example, the 10 year risk of coronary heart disease for an individual with a diastolic blood pressure over 110 mm Hg is about 4.5% and the risk of stroke in this group is about 1.4%.[2] The 10 year death rate from coronary heart disease for men with cholesterol levels of 250 to 300 mg/dl is about 2.5% to 4%.[3]

The third distinction between genetic testing and other sorts of new technologies is simply that the risks involved are psychosocial rather than physical. This has led a number of commentators to downplay the risks associated with the introduction of this technology. Indeed, early research results suggest that individuals in high risk families manage to deal with predictive testing for cancer susceptibility without serious psychological impairments.[4] Nevertheless, the impact on people's lives is profound. Therefore approaching testing with the utmost care, both in terms of accuracy of information and complete informed consent is essential.

Finally, the limited ability to respond to genetic test results with interventions to reduce morbidity and mortality is a distinction between some genetic tests and other predictive tests. We have confidence that we can do something about cholesterol and hypertension to reduce risk, but the data is still out on whether preventive surgery or early detection measures will substantially reduce the risk in a number of hereditary cancer syndromes such as BRCA1/2[5] or for hereditary nonpolyposis colon cancer.[6] This ability to diagnose risk before the ability to do something about it is the basic factor behind many of the ethical dilemmas in genetic testing.

Do these differences make genetic testing unique in medicine? No—there is no bright line between genetic testing and other sorts of testing just as there are no simple criteria that will separate genetic diseases from non-genetic conditions. The argument here is that there are aspects of genetic testing that make this form of testing sufficiently different to justify additional care and scrutiny. But there are also risks involved in overemphasizing distinctions between genetic testing and other forms. This has been termed "genetic exceptionalism."[7] The risk is that by overemphasizing genetics, we will be fashioning a self-fulfilling prophesy. Genetics may become special because we repeat over and over again that genetics is special. Genetic determinism, the belief that we are what our genes dictate, is both the cause and result of genetic exceptionalism and many of the concerns about genetics—stigmatization, discrimination, racism—have their root cause in genetic determinism.

Time will tell what contemporary research finds to be the role of genes per se in our understanding of life processes and disease. A number of critics are suggesting that we have gone too far in our rhetoric, that genes and molecular genetics dominate our thinking, our research funding, and the biotechnology industry because we have some understanding of DNA and the tools to dissect it. As the old saying goes, when your only tool is a hammer, all your problems look like nails. Richard Strohman suggests that as we learn more about the multiple layers of complexity in biologic systems, our current infatuation with genetic testing will dissolve.[8] It may be, he says, that genetic testing will remain valuable only for the relatively rare single gene disorders which comprise only 2% of the disease afflicting the population. If he is right, the genetic revolution may have a much more limited impact on medicine than is often predicted.

For clinicians trying to get up to speed on genetic testing for cancer susceptibility, the thrust of this argument is that we must pay special attention to genetic testing because it is technically complex requiring careful attention to when testing is indicated, how to order and interpret the test and how to adequately inform patients about the risks and benefits. Further, the family and psychosocial implications are issues that must be confronted in the clinical environment.

III. RIGHTS TO GENETIC INFORMATION

Let's take a step back for a moment and ask a more preliminary question to the ones raised in the case scenario. Should the physician in this case have offered genetic testing to Ray at all? BRCA1/2 testing is commercially available from several vendors but the commercial use of the test has been a focus of controversy over the past four years. In 1994 following the identification of the BRCA1 gene, the National Advisory Council for Human Genome Research published a statement advising: "Until more information is available to address these critical issues, it is premature to offer DNA testing for screening for cancer predisposition outside a carefully monitored research environment."[9] The statement outlined five concerns:

(1) Uncertainty about the number of genetic mutations for BRCA1 and MSH2 and the risk associated with each mutation
(2) Uncertainty over false-positive and false negative results for genetic testing
(3) Uncertainty over the prevention of cancer in high risk individuals
(4) Uncertainty over appropriate methods for education, informed consent and counseling, and
(5) Uncertainty over how to avoid genetic discrimination.

It is notable that none of these concerns have been resolved at the present time. Francis Collins, the current director of the National Human Genome Research Institute has reinforced this position, stating "[I]t is critical that we create safeguards to ensure that the benefits of testing exceed the risks. The technical ability to perform tests for mutations should not be confused with a mandate to offer them."[10]

The American Society of Human Genetics (ASHG) also published a statement in 1994 which states: "While the cancer risks associated with different BRCA1 mutations are being determined, testing should initially be offered and performed on an investigational basis by appropriately trained health care professionals who have a therapeutic relationship with the patient and are fully aware of the genetic, clinical, and psychological implications of testing, as well as of the limitations of existing test procedures."[11] The ASHG has yet to offer a statement promoting clinical testing for breast and ovarian cancer susceptibility. This concern about premature clinical application of testing by geneticists and the genetic research community is paralleled by concerns in the breast cancer advocacy community. The National Breast Cancer Coalition (NBCC), a coalition of some 350 organizations and 41,000 individuals dedicated to fighting breast cancer, stated in 1996 that: "genetic testing should only be available within peer-reviewed research protocols."[12] The statement goes so far as to request prohibition of commercial testing by the FDA. The concerns raised by the NBCC mirror those of the professional organizations—test sensitivity and specificity, education of providers and inadequate knowledge of appropriate counseling protocols.

The principal professional organization which has been open to the clinical application of genetic testing for cancer susceptibility is the American Society of Clinical Oncology (ASCO). A 1996 ASCO statement suggests that "genetic testing should be made available to selected patients as part of the preventive oncology care of families . . ."[13] ASCO specifically indicates that genetic testing for breast and ovarian cancer susceptibility is appropriate for clinical use. It also goes without saying that companies in the biotechnology industry that are selling the test believe that the technology is ready for clinical application. Further, there is a clear philosophical position supporting consumer choice that has been voiced by Mark Skolnick at Myriad Genetics: "We can attempt to turn back the clock and ignore the ability to provide knowledge to women who seek it; to me this is unethical. Alternatively, we can recognize that testing has value today, and we can work together to ensure that genetic testing for cancer susceptibility is introduced to society in the most responsible fashion possible."[14]

This debate also is not unique to genetic testing. There is a basic tension with new drugs and technologies between the individual's prerogative to accept risk in pursuit of personal gain with new interventions and the social need to protect individuals from exploitation. The demand of many in the AIDS advocacy community to be permitted to take drugs of their choice independent of FDA restrictions illustrates the same tension. On the one hand there is the perceived need to move slowly with this new kind of testing until we can determine whether individuals benefit from it, or, more specifically, how to help assure that benefit will result. Benefit will occur only if morbidity or mortality are reduced or if there is psychological benefit to testing. It still remains to be shown that either of these benefits are realized through BRCA1/2 testing. On the other hand, there is a legitimate argument to be made that individuals should be able to make these assessments for themselves and, with full knowledge of the uncertainties, pursue testing if they desire. We are open to criticisms of paternalism if we prohibit testing of individuals who are highly interested in pursuing this personal information. Perhaps it is up to the knowledgeable consumer to decide whether testing will be beneficial or not.

The FDA currently is not required to regulate genetic tests unless they are marketed as kits. When genetic tests are conducted by university laboratories or commercial vendors, FDA approval is not required. Therefore new genetic tests can move rapidly into commercial use without formal review by governmental or local agencies like IRBs. To address these concerns, the National Human Genome Research Institute and the Department of Energy established a Task Force on Genetic Testing in 1994.[15] Its 1997 report recommends formal scrutiny of new genetic tests before they are available for routine clinical use. It also recommends the establishment of a new office for genetic testing in the office of the Secretary of Health and Human Services. This office has been created and will advise the secretary on, among other things, the safety and effectiveness of new genetic tests. Before tests are available clinically, the task force recommends that the following criteria be satisfied:

(1) The genotypes to be detected by a genetic test must be shown by scientifically valid methods to be associated with the occurrence of a disease. The observations must be independently replicated and subject to peer review.
(2) Analytical sensitivity and specificity of a genetic test must be determined before it is made available in clinical practice.
(3) Data to establish the clinical validity of tests (clinical sensitivity, specificity, and predictive value) must be collected under investigational protocols.
(4) Before a genetic test can be generally accepted in clinical practice, data must be collected to demonstrate the benefits and the risks that accrue from both positive and negative results.

In addition, the Task Force recommended that genetics curricula be developed for medical schools, residencies and practicing physicians, and for nurses, public health officials and social workers. The report also encourages hospitals and managed care organizations to require evidence of competency before permitting providers to order genetic tests or counsel about them.

The difficulty in fulfilling the above criteria should not be underestimated. Hundreds of mutations in BRCA1 and BRCA2 have been identified, making it difficult to determine the sensitivity and specificity of each. It is also likely to take quite a few years to demonstrate the benefits and burdens of testing since all the psychosocial effects are not immediate and the effects on disease prevention or early detection will take much longer to observe. If a test proves to be highly beneficial, then the time and, potentially, lives lost through a slow regulatory process may be substantial. The problem of deciding how best to regulate predictive genetic tests without stifling beneficial interventions is considerable.

In the meantime, clinicians are left without regulatory guidance in deciding when to implement genetic tests. Is it time now to offer BRCA1/2 testing and, if so, to whom should testing be offered? One clear conclusion that flows from the above considerations is that there is no *obligation* to offer genetic testing for breast and ovarian cancer susceptibility at the present time. Patients do not have a right to be tested. However, the physician does have an emerging obligation to recognize high risk individuals, make those individuals aware that testing is possible, and to refer interested patients to knowledgeable experts. If the physician wishes to proceed with testing, she must be sure that she can adequately provide informed consent, interpret the results of the test, and provide appropriate recommendations for mutation positive and negative individuals.

The first priority in a decision to offer testing is to make sure that people are making fully informed choices. Whether benefits will flow from testing is often uncertain in medicine. Our own research in BRCA1 testing and the research of others is clearly showing that some individuals benefit from such testing and others are experiencing significant distress.[16] It is notable, however, that the Task Force does not require that net benefit be shown for a test before it becomes clinically available. It only requires that the benefits and risks be studied so that individuals can make informed choices. What must be minimized is the number of physicians and patients who misinterpret results—whether positive or negative—and make critical health care decisions based on confusion or false information. The track record to date is not encouraging. Giardiello's paper from March of 1997 in the *New England Journal of Medicine* found that 31.6% of the physicians ordering a genetic test for APC mutations misinterpreted the results.[17]

IV. GENETIC PRIVACY

Genetic testing for cancer susceptibility is about obtaining small bits of information which may have profound implications for our health and welfare. The information itself has direct implications in terms of risk of future disease and, as has been noted, the force of the information is due in large measure to the limited options available for preventing or ameliorating cancer. The information also has indirect implications. It has been said that human genetics is the science of human differences. Of course, this is only true to a limited extent because there are many sources of differences between any two individuals beyond genetics. Nevertheless, finding that one is at high risk for cancer is a distinct difference about which others care. Family members care because of the implications for their own health and because of the foreboding of future suffering and loss of a loved one, and the anguish and burdens that will place on the family. Friends care, not for their health, but for the welfare of the one at risk and for their own anticipated loss of friendship. Employers may care due to the loss of skills and the financial burden of illness. Insurers may care as well since they are in the business of covering loss of health and life. The biomedical community cares because those with interesting mutations make valuable research subjects to better understand disease.

From the tested individual's perspective, all of this indirect impact may constitute collateral damage. Hard enough to deal with your own struggle with mortality without seeing the fear and pity in the eyes of others—or perhaps the subtle disdain from those who are not so genetically flawed. How does one develop new relationships, new passions, new directions in life if others withdraw from your story, scripted to run tragically short? Sometimes the risks from testing run the other way. In high risk cancer families, some have clear expectations from early in life that *they* are the sibling who will be struck down with cancer. This may give some individuals a liberty to lead a life of limited expectations, self-indulgence and perhaps self-pity. This structured lifestyle also can be brought down with genetic testing, albeit with "good news" that proves not to be an unmitigated good.

It is little wonder that many choose not to be tested, perhaps both to protect their own psychological welfare but also to protect themselves from a new role in the eyes of others. Caryn Lerman's study found that about 48% of those at risk for being BRCA1 mutation carriers chose to be tested.[4] It is notable that this contrasts with the much lower number of individuals at risk for Huntington disease who have pursued testing—estimated to be about 15% to 20%. Precisely what the difference is between these two conditions remains to be determined, although we can surmise that there is more perceived benefit from genetic testing for cancer.

Genetic privacy is a term that has arisen in recent years to reflect the concern over how to control the impact of genetics on people's lives. Anita Allen[18] distinguishes four kinds of privacy:

> (1) informational privacy concerns about access to personal information; (2) physical privacy concerns about access to persons and personal spaces; (3) decisional privacy concerns about governmental and other third-party interference with personal choices; and (4) proprietary privacy concerns about the appropriation and ownership of interests in human personality. "Genetic privacy" typically refers to one of these same four general categories.

The dilemmas presented in the case scenario involve several of these privacy considerations. As Allen notes, many authors writing about genetic privacy focus on informational privacy—one's prerogative to control genetic information about oneself. One proposed principle is that individuals should have informed choice over whether to have genetic testing or not. Exceptions to informed choice in genetic testing are relatively few. Most states mandate newborn screening tests and, in some circumstances, genetic testing is required in the context of criminal investigations. For genetic testing for cancer susceptibility, a clear principle that individuals should not be tested without their informed consent appears basic (aside from situations where the individual is incompetent or dead). A second principle is that genetic information should not be disclosed to others without the informed consent of the individual (again assuming the individual is alive and competent). The second principle is simply a statement of the principle of confidentiality.

A model Genetic Privacy Act developed by George Annas, Leonard Glantz and Patricia Roche articulates these principles clearly.[19] It states ". . . no person may collect or cause to be collected an individually identifiable DNA sample for genetic analysis without the written authorization of the sample source or the sample source's representative." Further, any offer of testing must be accompanied by informed consent, to include at least 11 points of disclosure. With respect to confidentiality, the Genetic Privacy Act states ". . . no person who, in the ordinary course of business, practice of a profession, or rendering of a service, creates, stores, receives or furnishes private genetic information may by any means of communication disclose private genetic information except in accordance with a written authorization . . ." The Genetic Privacy Act has not been passed at the federal or state levels, although an increasing number of states are passing legislation to protect individuals from genetic discrimination—principally insurance and employment discrimination. There are also more than a dozen federal bills pending as of this writing that seek to address some aspect of genetic privacy.

The basic question that is at the center of this kind of legislation, and at the center of the case scenario presented above, is how much we as a society, and we as practitioners, want to respect genetic privacy. There are, of course, competing considerations. As we have seen, genetic information of one individual has implications for other family members. Information will have financial implications for employers and insurance companies. Information may have health implications for others if the genetic condition potentially makes an individual unsafe in the workplace or unsafe to drive a car. The firm and clear stand taken by the model Genetic Privacy Act is not shared uniformly by commentators, clinicians or judicial decisions. A number of committees and professional organizations support the prerogative of the clinician to disclose genetic information to family members in exceptional circumstances. The President's Commission for the Study of Ethical Problems in Medicine and Biomedical and Behavioral Research, the Institute of Medicine, The Social Issues Subcommittee on Familial Disclosure of the American Society of Human Genetics and the NIH/DOE Task Force on Genetic Testing support a position in which disclosure to family members "is appropriate only when the person tested refuses to communicate information despite reasonable attempts to persuade him or her to do so, and when failure to give that information has a high probability of resulting in imminent, serious, irreversible harm to the relative and when communication of the information will enable the relative to avert the harm."[20] This position permits physicians to disclose in some circumstances but does not require that they do so. A similar standard has been supported internationally by the World Medical Association, the World Health Organization, the Council of Europe, the Health Council of Netherlands, the Privacy Commissioner of Australia and the Japan Society of Human Genetics.[20] In contrast, the Swiss Academy of Medical Sciences and the French National Ethics Committee do not support disclosure without the patient's consent.[20]

Case law has addressed the issue to only a limited extent. The most famous "duty to warn" case is the Tarasoff Case in California in 1976.[21] A psychologist's patient threatened his girlfriend and the psychologist chose not to warn the young woman or her family directly. When the young woman was murdered, her family sued the University of California. The court found in a closely split decision that the psychologist did have a duty to warn when imminent, serious harm could be averted to an identifiable individual. More recent cases have addressed the duty to warn in the context of genetic information. In a 1995 Florida case, Pate v. Threkel, a daughter with medullary thyroid carcinoma sued her mother's physician for failing to warn her, the daughter, that her mother's cancer was hereditary.[22] Based on state law protecting confidentialty and the standard of medical care, the court found that the physician had a duty to warn the mother of the hereditary nature of the disease, but not the daughter. In contrast, a New Jersey case in 1996, Safer v. Estate of Pack, found that physicians do have an obligation to warn offspring of a genetic risk of cancer.[23] In this case, a daughter was diagnosed with colon cancer secondary to familial adenomatous polyposi. Her father had died 26 years earlier from the disease and the treating physician had failed to warn his offspring. This case may prove to be an anomaly since, due to procedural rules, the appelate court was required to accept the daughter's claim that disclosure was the standard of care in medicine at the time. Neither of these cases deal with a circumstance in which the initial patient refuses consent for disclosure of information to offspring. These expert opinions and legal cases suggest that disclosure over the objections of the patient are permissible in a narrow range of circumstances, disclosure may be mandatory in some circumstances with the consent of the patient, but it is debatable whether disclosure is ever ethically mandatory without consent.

The extent to which physicians behave in accordance with these principles is unclear. In a survey published in 1989 by Wertz and Fletcher, 60% would disclose a risk of Huntington disease to a relative without the patient's consent and 58% of geneticists said they would disclose a diagnosis of Hemophilia A.[24] How physicians actually behave in these sorts of circumstances is unknown.

A third position on the disclosure of genetic information is offered by Fost.[25] Fost suggests that such dilemmas are preventable by disclosing to the patient *before* genetic testing that the physician will be compelled to disclose results to certain family members without the permission of the patient, if necessary. The patient can therefore decide whether to proceed with testing or not based on this disclosure. This approach is supported by the NIH/DOE Task Force on Genetic Testing. This practice also is consistent with how many pediatricians approach confidentiality in the care of adolescents. If the physician does not believe that confidentiality is absolute in some circumstances, then warning the patient prior to the sharing of sensitive information will avert a serious dilemma. In the context of genetic testing, circumstances that involve a potential duty to warn are predictable, based on the nature of the disease involved and the structure of the patient's family. Therefore the clinician can anticipate this dilemma and prepare accordingly.

V. FAMILY IMPLICATIONS

V.1. Rights Not to Be Tested Without Consent

With this discussion as background, let's return to the case scenario of Ray. The first dilemma posed was how to deal with Ray's request for testing with the knowledge that Ray's mother had refused genetic testing. If Ray tests positive for the family BRCA1 mutation, then his mother is an obligate mutation carrier. Does the physician have an obligation to Ray's mother? Should the ethical physician forego testing of Ray so that Ray's mother does not receive results contrary to her wishes? Whose rights prevail here—Ray's right to be tested or Ray's mother's right of privacy, the right not to have genetic results forced upon her?

Ray's mother is not a patient so there is no physician-patient relationship and no formal obligation. Yet the very nature of genetic information is forcing a broader understanding of the physician's responsibility. If, as we have seen, there is an emerging responsibility to warn family members in some circumstances, so there is plausibly some responsibility to avoid harming family members by blundering through the family genome. The ripple effect of testing through a family can be anticipated and therefore should be considered in deciding how to manage genetic testing. A basic principle discussed above is that individuals must consent to genetic testing. Indeed, the proposed Genetic Privacy Act would prohibit testing without consent, consistent with our notion that such powerful information should not be foisted upon individuals who do not desire it. Ray's mother's desire not to be tested must have some pull on our deliberations.

A further consideration is that the genetic testing of Ray in a non-research environment is contrary to the recommendations of most organizations and interest groups. Certainly the physician is not obligated to offer or conduct testing on Ray in any circumstance, and particularly if there are additional complicating factors that suggest the harms in testing may outweigh the benefits for all concerned. Finally, Ray has little direct benefit to gain from the genetic information, other than to better clarify the risk status of his children. The current recommendations for male BRCA1 carriers is to follow the prevailing American Cancer Society recommendations for prostate and colon cancer offered for all men of his age.[5] The physician's obligation to Ray's sister would be stronger if she was the patient since there are a variety of preventative or early detection strategies that she should consider if she were a mutation carrier. Of course, she could pursue measures like mammography without knowing her genotype, although, of course, prophylactic mastectomy or oophorectomy would not be appropriate without testing for a known family mutation.

The resolution of this type of conflict should not come through an abstract determination of whose rights prevail. One aspect of genetic testing not discussed is a certain luxury of time. There is no compelling reason for Ray to be tested today or this month or this year. (Ray's sister may have a stronger claim to urgency, particularly if she is highly anxious, yet there is still the option of waiting weeks, months or even years depending on her age.) This time provides the opportunity to pursue a discussion with Ray's mother and Ray to see if an agreement can be reached on testing. In our own BRCA1 testing protocol, we attempted to avoid this problem by offering testing from the older generations to the youngest.[26] In a few instances, an older parent did not want testing, forcing us to decide how to proceed with their offspring. In all cases, a discussion between the family members involved resolved the conflict—usually in favor of the adult child who desired testing.

The important issues for clinicians in this context is, first, to recognize the implications and the responsibilities to other family members in genetic testing. Second, physicians can proceed slowly into testing, if at all, when such conflicts exist in order to allow time for a negotiated resolution.

V.2. Confidentiality and the Physician's Duty to Warn

The second dilemma posed concerned the physician's duty to warn Ray's daughters without his consent. While a few of the positions outlined above argue for strict confidentiality, most of the authoritative statements support a limited duty to warn. The duty materializes when there is serious, imminent harm that can be averted only through disclosure. If we adhere to this standard, will notifying his daughters of their 50% risk status for a BRCA1 mutation prevent serious, imminent harm? If one or both daughters are mutation carriers, their risk of breast or ovarian cancer is substantial over their lifetime, but the risk does not begin to rise until at least the late twenties or early thirties. Further, they may never develop cancer despite the mutation. Cancer is obviously serious, but the risk of cancer is not imminent. There also remain substantial uncertainties about the ability of BRCA1 mutation carriers to reduce the morbidity or mortality of the disease by preventative or early detection strategies. Thus there is no certainty that disclosure will avert the anticipated harm.

These considerations suggest that there is no solid justification for breaching the respect for Ray's confidentiality. Further, it is not clear that there are any circumstances in which the risk posed by BRCA1 or BRCA2 would meet the emerging standard of preventing serious, imminent harm. (Of course, each form of genetic testing for cancer susceptibility should be evaluated separately by this standard. Rarely, however, could the development of cancer be considered imminent.) The physician can still exert substantial effort over time to convince Ray of the unethical nature of his decision not to share this information with his daughters. If evidence emerges that there are effective strategies for mutation carriers to reduce disease, then there will be a stronger obligation to warn. However, an affirmative decision about a duty to warn should trigger a disclosure of this duty to the patient prior to testing.

There is one additional alternative in this situation that deserves consideration. The duty to warn is discussed almost exclusively in terms of the disclosure of personal genetic status. In some circumstances, what relatives may need to know is not the personal results of one family member, but the general information about the family's risk status. Ray's daughters, for example, might benefit from knowing that their great aunt who died of ovarian cancer was a BRCA1 mutation carrier. As we have seen, the great aunt's physician may have a duty to advise the great aunt to warn others or the physician herself may have a duty to warn kindred members of the risk. It may be possible therefore for Ray's physician to promulgate a warning to all individuals in the kindred, including Ray's daughters, without disclosing Ray's personal genetic results.

VI. CONCLUSIONS

Genetic research in cancer will produce substantial benefits in the future through a more thorough understanding of the pathophysiology of cancer. In the mean time, genetic research will enable testing for cancer susceptibility in a growing number of clinical circumstances. As gatekeepers for this technology, physicians have a substantial responsibility to assure that testing is conducted with careful attention to patient education and informed consent and with a sensitivity to the complex family environment in which genetic testing is conducted.

REFERENCES

1. Geller G, Botkin J, Green M, Press N, Biesecker B, et al: Genetic testing for susceptibility to adult-onset cancer: the process and content of informed consent. JAMA 277:1467–1474, 1997
2. MacMahon S, Peto R, Cutler J, et al: Blood pressure, stroke, and coronary heart disease: Part 1, prolonged differences in blood pressure: prospective observational studies corrected for the regression dilution bias. Lancet 335:765–774, 1990
3. Anon: Classification, Prevalence, Detection, and Evaluation. Circulation 89:1344–1356, 1994
4. Lerman C, Narod S, Schulman K, Hughs C, et al: BRCA1 testing in families with hereditary breast-ovarian cancer. JAMA 275:1885–1892, 1996
5. Burke W, Daly M, Garber J, Botkin J, et al: Recommendations for follow-up care of individuals with inherited predisposition to cancer: BRCA1 and BRCA2. JAMA 277:997–1003, 1997
6. Burke W, Petersen G, Lynch P, Botkin J, Daly M, et al: Recommendations for follow-up care of individuals with inherited predisposition to cancer: hereditary nonpolyposis colon cancer. JAMA 277:915–919, 1997
7. Murray T: Genetic exceptionalism, and "future diaries": Is genetic information different from other medical information? in Rothstein M (Ed) *Genetic Secrets: Protecting Privacy and Confidentiality in the Genetic Era*. Yale University Press, New Haven, 60–73, 1997
8. Strohman RC: The coming Kuhnian revolution in biology. Nature Biotechnology 15:194–200, 1997
9. National Advisory Council for Human Genome Research. Statement on use of DNA testing for presymptomatic identification of cancer risk. JAMA 271:785, 1994
10. Collins FS: BRCA1—Lots of mutations, lots of dilemmas. N Engl J Med 334:186–188, 1996
11. American Society of Human Genetics. Statement of the American Society of Human Genetics on Genetic Testing for Breast and Ovarian Cancer Predisposition. Am J Hum Genet 55:i–iv, 1994
12. Visco F: Commentary on the ASCO statement on genetic testing for cancer susceptibility [press release] Washington, DC, National Breast Cancer Coalition
13. Statement of the American Society of Clinical Oncology: Genetic Testing for Cancer Susceptibility. J Clin Oncology 14:1730–1736, 1996
14. Mark Skolnick, Ph.D., Myriad Genetics, 1996
15. Task Force on Genetic Testing. Promoting Safe and Effective Genetic Testing in the United States: Final Report of the Task Force on Genetic Testing. Holtzman NA, Watson MS (Eds) available at http://www.nhgri.nih.gov/ELSI/TFGT_final/
16. Croyle R, Smith K, Botkin J, Baty B, Nash J: Psychological responses to BRCA1 mutation testing: preliminary findings. Health Psychology 16:63–72, 1997

17. Giardiello FM, Brensinger JD, Petersen GM, et al: The use and interpretation of commercial APC gene testing for familial adenomatous polyposis. New Engl J Med 336:823–827, 1997
18. Allen A: Genetic privacy: emerging concepts and values. In Rothstein M (Ed) *Genetic Secrets: Protecting Privacy and Confidentiality in the Genetic Era.* Yale University Press, New Haven, 31–59, 1997
19. Annas GJ, Glantz L, Roche PA: The Genetic Privacy Act. 1995, Boston: Boston University School of Public Health
20. The American Society of Human Genetics Social Issues Subcommittee on Familial Disclosure. Professional Disclosure of Familial Genetic Information. Am J Hum Genet 62:474–483, 1998
21. Tarasoff V: Regents of University of California 551 P.2d 334
22. Pate V: Threkel, 661 So. 2d 278 (1995)
23. Safer V: Estate of Pack 677 A. 2d 1188
24. Wertz D, Fletcher J. An international survey of attitudes of medical geneticists toward mass screening and access to results. 1989 Publ Health Reports 104:35–44
25. Fost N: Genetic diagnosis and treatment: Ethical considerations. AJDC 147:1190–1195, 1993
26. Botkin J, Croyle RT, Smith KR, Baty B, Lerman C, Goldgar D, Ward J, Flick B, Nash J: A model protocol for evaluating the behavioral and psychosocial effects of BRCA1 testing. JNCI 88:872–882, 1996

INDEX

Acral keratosis, 59
AFAP (Attenuated Familial Adenomatous Polyposis), 81, 158, 159
American Board of Genetic Counseling, 6
American Society of Clinical Oncology (ASCO), 2, 193
APC gene, 17, 73, 158, 159, 195
Ashkenazi Jew, 2, 50, 59, 69, 72
Atypical hyperplasia, 42, 44
Autosomal dominant (AD) trait, 51, 57, 60, 68

Behavioral medicine–cancer, 19, 21, 29, 32, 35, 71, 88
Billing, 8, 9
BRCA1, 1, 2, 16, 20, 32, 40, 41, 48, 51, 58, 59, 62, 65, 66, 67, 68, 69, 72, 73, 74, 75, 76, 91, 94, 95, 96, 97, 98, 100, 101, 103, 104, 105, 106, 108, 109, 111, 120, 121, 123, 124, 125, 127, 128, 129, 144, 145, 176, 189, 190, 191, 192, 193, 194, 195, 198, 199, 200
BRCA2, 2, 40, 41, 48, 51, 58, 59, 62, 65, 66, 67, 68, 69, 72, 73, 74, 75, 76, 91, 94, 95, 96, 97, 98, 100, 101, 103, 104, 105, 106, 108, 109, 111, 120, 121, 123, 124, 125, 127, 128, 129, 144, 145, 176, 189, 190, 191, 192, 193, 194, 195, 198, 199, 200
Breast cancer, 39, 40, 56, 59, 81, 94, 95, 96, 97, 100, 101, 103, 104, 105, 106, 108, 109, 111, 120, 123, 126, 127, 136, 137, 140, 141, 142, 147, 160, 176, 177, 178
Breast Cancer Detection Demonstration Project (BCDDP), 39, 40, 42, 43, 44, 46, 47, 48, 49, 50, 106

Cancer and Steriod Hormone Study (CASH), 45, 47, 48
Cancer genetics, 7, 65
Cancer registries, 184
Cancer risk assessment, 1, 28, 29
Chemoprevention, 2, 61, 103, 104, 105, 109, 130, 135, 136, 141, 142, 146, 167
Claus model, 39, 42, 50, 70
Cloning, 5, 8, 14, 17, 18, 71, 72, 93, 94, 95, 97, 98, 99, 137, 161, 162, 165, 168, 173, 176, 182, 192, 196
Colon cancer, 2, 159, 164, 166, 167, 197
Colonic polyposis, 158

Colorectal cancer (CRC), 69, 75, 76, 82, 153, 158, 159, 160, 161, 162, 163, 164, 165, 167, 168
Confidentiality, 10, 173
Cowden syndrome, 4, 14, 16, 51, 59
COX-2 inhibitors, 167

Discrimination, 88, 173, 174, 178, 179, 180, 181, 182, 183, 184, 185, 186, 196, 197, 200
DNA, 5, 8, 14, 17, 18, 71, 72, 93, 94, 95, 97, 98, 99, 137, 161, 162, 165, 168, 173, 176, 182, 192, 196

Employment discrimination, 6, 88, 147, 148, 173, 174, 178, 179, 180, 181, 182, 183, 184, 185, 186, 196, 197, 200
Endometrial cancer, 140, 141, 144, 160, 165
Estrogen therapy, 61, 76
Ethics, 6, 147, 148

Familial cancer risk, 56, 58, 59, 91, 92, 94, 100, 164, 165, 177
Family history, 56, 58, 59, 100, 165, 177
FAP (Familial Adenomatous Polyposis), 153, 158, 165
Fiduciary duty, 88, 173, 174, 178, 179, 180, 181, 182, 183, 184, 185, 186, 196, 197, 200
FJP (Familial Juvenile Polyposis), 160

Gail model, 43, 70
Genetic counseling, 1, 2, 6, 10, 12, 13, 16, 18, 21, 28, 30, 31, 33, 35, 70, 71, 82, 83, 85, 86, 87, 88, 177, 178
Genetic education, 1, 11, 15, 16, 17, 18, 21, 28, 29, 30, 32, 33, 56, 60, 65, 82, 83, 91, 129, 144, 148, 168, 173, 175, 176, 178, 179, 181, 182, 184, 185, 187, 189, 190, 191, 192, 193, 194, 195, 196, 197, 198
Genetic susceptibility testing, 1, 11, 15, 16, 17, 18, 21, 28, 29, 30, 32, 33, 56, 60, 65, 82, 83, 91, 129, 144, 148, 168, 173, 175, 176, 178, 179, 181, 182, 184, 185, 187, 189, 190, 191, 192, 193, 194, 195, 196, 197, 198
Genetic syndrome, 91, 92, 94, 164

Hamartomatous polyps, 59
Health insurance discrimination, 2, 173, 174, 175, 176, 177, 178, 179, 180, 181, 182, 183, 184, 197

The manufacturer's authorised representative in the EU is Springer
Nature Customer Service Centre GmbH, Europaplatz 3, 69115 Heidelberg,
Germany. If you have any concerns regarding our products, please
contact ProductSafety@springernature.com

Printed and bound by CPI Group (UK) Ltd, Croydon, CR0 4YY
24/04/2026
02096348-0016